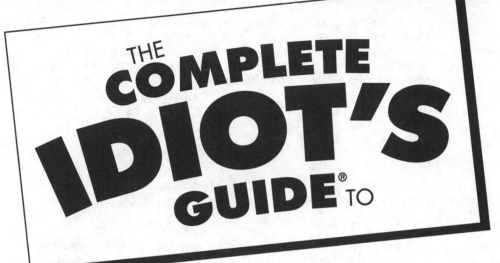

THE COMPLETE IDIOT'S GUIDE® TO

Living with Breast Cancer

*by Sharon Sorenson
and Suzanne Metzger, D.B.A.*

alpha
books

Macmillan USA, Inc.
201 West 103rd Street
Indianapolis, IN 46290

A Pearson Education Company

International Standard Book Number: 0-02-863938-3
Library of Congress Catalog Card Number: Available upon request.

02 01 00   8 7 6 5 4 3 2 1

Interpretation of the printing code: The rightmost number of the first series of numbers is the year of the book's printing; the rightmost number of the second series of numbers is the number of the book's printing. For example, a printing code of 00-1 shows that the first printing occurred in 2000.

Printed in the United States of America

Note: This publication contains the opinions and ideas of its authors. It is intended to provide helpful and informative material on the subject matter covered. It is sold with the understanding that the authors and publisher are not engaged in rendering professional services in the book. If the reader requires personal assistance or advice, a competent professional should be consulted.

The authors and publisher specifically disclaim any responsibility for any liability, loss, or risk, personal or otherwise, which is incurred as a consequence, directly or indirectly, of the use and application of any of the contents of this book.

Publisher
Marie Butler-Knight

Product Manager
Phil Kitchel

Managing Editor
Cari Luna

Senior Acquisitions Editor
Renee Wilmeth

Development Editor
Suzanne LeVert

Senior Production Editor
Christy Wagner

Copy Editor
Erica Rose

Illustrator
Jody P. Schaeffer

Cover Designers
Mike Freeland
Kevin Spear

Book Designers
Scott Cook and Amy Adams of DesignLab

Indexer
Mary SeRine

Layout/Proofreading
Angela Calvert
John Etchison

Contents at a Glance

Contents

Foreword

When I was in college, one my favorite professors, Dr. Ethel Trice, used to say, "I don't expect you to have all the answers, but I do expect you to know where to find them." As an educator, she was talking about "resources" and the critical role they would play in my future ability to be successful and truly effective in helping others through my work.

During my career as a professional health educator and long-time breast cancer advocate, I have sifted through a mountain of educational materials and resources to find the best of the best. I have made thousands of referrals, handed out a warehouse of brochures and pamphlets, recommended countless books and Web sites, worked with numerous patients and families through support groups and retreats, recruited dozens of expert guest speakers for seminars and symposiums, and made hundreds of presentations—all with an eye toward connecting cancer patients and their families with the best and most appropriate information to help them through their journey toward health and healing.

With this book, *The Complete Idiot's Guide to Living with Breast Cancer*, Sharon Sorenson and Suzanne Metzger have synthesized what is for most an insurmountable amount of information about breast cancer and delivered the closest thing I've seen to Breast Cancer 101. It's a simple yet comprehensive, user-friendly guide that's written in a clear, easy-to-understand common language, avoiding the ultra-sophisticated terminology that often permeates other publications. It fills an unmet gap between information provided by doctors, nurses, and other health professionals and material available in medical books and journals so filled with technical jargon they are of little help to those who need it the most.

As part of an ever-growing sisterhood of survivors, Sharon Sorenson and Suzanne Metzger bring an important and much-needed perspective to each page, because when you're fighting breast cancer, you need someone who understands, someone who has walked in your shoes, and someone who is still around leaving footprints. This book, however, isn't just for survivors or those newly diagnosed. It will connect with a new and much broader base of readers, including husbands, lovers, children, close friends, and caring neighbors. The authors have made the subject of breast cancer approachable. They have written an inspiring and upbeat "everything you need to know" book that can help everyone involved in the cancer experience. It's full of love, hope, wisdom, and realistic, practical advice. It has the right blend of concrete information and real-life anecdotes, and it's filled with tongue-in-cheek humor—the kind you need to break the tension and ease the stress, regardless of your role in the experience.

We owe a debt of gratitude to these two women for helping simplify a very complex subject!

Jody Brennan, MA, CHES
Vice President of Communications, ContourMed, Inc., and past Vice Chair of education committee, Susan G. Komen Foundation.

Introduction

One of the biggest shocks in life is the news that you have breast cancer. Nothing hurts; you don't have a fever; you feel just fine, thank you. But you found this lump, and your heart jumps to warp speed. Or the doc jabs his finger to a spot on your mammogram. "Right there. That looks suspicious." And the room spins.

The shock of learning that you have breast cancer puts the world on hold until you can regain your balance. This book will help you through this process. In fact, we've written it to give you the help we wish we'd had when our own worlds went into a spin. The old saw that hindsight is 20/20 makes us—and the more than 70 survivors we interviewed—the experts. We're not medical folks; rather, we've been through the battle of surgery and treatments. We've walked in your combat boots, and we're here to help you with your battle plan.

What You'll Learn in This Book

This book is divided into five sections that take you from the first skirmish of the battle with breast cancer through the front-line attacks and on to the victory field. Here's how the book is arranged:

Part 1, "The Big Shock: First Events," begins where we all begin—with the discovery of a lump or a suspicious mammogram. Then you'll learn ways to prepare for battle by sharing your news with family and friends, learning what your diagnosis means, finding your medical dream team, making decisions about your treatment, and figuring out what to do about your job.

Part 2, "Shock Waves: Dealing with Treatment," describes the how and why and aftereffects of the surgeries and treatments you may face—from lumpectomy to mastectomy and on to chemo, radiation, and hormonal therapy.

Part 3, "After Shock: Dealing with the Tremors," focuses on the ups and downs you may face when you think the battle is over. You'll discover ways to take care of yourself now and forever more by protecting yourself against lymphedema, keeping regular follow-up appointments, recognizing risk factors you may face, and dealing effectively with the emotional shake-ups from this series of tremors.

Part 4, "Shock Absorbers: Finding Support," points the way toward getting the support you need so that you never have to fight this battle alone. You'll find out how you can find support from others in the sisterhood, from spiritual guidance, and from self-help strategies or professional counselors. And you'll learn, too, where to find the support that your family and friends need so they, in turn, can support you through the battle.

Part 5, "The Aftermath: Its Many Parts," explores the issues of breast reconstruction and breast prostheses and what the happy—and not so happy—customers say. You'll learn about ways you can make yourself feel and look better and how you can dress more comfortably in terms of your physical changes. You'll follow along the path through possible recurrence and the potential agony of leaving your family alone. Finally, you'll learn how survivors move forward, many of them volunteering to help others in their fight against breast cancer or assuming advocacy roles to educate the world and eradicate the disease. It's a path on which most survivors march to the victory field.

Finally, at the end, you find several appendixes, including a glossary and lists of further readings, support groups, sources of prostheses and post-surgical clothing, and informational Web sites.

Extras

In addition to the facts and figures, technical details, and tell-it-the-way-it-is descriptions, we make it easy for you to pick up the tidbits that we survivors learned in the school of hard knocks. Here's how you can recognize these features:

From the Book

You'll find yourself surrounded by a whole new vocabulary, but you'll learn the meanings painlessly—by checking these boxes.

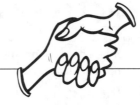

Helping Hand

We survivors offer our collective hand to share information about routine matters that the medical folks sometimes forget to mention.

Take It from Us

These warnings let you know about the minefields and how to avoid a wrong step. In short, they're important bits of advice and warnings that we survivors think will make your battle easier.

Tales from the Trenches

These real stories come from over 70 battle-scarred survivors who range from folks who were diagnosed 20 years ago to those currently fighting on the front lines. Their stories simplify and help you make sense of all the medical mumbo jumbo.

Acknowledgments

We owe a tremendous thank-you to well over 100 folks who graciously shared their time, experiences, and expertise. Their stories made us laugh and cry, grimace and grin, and every single survivor left us in awe. We shared hugs with instant friends; we heard messages of resounding support.

To protect their privacy, the 70 or so survivors' real names never appear in the text of our book, and we honor the request of many to acknowledge them here only by their first names. Their names hardly matter; their stories do. To each of them, our sincerest thanks.

Our humble gratitude for their extraordinary support goes to survivors and their friends and families, healthcare providers and professionals, political advocates, folks in the related business communities, and manuscript readers and editors who rapped our knuckles when we muddied our message. Our thanks, in alphabetical order, to Kay Anderson (Regional Contact, Komen Foundation), Patricia J. Anderson (Registered Nurse and author), Andrea, Elwood Arnold, Nancee Baldwin, Gail Behrens, Jody Brennan (Vice-Chair of Education, Komen Foundation; Vice-President of Communication, ContourMed), Sue Ann Brown, Cindy Booth (JD, Executive Director of Child Advocates, Inc.), Donald Burck (owner of a mastectomy boutique), Pauline Burgdorf, Janet Burkley (owner, Close to You; organizer of lymphedema support group), Lisa Caplan-Melnick (founder, Magic and Vanity), Cheryl, Kathi Clark (North Jersey Affiliate, Komen Foundation), Connie, Thelma Cooper, Beverly Coram, Barb Darbos (Information Systems Manager, Deaconess Breast Center), Linda M. Deig, Candace Dempsey (editor, *Underwire*), Kathy Dockery (Administrator of Deaconess Breast Center), Dr. J. Frederick Doepker Jr. (plastic surgeon), Dorothy, Dot, Kristen Duffy, Deborah Erwin (Advisory Board Member, ContourMed; Associate Professor of Surgical Oncology, UAMS; and Associate Director of Education, ACRC), Michelle Fouts (organizer of Bald Is Beautiful Day), Karen Gangel, Beth Garry, the Reverend Joy Bilger Gehring, Judy Gianelas (Oncological Nurse and Reach to Recovery volunteer), Susan Goldberg, R. Graham (Classique), Bettye Green (founder, African-American Women in Touch), Laurie Guitteau, Bridget Hadley, Claudia L. Hickey (Director of Colesce Couture), Felicia Hodge (Center for American Indian Research and Education), Patricia Holcomb (Registered Occupational Therapist), Rosalind Hunt, Alexandra Jackiw, Karen Jackson (founder, Sisters Network), Jo, Joan, Sandra Johnson (Medical Secretary), Ralph Kahn (Jodee Post-Mastectomy Fashions), Karen Kuebler, Christine Lammers (Oncological Nurse), Linda, Yvonne Lingo, Pat Edwards Loge (speaker, Evansville Race for the Cure), Lois, Madeline, Margret, Mary, Joan Maryniak (Facilitator, CHESS: Comprehensive Health Enhancement Support System; founder, cancer support group), Jackie Manthorne (Executive Director, Canadian Breast Cancer Network), Dianne H. McCabe (BSN and Registered Nurse), Martha McCaffrey (Certified Plastic Surgical Nurse), Fiona McTavish (Project Director of the Breast Cancer Module of CHESS: Comprehensive Health Enhancement Support System, developer and facilitator), Stan Metzger (Administrative Director of Radiology, Clarian Health), Carol Miley, the Reverend Kent Millard, Donna Miller (Esthetician and Owner,

DM Designers), Kathy Moore (Registered Dietitian, Clarian Health), Margaret Lynn Murrell, Debbie Nagel (Administrative Director of Radiation Oncology, Clarian Health), Staci Neely (President, B&B Company, Inc.), Vikki Newman, Linda Nielson, Carol Outland (founder of Care Products), Autumn Owens, Pam, Paula, Dr. Robert Penkava (Radiologist), Jamie Pensly (Boston Women's Health Book Collective), Monica Perdue, Judy Perotti (Director of Patient Services for Y-Me), Carol Pettys, Melanie Powell (Registered Pharmacist), Jay Dee Prohosky, Dr. William Rate (Radiation Oncologist), Jean Ripple, Lou Robichand (Certified Prosthetic Fitter), Carol Rogers (co-founder, Woman to Woman; NBCC lobbyist; and lay committeeperson for American Cancer Society grant review process), Michael Ross, Laurie Rozakis, Connie Rufenbarger (Indiana Coalition), Barbara Russell (Executive Director, American Cancer Society, District 8), Leslie Sallee (founder, Mastique Lingerie), David Sammet, Nicolette Sammet, Linda Saunders, Mary Katherine Schnitz (Director, Stephen Ministers, St. Luke's United Methodist Church), Wanda Schultz, Dr. Brian Schymik (surgeon), Marian T. Seibert, Judy Seeley, Judi Simon (owner, Capital Marketing), Bette Slutsky (Reach to Recovery volunteer), Charles E. Sorenson, Moli Steinert (LunaTours Outdoor Adventures for Women, sponsoring Bike Against the Odds), Nancy Sweeney (Director, Grief Ministry, St. Luke's United Methodist Church), Susan Thomas, Julie Thorpe, Mary Unfried (Deaconess Breast Center), Janet Voelkle, Wanda, Bobbie Warnock, Eileen Weinzapfel, Kathy Weinzapfel (Supervisor of Physical Medicine, Deaconess Hospital), Judy White (MSN and Registered Oncological Nurse), Marilyn Williams, and Robynn Working (Deaconess Breast Center).

A special word of thanks to our incredibly keen and patient Development Editor, Suzanne LeVert. We thank you for your insights and faith in our project. And finally, of course, hats off to Renee Wilmeth, our Senior Acquisitions Editor who approached us to do this book. Thank you for believing in us, and know that we've desperately tried to measure up to your high expectations.

We fervently believe that no one can write a book without the support of immediate family and close friends. They accepted leftovers night after night, put up with grouchy requests to "Do something with this house; it's a disaster," and shrugged off tolerantly the "I can't go this week; I have a deadline Friday." Hugs and kisses, all. You're precious to us.

Editor's Acknowledgements

The creation of a *Complete Idiot's Guide* is always quite an undertaking. However, we could never have conceived of and executed this powerful title without the help of many, many people who lent their opinions, their knowledge, and their support. As the acquisitions editor, I'd like to thank the many survivors, doctors, and advocates who helped in developing this groundbreaking project: Dr. Bill Shiel, Shelley Barsanti, Linda Birnbach, Jody Brennan, Debbie Long, Joann Schellenbach, Barbara Russell, Gary McMullen, and—of course—the authors, Sharon and Suzanne.

Special Thanks to the Technical Reviewer

The Complete Idiot's Guide to Living with Breast Cancer was reviewed by numerous experts who double-checked the accuracy of what you'll learn here, to help us ensure that this book gives you everything you need to know about living with breast cancer.

Special Thanks to the Cover Models

Special thanks to the breast cancer survivors who volunteered to be our cover models (in alphabetical order): Joyce Boice, Terri Cable, Jolee Chartrand, Chris Cianciolo, Jennifer Doss, Marian Elliot, Sandy Fink, Marge Frantzreb, Shannon Hamerin, Patti Houtman, Marylin Huckleberry, Mary Jones, Mary Larson, Pat Logan, Janet Lome, Suzanne Metzger, Michey Mills, Judy Moon, Karen Morris, Linda Nourse, Joan Overholser, Amy Patton, Connie Ruch, Michal Shutz, Judy Simpson, Sharon Sorenson, and Merle Stoughton.

Trademarks

All terms mentioned in this book that are known to be or are suspected of being trademarks or service marks have been appropriately capitalized. Alpha Books and Macmillan USA, Inc., cannot attest to the accuracy of this information. Use of a term in this book should not be regarded as affecting the validity of any trademark or service mark.

Part 1
The Big Shock: First Events

Getting the word that you have breast cancer is surely one of the biggest shocks in your life. You feel fine. Nothing hurts. You have no fever. But with the four simple words "You have breast cancer," your life's path takes a sharp turn. You're dumped unceremoniously into the midst of another world. The folks in this new world come dressed in white jackets and green scrubs and throw words at you that surely come from some foreign dictionary. Still, you have the clear understanding that, whatever the words mean, they all apply to you. And they sound fairly frightening.

As survivors, we're standing beside you to chant in your ear the mantra we know from the bottom of our hearts to be true: "You can do this. Yes, you CAN do this!"

This part of the book tells you how the docs determine that you have breast cancer. Then we'll help you through sharing your news with family, friends, and colleagues. Next we'll work really hard at taking away some of the fears (we hope!) by helping you figure out what your diagnosis means, suggesting how to put together your medical dream team, and sharing the nitty-gritty about treatment options. Then you'll be better prepared to know what to do about your 9-to-5 job.

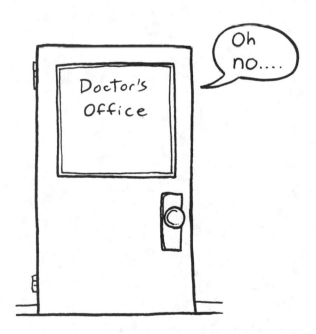

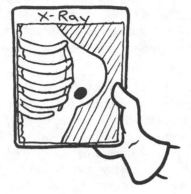
It Ain't Gold in Them Hills

In This Chapter

➤ Breast cancer—the big picture

➤ First clues in lumps and pictures

➤ Diagnosis with a biopsy

➤ When the shocking news comes

At this moment, more than two million breast cancer survivors are hugging their kids and grandkids. They're trotting off to work or trekking the Rockies, chairing a fund-raiser or a family reunion. We breast cancer survivors make up a huge sisterhood (and a tiny brotherhood). In this chapter, we'll look at the big picture of breast cancer and how it's changing. We'll outline the telltale signs of breast cancer and explain how doctors know whether the signs are for real or not.

Finally, we'll prepare you for the possible news that you have suddenly become a member of the club nobody wants to join. Not one of us in the sisterhood is ever glad to learn that another one of you is newly initiated. But we will extend a long arm of support should you find yourself eligible. There is no trial membership. The initiation rites are the pits. The dues are way too steep. But the membership is for life. There is no past tense to having breast cancer.

Breast Cancer: The Big Picture

The statistics sound like a bad movie plot. By the time a given group of women is 85 years old, one in eight of them will have breast cancer. The older you get, the more likely it will be you. Fortunately, however, what used to be a doomsday diagnosis is

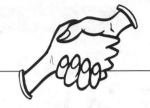

Helping Hand

It helps to share! Karlene, eight-year breast cancer survivor, pointed out that we survivors share a private and highly personal humor. We can share the laughter because we also share the fear and the pain. Sure, our breast cancers are not exactly the same, but we can all relate to the feelings that go along with the diagnosis.

today not nearly as serious. Not that breast cancer isn't serious. *It is.* Not that breast cancer can't be fatal. *It can.* In fact, 43,000 women died last year from breast cancer. That's more deaths in a single year than the total U.S. Army and Marine casualties in the extended war in Southeast Asia.

This year, doctors will diagnose another 175,000 to 185,000 American women with breast cancer. That's equal to the entire population of a fair-sized city. Another 30,000 will be diagnosed with a pre-cancerous condition that, if ignored, almost always turns into breast cancer. The good news, however, is that with early detection and routine treatment, most women go on to lead long, happy, healthy lives.

I've never ever heard a woman out there say, "Oh, yeah, I'll be the one in eight. I'll be the one to get breast cancer." We all assume bad things happen to other people. Breast cancer will never threaten our lives or reduce our families to tears. So when it happens, it's a terrible shock. Big time. With aftershocks and shock waves.

What It Means—Then and Now

A 37-year survivor described her surgery and treatment by radioactive radium. Confined to the hospital for six weeks and in isolation for most of that time, she underwent what by today's standards would be a brutal regimen. You had to wonder, having heard her story, if she still glows in the dark.

Take It from Us

Don't feel alone. One in eight women in a lifetime will have breast cancer. So if you face the misfortune of finding yourself initiated into the club, know that you will find tremendous support from everyone who went before.

Twenty-five years ago, my mother-in-law called in tears. The doctor had found a "highly suspicious" dimple in her breast. Without any tests, no questions asked, she went to surgery. They cut out a portion, tested it, and, having found cancer, removed her breast. She had no input, no opportunity to ask questions or make decisions. When she woke up, her only question was, "Did they take it all?"

These two women and hundreds of thousands like them were the pioneers whose treatments paved the way for us. Some paid a dear price. Many lost their lives. Their sacrifices, however, have resulted in heartening statistics from the National Cancer Institute. For the first time ever, breast cancer survival rates are increasing. The improved survival rates are in large part the result of women conscientiously doing their monthly breast self-exams and getting annual clinical exams and mammograms.

But it's a good-news-bad-news situation. The bad news is that the increase in survival follows hard on the heels of an increase in the number of breast cancer diagnoses. Most authorities agree, however, that the cases aren't really increasing. We're just better at detection. Early detection, in turn, improves survival rate.

The long and the short of it is elementary, my dear Watson: Not only have there been significant strides in the detection of breast cancer but also in its treatment. What it meant when Aunt Minnie had breast cancer is not what it means today—to you. After diagnosis, you can still buy long-term stocks and bonds with high hopes of cashing them in, but the secret is early detection.

First Clues: Yours and Theirs

Since everything we know about breast cancer leads us to know that early detection is the real secret to successful treatment, what are our first clues? How do we first know that we may be one of the eight? Is it pain? A lump? An irregular mammogram?

Peas and Marbles: Finding a Lump

Since only rarely does a woman feel any pain with breast cancer, the American Cancer Society and others have emphasized breast self-exams (BSEs). We're told to examine ourselves monthly, preferably in the shower. For some women, the hype about BSE makes them feel guilty. Guilty because we forget on the first of the month to do the exam. Guilty because we haven't joined a buddy system to remind each other to do the exam. Guilty because we tell the doctor we do it when we really don't.

Okay, so quit the guilt trip. *Do it!* Women regularly discover lumps in their breasts in just this way— a routine monthly BSE. After all, you know your body better than anyone else. Why wait for someone else to poke and prod just once a year? Truth be known, however, some women don't discover the lump themselves. Their husbands or lovers find it. Kathy Dockery, administrator of the Deaconess Breast Center told me, "We hear this more than any other story, that their husbands found the lump, and that they may not have noticed it otherwise."

Then what if you—or someone—finds something? If you find a *palpable* lump, no matter its size—pea or marble—there's no need for panic. The good news is that roughly 80 percent of all lumps are *benign*. That is, they are not *malignant*. They have no cancer cells in them.

Take It from Us

Don't delay! Some women, after finding a lump or visible clue, go into denial. They prefer to ignore the symptom, hope it will go away, or wait and see. That's precious time wasted. Call your doctor immediately. Not tomorrow. Today.

The bad news is that you must—absolutely must—call your doctor immediately. The doc will check you over to see if you have a problem. Maybe you will hear "I think it's just a *cyst*." To validate what he thinks, he will likely *aspirate* it. Cysts are mostly fluid-filled, and aspiration is a simple, generally pain-free procedure in which the doctor deadens the tissue with an anesthetic, inserts a needle into the lump, and tries to draw out fluid. If he can withdraw fluid, you have a cyst, and cysts are most often, but not always, benign. In cases where the results of the aspiration are inconclusive, your doctor will have a pathologist take a look at the fluid and/or cells withdrawn.

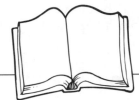

From the Book

Palpable means that you can feel it. **Benign** means not cancerous. **Malignant** means cancer cells are present. A **cyst** is a fluid-filled lump, not usually cancerous. To **aspirate** means to insert a needle and withdraw any fluid/cells, especially from a cyst.

Using the Eagle Eye

We've also been taught that we should study our breasts in the mirror. So, what do you look for? There are three clues:

➤ A dimpling anywhere on the breast (looks just like a smile dimple in a cute little kid's cheek)

➤ A change in the nipple, especially if it seems to be drawing inward or looks scaly

➤ Any drainage from the nipple

If you spot a visible clue, there's no need for panic. But you absolutely must call your doctor. Immediately.

Get the Picture: Mammograms

Okay, so you've called the doctor. You have an appointment. What happens then? Chances are, in addition to a clinical breast exam, you'll be scheduled for a *mammogram*.

Why are mammograms so important? They can detect cancer that can neither be seen nor felt, thus identifying the earliest forms of breast cancer. The *radiologist* who reads the film can see suspicious spots smaller than the head of a pin. Depending on where these spots are, it could take several years before they're large enough to feel or see.

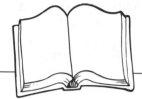

From the Book

A **mammogram** is a series of really low-dose x-ray pictures of the breast from the top and side. A **radiologist** is trained to read the pictures and decide which shadows and dots are suspicious and which are not. A **diagnostic mammogram** is a mammogram used to examine a lump or visible abnormality. A **baseline mammogram** is a first mammogram, usually made between ages 35 and 40, used as a frame of reference for later mammograms in order to detect changes in the breast. A **screening mammogram** is an annual, routine examination for women over 40.

Thus, mammography involves two purposes:

1. A *diagnostic mammogram* usually follows if you find a lump or visible abnormality.

2. A *screening mammogram* is usually an annual routine for women over 40 (although some experts still argue over age).

Based on family history and personal health, you and your doctor should decide when to do a first or *baseline mammogram*. The baseline serves as a frame of reference so future mammograms can identify change. You and your doctor must also decide how frequently to have routine mammograms. While annual mammograms are typical after age 40, those of us at high risk may have them every six months (more on risk factors in Chapter 15, "Caution Flag: Risk Factors"). And some doctors recommend only every other year if you're between 40 and 50. If you're low income and age 40 or over, ask your doctor about free or low-cost breast screening. With the hundreds of local and state programs available, there is no reason for a person not to have a mammogram because she can't afford it.

Some women complain about how much a mammogram hurts. But, really, folks, it's not that bad.

Tales from the Trenches

The irregularity on Clarine's routine mammogram was five dots in an area smaller than a pea, located behind the nipple and against the chest wall. Just think how large that lesion would have had to become before she—or anyone—could have felt it (especially if you're a C cup). Now that's early detection!

Yes, those little plates on which the breast rests always seem a little cold (no, they don't have refrigeration coils in them). Yes, the plates squeeze the breast as flat as possible in order to get a clear picture (no, they aren't the hinges of hell). But many clinics now use heating pads to warm the plates and allow the patient herself to determine how much pressure the plates exert. It may be temporarily uncomfortable, but it can also save your life. It did mine.

Like all areas of medicine, mammography is an ever-improving science. New equipment, like digital mammography machines, projects the breast image on a screen and allows for manipulation to give the best view. It virtually eliminates the need for any repeat mammograms. Just make sure whatever equipment they use for your mammogram is accredited by the American College of Radiology. Ask your doc or, if you really want to check it yourself, you'll find a label attached to the machine that gives its accreditation number.

In certain cases, your doctor may use an ultrasound with or without a mammogram. The doc will usually use an ultrasound, a painless exam using sound waves, if he or she needs to distinguish between a solid and fluid-filled lump (sound waves go through fluid but bounce off solid lumps). He or she will also use ultrasound if you're pregnant (radiation may harm the fetus) or if you can feel a lump that doesn't show on a mammogram (usually because of dense breast tissue, typical in younger women).

Dreaded Word: Irregular

Some of us have had lots of "irregular" mammograms. The call comes, saying "We need to do another mammogram. There's a questionable area we need to re-check." So we trudge in, scared witless about what's wrong, only to discover that it's nothing after all. But then one day a different call comes. You may be told your mammogram shows a lump or *microcalcifications*, tiny specks of calcium. Scattered specks aren't likely to be a problem, but a tight cluster of such deposits is most likely pre-cancerous. (More on this in Chapter 3, "Learning a New Vocabulary.") But a mammogram can't diagnose for certain that a lump or a cluster of microcalcifications is breast cancer. Only a biopsy can do that.

Take It from Us

Remain vigilant! Mammograms aren't foolproof. They miss about 25 percent of cancers. Rhonda found a malignant lump in her breast only two months after her "all clear" mammogram. Still, they're the best diagnostic tool we have. They reduce the risk of death from breast cancer by 30 percent.

Tales from the Trenches

Syndicated newspaper columnist Molly Ivins discovered she had breast cancer and wrote in her column that day, "I don't need get well cards, but I would like the beloved women readers to do something for me: Go. Get. The. Damn. Mammogram. Done."

It's Biopsy, Not Autopsy

In ignorant bliss, I assumed a biopsy was no big deal. I'd heard the term "needle biopsy." It sounded pretty much like getting a shot. Wrong! In fact, a *biopsy* is a surgical procedure in which tissue is removed and examined by a *pathologist*. In addition to the fine needle aspiration discussed earlier (which can be and sometimes is biopsied) there are two kinds of biopsies: core needle and surgical.

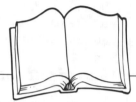

From the Book

Microcalcification refers to tiny calcium deposits. Scattered deposits are likely benign. A tight cluster often indicates malignancy. A **biopsy** is the removal of tissue to be examined for malignancy. A **pathologist** is a medical doctor who specializes in analyzing tissue to determine the presence of disease. A **radiological technologist** is someone who specializes in the use of x-ray equipment. A **core needle** biopsy uses a large needle to take out a core of tissue for examination and is either **stereotactic guided** (using x-rays from two directions to guide the needle) or **ultrasound guided** (using sound waves to guide the needle).

Core Needle—to the Heart of the Matter

A *core needle* biopsy uses a really big needle (borrowed from the veterinarian?) to withdraw a core specimen of tissue. The core can be taken with *stereotactic guidance* or by *ultrasound guidance*. A stereotactic biopsy is usually used when the mammogram shows a microcalcification cluster. The ultrasound guidance is usually used when a lump is felt or seen on a mammogram. In either case, the core biopsy gives the pathologist actual tissue, not just a few cells as with an aspiration. Sure, you get a local anesthetic, but the process is very exacting, takes an hour or more, and is generally uncomfortable.

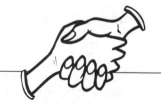

Helping Hand

Always ask questions! While your doctor will recommend the kind of biopsy you should have, don't hold back the questions. Make sure you understand why you're having a biopsy and why your doctor recommends the kind he does.

The stereotactic biopsy requires you to lie on your stomach with your breast hanging through a hole in the table. What's more, you must remain perfectly still for the duration. Using computers and x-ray pictures, the *radiological technologist,* whose expertise is using x-ray equipment, locates the spot to be biopsied. Then the radiologist inserts the needle and an attached suction pump withdraws the cores, usually several. A Steristrip closes the quarter-inch cut where the needle was inserted, you're sent home bound up like a mummy, and a nurse reminds you to use ice packs for the next 24 hours to limit bleeding and/or swelling and general discomfort.

Take It from Us

Don't go it alone. While there's nothing about a core needle biopsy that will keep you from driving home, it's an experience that can leave you shaky and weak. Accept company.

Surgical Snip-Snip

A surgical biopsy is just that—surgery. The surgeon removes a small lump of tissue, much like a lumpectomy. (See Chapter 7, "Taking Your Lumps: Lumpectomy," for all the details.) Sometimes the surgical biopsy follows a needle biopsy.

It's Not the Avon Lady Calling

The biopsy results give the final word. Malignant or benign. Up until now, you had "maybe," "probably," "possibly," or "suspicious." You've also probably worried yourself into a frenzy. You've waited for the appointment to get the biopsy. You've waited for results from the biopsy. The waiting seems interminable. Keeping busy is the best remedy, but quite frankly, not knowing is in many ways worse than knowing the worst. Kind of like a Chinese water torture.

Getting Psyched

Not every doctor handles the telltale call the same way. Some insist you come to the office for the results of a biopsy because they don't want to give bad news over the phone. Others prefer to call you in the comfort of your home where you don't have to compose yourself to walk out through the waiting room or try to be courteous to strangers around you. Find out ahead of time what your doctor will do. Know the plan.

Fortunately, these folks work with the agony and ecstasy of biopsies every day and are usually sensitive to your feelings. So what are the next steps?

➤ Find out who's going to give you the results.

➤ Find out when to expect the results.

➤ Find out if you must go in or if someone will call.

➤ If you must go in, take someone with you who can listen and take notes.

➤ If someone will call you, have the call come wherever someone can listen with you, such as on an extension phone.

➤ Prepare yourself for the worst possible news. That way, you'll be able to listen to what the doctor tells you even if the news is bad.

➤ When the news comes, listen carefully, and don't hesitate to ask questions.

➤ Write down exactly what you're told—what the results show, what kind of malignancy, etc.

➤ If the doctor or nurse uses words you don't understand, ask for spellings, definitions, and explanations.

➤ Have your husband, friend, or relative (whoever is listening with you) take notes.

➤ Clarify with the doctor or nurse what your next step should be.

➤ Clarify who makes what appointments with whom.

Pow! Just like that, your life changes and everything goes into a spin.

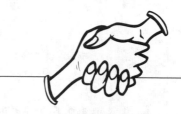

Helping Hand

Prepare for the worst; hope for the best. If you have planned for the worst possible news, anything less will be a big relief. Shock is easier to absorb when you have the opportunity to get yourself mentally prepared.

Now You Know: Tears and Fears

The call has come. The diagnosis is in. You have breast cancer. If you're like most of us, your first reaction is shock. Shock that without warning, your life has gone out of control. Shock that even though you feel fine, nothing hurts, and you have no fever, you have a life-threatening disease. Shock that you know someone who died of breast cancer and now you have it, too. Shock that your family will be dramatically affected by what's happening to you. Shock that you don't really have a clue about what's going to happen to you next. Shock that now you're that "one in eight." Shock that turns to fear.

Okay, hit it. Bawl your eyes out. It's good release. It's okay, too, if you and your husband or partner cry together. But at some point you have to toss the tissues and get on with the next steps. The first step is to stop immediately the use of any kind of estrogen—estrogen replacement therapy (like Premerin) if you're in menopause or estrogen creams for vaginal dryness. Your doctor will probably tell you, but if not, ask immediately. Depending on the kind of cancer you have, the estrogen may be feeding its growth.

Next, you have real fears that need to be addressed. The bottom line for every woman with breast cancer is almost always, "Am I going to die?" Well, everybody dies sooner or later, but most likely you aren't going to die from breast cancer. But you will likely have surgery, or even more than one surgery. And you may have other treatments to save your life. It's time to go to battle. Bring out the troops.

Tales from the Trenches

Eight years ago, Kate was diagnosed with breast cancer and given a year to live. Today she writes, "I believe I always have a choice. I can sit on the couch and suck my thumb, or I can get on my horse and ride." She chose to ride. And when I called her last night to say hello, she answered the phone breathlessly. "I'm riding my bike," she explained. She's 64.

If you're new to the club, know that we would like to be with you right now to dry your tears and give you hugs. Having been in your shoes, we know that no one other than another survivor can understand what you're going through. Hundreds of thousands of women have been through this. You can do it! Just keep reminding yourself that whatever battles you must go through to conquer this disease—the surgery, the treatments—it's all temporary. It's. All. Temporary. Life goes on. You'll come out the other side a different person, but life goes on. And we're here for you. So consider yourself hugged.

The Least You Need to Know

➤ Perform regular self-exams to feel any lumps or see any visible abnormalities.

➤ Receive regular screening mammograms and clinical exams, for they usually offer the earliest detection.

➤ Follow your doctor's advice about the best biopsy for you—a fine needle, core needle, or surgical biopsy.

➤ Plan for the news and the possibility that it will be bad news.

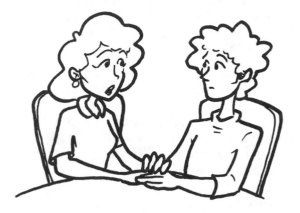

Chapter 2

We Need to Talk

In This Chapter

➤ Picking the right time

➤ Understanding what others might be thinking

➤ Family matters: telling the kids

➤ Sharing fears with loved ones

➤ Making a temporary shift in the day-to-day

Cancer. It remains one of the most difficult words in the English language to hear or to say. At the same time, out of necessity, it's become a pretty common topic of conversation because of it's pervasiveness in our society. Consider this statistic: The risk of cancer in men is one out of two and for women one out of three. The men and women who develop the disease as well as their family and friends will also be affected by it. Needless to say, cancer touches almost everyone's life these days.

Nevertheless, cancer is a difficult topic to discuss. In this chapter, we'll show you how to talk to the people in your life who need to know about your diagnosis and your treatment plan. It won't be easy, but we'll help you through it.

Things Are Going to Be Different

Different? Well, that is certainly an understatement about what a cancer diagnosis does to our lives! You've just been thrown into a card game that you really don't want to play. Although you can't choose the cards you're dealt, you can choose how to play them.

When it comes to letting the people you love know of your new situation, you also have lots of choices. You can choose whom to tell, when to tell them, and how much you want to reveal at any given time. It's important to remember, always, that you're in control of your half of the relationship equation.

At the same time, the one thing you can't control is another person's feelings or reactions—and you'll no doubt be surprised by some of them. You might find that a few of your friends will actually compete for the "most favored position" and want to be the one you reveal all of your confidences to; others will simply walk away. Still others might withdraw at first, but then quietly become your strongest supporters. For better or worse, navigating through the relationship waters will be another challenge for you!

No doubt there will be changes in your normal daily routine, and your family and friends may feel threatened because of these changes. You yourself will change, too—perhaps physically, certainly emotionally—and your loved ones might not know how to react to those changes either. In fact, they may wonder if you're really the same person inside. You may wonder that, too. Indeed, things will never be quite the same again. That doesn't mean things will be worse, or better, but they will be different. And they'll start to change as soon as you choose to tell the people around you what you've learned about your medical condition.

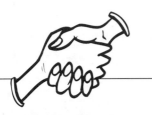

Helping Hand

Know your limits. Please remember that breast cancer is a very personal disease, and you are not required to share intimate details with anyone (other than your doctor!). If you feel like sharing, do. If not, feel free to keep your personal business private.

Take It from Us

Don't be afraid to be annoyed! Anything that disrupts our normal routine is irritating. Think of how exasperated you become when just a minor inconvenience interrupts your day. It might help, at least at first, to think of cancer as a temporary roadblock that will exasperate you and your family.

What's Good for the Goose ...

When it's time to start thinking about how to inform your loved ones, try to figure out how much—in general—you want to relate about having breast cancer. Then decide the point of view you'll take when telling particular individuals in your life. You probably won't say the same things in the same ways to your partner and to your children, for instance, or to your best friend and to your co-worker. Let's explore the general considerations first.

Finding the Words and Voice

How do I tell them? When do I tell them? What do I say? Do I get them together or tell them separately? Can I do this by myself? Where can I find someone to help me?

These are just a few of the questions that will run through your mind, and you may feel a desperate need for answers for them. You have to find the words and the voice before you begin to share with those who you care for and who care for you. One idea is to write down what you're going to say and then read it back to yourself out loud. This method might help you to judge the impact of your words and gain some composure when you say them to others.

There are several key elements that may help you sort things out and give you a good, solid head start:

➤ **Accept your emotions.** To say that you will be upset is an understatement. Let's face it: You've just learned that you have breast cancer. This is an emotional time.

➤ **Compose yourself.** Take whatever strength you need to calm yourself before you tell others. If you're out of control emotionally, your friends and family will be, too. If you're terrified, they will be, too. Needless to say, there's no benefit in spreading panic and fear at this point.

➤ **Reach out for support.** If you have any doubt about how to approach telling others, seek help from members of a support group who can give you some suggestions on how to break the news. (See Chapters 17, "Groupies: Yea or Nay?" and 19, "Support Tools," and Appendix E, "Informational Web Sites.")

➤ **Get a handle on vocabulary.** Determine what terminology you want to use with others. If the word "cancer" is too direct and scary, try words like illness, malignancy, tumor, or even problem. Tailor your words to whom you are speaking. A child may understand "Mommy's sick" better than "Mommy has cancer."

> **Helping Hand**
>
> *Silence is golden. Claire said talking was only half of it. Silence was the other half. The closeness she felt with her husband was so intense that there were times when they simply didn't need words. Just sitting together in the backyard or in front of the fireplace, walking down the lane holding hands, and cuddling in bed were great forms of communication.*

With these basics out of the way, let's proceed to more general information points.

Get Ready for the 180 Degrees

Let's talk variety here. Remember one of your high school math teachers talking about a 180-degree turnaround? Now you get to see this in action! Here are just some of the 180 degrees you might expect:

- ➤ From anger to tears
- ➤ From closeness to distance
- ➤ From numbness to frantic
- ➤ From grieving to not grieving
- ➤ From questions to silence
- ➤ From compassion to stone

Not everyone in your life will react in the same way or at the same time to your news. Each of us has many variables that affect our reactions. The better you know the person, the more likely you are to know how they will react. We'll talk more about this matter a little later in the chapter.

First Things First

You've delivered the news. One person is angry and rages at the unfairness of it all. One has just become numb and withdrawn. One has tears rolling down his face and wants to hold you. Where do you go from here?

The only option open to you at this point is to accept each person's reaction as best you can. Know that, like you, he or she will eventually adjust to the news in his or her own way. Remember that your attitude and way of coping will probably continue to change on a daily basis. Your friends and family will need time, too.

Tales from the Trenches

Evelyn's family ran the gamut of emotions: crying, swearing, raging, and denying. Actually, they were feeling the very same emotions as she did, only she felt them first. As she watched her family react, she consoled them. In fact, she found that she became strong—if not for herself, then for them. She remembered the adage her mother always related to her: "We all rise to the occasion." Now she knew what her mother meant.

And there will be questions—questions they expect you to answer. Our best advice: Think before you answer. Once words leave your mouth it is impossible to take them back, no matter how badly you would like to.

No, you are not going to die tomorrow. No, you are not contagious. No, it is not anybody's fault. Yes, bad things do happen to good people. Yes, in most cases, it is a curable disease not a death sentence. And, yes, some things will have to change temporarily.

Speak Up and Speak Out

For the next 6 to 12 months you will need some extras. You will not be able to participate fully in day-to-day activities. Will everything go smoothly? Probably not. But in what family do all things go smoothly under normal circumstances? As far as I know, family perfection exists only on television commercials, Christmas plates, and reruns of *Father Knows Best*. Such "perfection" is artificial and lasts for 30 minutes or less with two commercial breaks. We're talking about having to cope with a serious illness for at least 6 to 12 months.

Under most circumstances, your family and friends will be considerate and supportive, so don't be afraid to ask them for help you could use. And be specific. "Pick the kids up from school." "Take me to the hospital for my treatment." "Help me with the housework or cooking." Sometimes help is just a request away.

In this un-normal time, try for as much normalcy as possible. Don't expect people to grieve all the time. Everyone's emotional mind needs a break. You can turn away from grief and come back to it at a later time. Work in some fun and laughter. Even be the one who starts it! Just as you cannot grieve all the time, you cannot be serious all the time. Make small talk and share in what's happening to other people. The world has never stopped turning because someone has breast cancer. Life does go on. Participate in others' lives, too.

Let's add some specifics to this general information, and plan on how to deal with those closest to us.

First Love: Telling Your Partner

"For richer, for poorer; in sickness and in health; until death do us part, so help me God." This is a *covenant,* a pact, and one that some people take to heart more than others do. For some partners, the relationship improves with the addition of the personal, intimate challenge of an illness. For others, the news sticks in the cracks of the relationship, widening them until the relationship gets worse and maybe even ends.

And, you don't have to be married for this to be the case. With boyfriends, girlfriends, and fiancés, you are also treading on uncertain ground. Yes, it can depend on how long you've been together, what future plans you have, or even the depth of your relationship. If a relationship is on shaky ground to begin with, a diagnosis of breast cancer may cause the ground to crumble; however, depending on what kind of bonds you share and how strong they are, you both can rise to the occasion and fight the battle together.

Remember, in this instance, that the person you're telling is the person you eat with, sleep with, make decisions with, the person with whom you're sexually intimate, and with whom you intend to grow old. You think you've built a foundation, but now that you have breast cancer that foundation may feel a little shaky. Just as "location, location, location" is the most important consideration in real estate, "communication, communication, communication" is the most important factor when it comes to maintaining a healthy relationship with your partner during this challenge. When breaking the news, be honest. Don't over- or underplay the situation. After all, this person probably knows you better than anyone else, and your partner will know if you're telling the truth.

From the Book

A **covenant** is a solemn vow serving as a binding agreement or contract between two or more parties.

Once you've communicated the news, you might want to consider having your partner join you at your doctor's appointments. That way, he (or she) can more fully understand what you're going through and what kind of help you'll need and when you'll need it. If you'd rather cope with your appointments on your own, take your journal along with you to jot down notes, questions, and concerns. Your journal can be your second set of ears.

It's important to talk to your partner about how your treatment makes you feel, and describe if your energy level drops or your appetite changes. That way, your partner can know what you might need in terms of physical or emotional help.

Tales from the Trenches

Sharon and I were both so well blessed in our husbands. Charlie, Sharon's husband, picked up the phone the same time she did when the call came. Sharon said she could hear choking sounds in the phone and knew Charlie was crying. After the phone call, they hugged and cried. You see, Charlie is a "fixer" and here was something he couldn't fix—not in his mother or in Sharon. Even though he couldn't fix it, he could be a soldier in her battle. He went to every appointment and learned all he could. Charlie walked with Sharon every step of the way. As Sharon said, "That's what happens when you marry your best friend."

Under normal circumstances, talking about sexual intimacy can be difficult, and your partner may feel uncomfortable bringing the subject up. You may need to begin this conversation. Talk to your partner about the importance of affection and how holding hands and cuddling mean so much to you. Or, if you are the type of person who prefers "hearing sweet things" as opposed to touching, inform your partner that you have not gone deaf, and you still need to hear "sweet things." You may look different on the outside, but on the inside you are still just the same.

If you're like most couples who face this challenge, your foundation may shake, but it should not crumble. Open and honest discussion will be the mortar that holds the marriage together.

Family Matters: Telling the Kids

With rare exceptions, you should tell your children about your condition. Have you ever tried to keep a secret from a child? It's impossible. They eavesdrop. They hear the news from other children or adult friends. If you need help in telling them the news, seek help from a support group, a therapist, or a school psychologist.

If your children are still young, your first job is to reassure them that no matter what happens, they'll be taken care of. If your children are adults, you may want to keep your grandchildren in mind.

With adult children, your relationship with them will dictate the approach you take. If you're very close, you'll probably know how to tell them and how they'll react. If you're not close, you may have more difficulty.

Let's see. What's a mom for? Laundry, cooking, hugging, teaching, and taking care of the kids. But what happens now, when you may need some taking care of yourself, when *you* need the hugs? If you're like most moms, learning to ask for such things from your children, even if they're adult children, may be very difficult.

Take It from Us

Don't let your children hear it from someone else. Survivor Heidi hadn't told her daughter, but she had told several of her friends with children who attended the same school. One afternoon, her daughter came home in tears asking, "Mommy, when are you going to die?" Heidi spent more time undoing the damage than she would have just explaining what was happening.

Age Matters

When you tell your children, do so in an age-appropriate manner. Generally speaking, the younger they are, the more comfort they'll need. Preschool children need the KISS (Keep It Simple, Sweetie) approach. Don't lie to them, but keep it very simple. Hug them. Let them know there will always be someone around to take care of them.

If it becomes necessary, you may also need to help them understand that death is a part of life. You can use the loss of a pet, the end of a day, or the withering of a flower as analogies. Let them tell you how they feel. For the very young, it is frustrating because they don't know exactly how to express what they feel. This is a good time to help them draw or paint what they feel.

School-age children also need a simple approach, but with one addition: They're sure to have questions. They've probably heard the word *cancer,* and will be naturally and sympathetically curious. If you help them understand, they'll help you in return. They've already begun to see themselves as people. They also see themselves as useful. Let them tell you what they can do to help. They are also much better at putting words to feelings. If they do have trouble talking to you about your illness, ask them to write you a letter about what they think and feel.

Teen comes from an Old English word that means "agitation," and you've probably already discovered how appropriate the word is. Indeed, the teenage years represent a time of great transition and can be very tough for all involved—even without the addition of a serious illness. A teen's life is all about trying to "fit in." Anything that causes them to stand out will be vexing. You'll want to make sure to protect their privacy. Don't talk about your illness in front of their friends unless they tell you they feel comfortable with it.

However, no matter how standoffish or even surly your teens may behave in front of you, chances are that they are just plain scared.

The biggest reason teens get scared is that they barely have control of their life as it is and now they could be about to lose a loved one. This problem is so great that sometimes they distance themselves from the parent in order to buffer themselves from the pain.

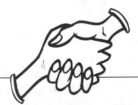

Helping Hand

Ask your teenagers for help. When Marion was diagnosed with breast cancer, she had two teenagers who were very curious about her disease. Marion also knew they surfed the Web, so she asked them to help her gather as much information as possible. By the time they finished their research, they knew more about breast cancer than she did. Not only did their involvement help her, it also made them feel part of her treatment plan.

They're also smart enough to understand the concept of genetics, and may be afraid that if cancer can strike you, it can strike them as well. It may be the first time they think of themselves as vulnerable in recognizing their own mortality.

The good news is that with age comes knowledge, and an older teen may be able to understand more difficult concepts when it comes to both the emotional and the medical challenge you face. A teen will typically ask more in-depth questions than a younger counterpart, and you'll be able to answer with more technical and clinical details.

Finally, do remember that as mature and intelligent as your teens may seem, they are in fact still children. Try to keep their lives as normal as possible and give them permission not to grieve or to worry, but to live as normal a teenage life as possible.

Gender Bender

Another thing to keep in mind is that your children's reaction may depend on their genders. Generally speaking, boys will tend to grieve at the news, to consider the loss of their mothers. Girls, on the other hand, will identify with their mothers and experience a mirroring effect, seeing themselves contracting the disease. Consider these gender issues, especially if your children are teenagers.

If you need more advice, and chances are you will, take the time to consult professionals about the best ways to break the news to a male or female child.

Folk Tales: Telling Your Parents

Age comes into play when telling your parents about your illness. If your parents are very old, physically ill, suffering from senility, or living far away, you may decide not to tell them at all.

If you do decide to tell—and if you're at all close to your parents we recommend that you do—understand that the news their child has a life-threatening illness violates the natural order of things. They are the ones that are supposed to become ill and face their mortality, not their children.

At the same time, no matter how old you and they are, you're still their baby, and most parents want the best for their babies. Breast cancer isn't the best. It will be difficult news for them to hear, to accept, and to cope with. The hardest part may be their feelings of helplessness—for once, there is truly nothing they can do to keep their child from being hurt.

Another issue to consider is the health and vitality of your parents. If they already lead sedentary, solitary lives, your news could increase their risk of developing depression. In this case, the best thing you can do for them is to let them do something for you! If there are ways that they can help you, please ask. Being active and involved will help them be part of your recovery.

Tales from the Trenches

Suzanne was 46 years old when she was diagnosed with breast cancer. Her mother was 74 years old, very healthy, and always very in tune with what was going on in her daughter's life. There was no way Suzanne could hide her diagnosis from her mother, and she didn't intend to. When she told her, her mother practically went into a state of shock that this could happen to her daughter. She said to Suzanne, "I'm 74 years old. You have most of your life ahead of you. I just wish it could be me." How many of your mothers have said that to you? Mothers give you the gift of life over and over.

Heart to Heart: Telling Your Friends

"A *friend* in need is a friend indeed." Those words ring especially true when it comes to coping with an illness like breast cancer.

For some of you, your friends are closer to you than your family and will want to help in whatever way they can. Because they are your friends and not your family, they may be easier to tell. Usually, friends are not as close as family, and this little bit of distance may make it easier for friends to cope.

Just as your family members acted differently, so will your friends. Because your friends are probably the same age and gender as you are, the way they are affected may be different than family members. They may be thinking that this could happen to them, too. And it could!

When it comes to telling friends, you might try remembering the five Ws and H you learned in writing class: who, what, when, where, why, and how. We already know the who (you and the individual you're ready to tell) and what (that you have cancer).

➤ **When.** Tell your friends when you both have some down time. Trying to relate difficult information when someone is answering phones or caring for unruly children or running off to meetings is not a good time. You want your friend to be able to focus on what you're saying.

➤ **Where.** Where do you want your friend to be when he or she learns your news? At a computer screen looking at an impersonal e-mail? Probably not. Face-to-face in a comfortable, private place is best, with a phone call at home running a close second. You have the ability to tune in on their tone of voice or facial expressions. This helps you determine the path you want to take when it comes to how much information they can handle.

➤ **Why.** Hiding information from friends, the people who know you so well, will be difficult. You may also want to forewarn them about mammograms and BSEs. You may need help. Friends do for one another. Now you may need them to do special things for you.

All that said, telling your friends individually is probably a good idea. Think, up front, of each friend and how they might react to this type of crisis. With some you can be blunt and rely on their strength to handle the news. With others you may have to break the news gently and be ready for tears.

From the Book

By definition, a **friend** is a person you know, like, and trust. In Ecclesiastes, a friend is referred to as "the medicine of life." Aristotle defines a friend as "a single soul dwelling in two bodies," and Cicero says a friend is "a second self."

Your multitasking friends will want to help. Once they have the news and know what you need, they can shop for both of you when they are at the store, pick up your kids when they are picking up theirs, and take care of your kids when they are taking care of theirs.

The most important thing friends can do is listen. When you are scared, sad, or disappointed or when someone in your family has accidentally said something to hurt you, you can turn to your friend.

A Tear to the Eye

I was speaking at a luncheon. During the meal, I began a conversation with the lady next to me. When she asked me about my current project, I mentioned the book. She told our table a story that put tears in everyone's eyes.

A single working mother in her town found out she had breast cancer. Her family and estranged ex-husband were several states away, and she knew she was going to need help. She got a baby-sitter for her children and asked all of her friends to join her for dinner at a local restaurant. After dinner, she told her friends that she had breast cancer and explained the treatments and timing of her disease. She said she needed their help desperately.

They made a list of all the things they could do for her and then created a schedule. For the next 12 months they were there with her and for her every step of the way. Whatever she needed, they did.

This group of fiends gained such a sense of fulfillment out of helping that they formed a special group. When any woman in their town was diagnosed with cancer, they rallied together, found out what the person's needs were, and helped out for as long as it took. Now that's a support group!

Take It from Us

A woman, whose family was a little less than supportive, turned to her friends for help. As most friends do, they came to her rescue. Her family, who was having difficulty with the fact that she had breast cancer, became even more difficult when friends arrived with meals and gifts. It made her family look bad. She suggests that when turning to friends, either have your family's support or be covert about their help.

When you are single, alone, and in need, friends are a special gift. And, never forget that you reap what you sow. There will be a time when you will need to help them.

Most of our family and friends are the mainstays of our lives. Where would we be without them? They are there for picnics, weddings, graduations, birthdays, and—more important—the little, normal, everyday things. Family and friends are the people we not only share our joys with but also our sorrows. Family and friends help us double the joys we share and cut the sorrows in half. Family and friends can be a big help in dealing with and getting through breast cancer.

A Final Word to the Wise

When we decide to share our news of being diagnosed with breast cancer, we have the very best intentions in how we relate it to others. And although our intentions are good, it does not mean that we will always be successful. No matter how long we have thought it through or how carefully we have selected our words, we still may not be able to help those around us cope or even understand.

If this is your case, don't hesitate to ask for professional help. Find a counselor who specializes in sharing this kind of news with partners or children. They may be more aware of what a child's or partner's need is, how to relate the information so that it doesn't terrify or worry them, and even what to expect from them down the road. Someone in a support group, a physician, or a member of a cancer society may be able to recommend a counselor with this type of expertise.

You don't want to suffer any more than you have to, and neither do your loved ones. This may be the most important ounce of prevention in your cure.

The Least You Need to Know

➤ You do not owe anyone the personal, intimate details about your illness. You choose what you want to share, when, and with whom.

➤ Try to compose yourself before telling others. They will pick up and reflect your state of mind.

➤ While there are general things to keep in mind when breaking the news, also think of specific concerns that different people will have.

➤ Seek professional help from those who know or have been there in helping you decide how to break the news.

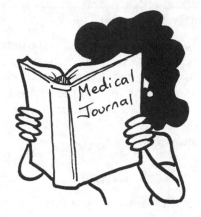

Learning a New Vocabulary

Once you've been diagnosed with breast cancer, you've entered a brave (or not so brave) new world. It's time to hit the information highway and become an informed consumer. Some folks listen to the doc's advice and go with it. Nothing wrong with that, if your doctor has his fingertips on all the up-to-the-minute details about your particular cancer. If he does, great. But what if he doesn't? Or what if he tends to pre-scribe a more aggressive treatment than the standard? Or less aggressive? How do you know what's best for you? How do you find out?

Sometimes those who listen to the doc's advice and go with it wonder later if they did the right thing. In this age of information, you owe it to yourself to dig up the details. You have one shot at this, and you don't want any regrets. The best news is that you don't have to dig very far, and you start here. In this chapter, we'll tune in to what the doctor's words mean, how to find more information about your diagnosis and op-tions, what to read—and what to skip—and how to learn from the sisterhood.

The Doctor's Word

Not knowing—a diagnosis, the meaning of a word, or the potential side effects of a treatment option—only feeds your anxiety. You feel helpless, hopeless. In this battle, you are what you know. The more you understand about your diagnosis and recommended treatment, the more you can do to make it successful.

The first step to becoming informed is to understand your diagnosis. Breast cancer comes in many different kinds, sizes, and stages, and doctors handle each one in a different way. When you got the word about the biopsy report, that moment put your mind in a whirl. So how can you remember exactly what the doctor or nurse said? Here's how.

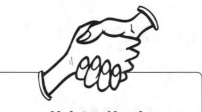

Helping Hand

Survivor Helen says, "When you know it's cancer, give yourself permission to grieve. I didn't know I could cry so much and so hard. But after the pity party, take charge of your life. Get the information you need."

Survivor's Notebook

As part of getting informed, start a survivor's notebook now. Get a loose-leaf notebook in an easy-to-carry size. On the inside front cover, create a "Return To:" box with your name and address so that if you lose it, the person who finds it can return it to you. (Even if you've never misplaced anything in your life, the current undue stress may cause you to lose track of details—like where you put your notebook.) Then, on the first page, list your doctors' and nurses' names and phone numbers. Use the notebook to keep all the details about your diagnosis and your treatment: questions, dates, names, responses, advice, and side effects of medications or treatments. As you become more informed, you'll also use it to summarize what you read, where you read it, and questions you have about it. So let's get started.

Take It from Us

You have time. Chances are, you've had the cancer two or three years already, maybe as long as eight or ten. Another week or so isn't a crisis, so take time to get informed.

Tell-All Diagnosis

The first document that goes into your notebook is a copy of your mammogram report. What does it show? How has it changed from your previous one(s)? Ask questions of nurses, doctors, or the radiologist who wrote the report. Keep asking until you understand everything there.

The next document is your diagnosis. Exactly what does the doctor say you have? What kind of cancer? Where is it located? What does the pathologist's report say? Get a copy of it; you're entitled to it. Keep asking questions until you understand exactly what it means. Here are some general terms for starters:

➤ **Ductal carcinoma in situ, lobular cancer in situ, or noninvasive carcinoma.** If your report lists these terms, you have what some medical folks today call a pre-cancerous condition. The most important detail is the "in situ" or "noninvasive" part. That means the condition is confined to the milk ducts (ductal) or the milk lobules (lobular); it hasn't spread anywhere. Of all the bad news you can get, this is best.

➤ **Invasive or infiltrating.** These words will be connected with either "ductal" or "lobular" and mean that your condition is no longer in situ, but has spread beyond the walls of the ducts or lobules.

Most other terms that may appear in your report are labels that tell how an invasive ductal carcinoma looks: tubular (looks like little tubes), medullary (has the color of the medulla, or brain tissue), mucinous (has mucus around it), papillary (has little fingers, or papules, that stick out). Other terms, however, may label a rare kind of malignancy, such as inflammatory breast cancer or Paget's disease.

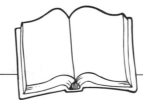

From the Book

Ductal carcinoma in situ, also called **intraductal carcinoma,** is usually considered a pre-cancerous condition and is confined to the milk ducts. **Lobular carcinoma in situ** is a pre-cancerous condition confined to the milk lobules. **Noninvasive carcinoma** is a term used to refer to either ductal carcinoma in situ or lobular carcinoma in situ. **Infiltrating** or **invasive cancers** are those that have grown outside the ducts or lobules. The **stage** of cancer indicates how far it has progressed.

All the World's a Stage

All kinds of cancer, including breast cancer, are categorized by *stage,* which generally indicates how far it has spread, which in turn determines treatment. The higher the stage, the more aggressive the treatment. So find out at what stage the pathologist has categorized your cancer. The report may use one of two staging systems, or even a combination. Here's a summary of them and what they mean:

The first staging system uses Roman numerals from I through IV, but begins with Stage 0:

➤ **Stage 0:** pre-cancerous (in situ) conditions

➤ **Stage I:** small, localized cancers, usually curable

➤ **Stage II:** small tumor with *positive lymph nodes,* or a larger tumor with or without positive lymph nodes

➤ **Stage III:** large tumor with positive lymph nodes

➤ **Stage IV:** tumor with obvious *metastasis*

Another kind of staging uses TNM, referring to Tumor, Nodes, and Metastases. In general, here's what it means:

➤ T refers to the size of the tumor, from T0 through T4, with T0 for in situ conditions and T4 for a very large tumor that has invaded other organs.

➤ N refers to the number of lymph nodes involved, with N0 meaning no positive nodes and N4 meaning extensive node involvement.

➤ M refers to the amount of metastases, from M0 to M4.

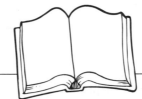

From the Book

Lymph nodes are glands found throughout the body that help filter bacteria. Cancer frequently spreads through the lymphatic system and shows up in lymph nodes. With breast cancer, many of these nodes are located in the armpit. **Positive lymph nodes** are those in which cancer is detected; **negative lymph nodes** show no cancer. **Metastasis** refers to the spread of cancer, as from the breast to some other part of the body.

Hotlines: Who You Gonna Call?

With your diagnosis in mind, you're ready to ask questions and search for answers. Many women turn first to a cancer hotline. Some are local, and if no one told you about a local hotline when you got your biopsy report, ask your doctor about it now. Even in small communities without a formal hotline, someone probably has made a standing offer to talk with newly diagnosed folks about the news.

Other hotlines are national. Some are staffed by survivors, those wonderful women of the sisterhood who have been where you are today and are now there to support you. They volunteer their time on the phone lines to help you with whatever questions you have.

Before you call, write down the questions that you want to ask. Do you want someone to help you understand your diagnosis or exactly what the doctor meant when he said such and such? Or someone to talk to about treatments? Want to hear about options for reconstruction? Need someone to help you cope now that your husband has ordered you to "quit that crying"? Want someone to help you overcome your fear, even though the statistics say you shouldn't be afraid? Need someone to bolster your spirits? All are typical hotline topics. There are no holds barred on what you can ask, so make a list of your questions, and leave space after each for the answer.

Okay. List done. Now, whom do you call? Check out the following popular hotlines, listed in alphabetical order, and then turn to Appendix E, "Informational Web Sites," for more sources.

➤ **American Cancer Society** at 1-800-ACS-2345 (1-800-227-2345) where trained cancer information specialists answer the phone in English or Spanish, 24 hours a day every day. At peak calling times, you may be on hold for a time, but eventually you'll always speak to a live person. The specialists can tap into a massive database, send documents through U.S. mail or e-mail, refer you to other national resources for support and financial assistance, and put you in touch with the local ACS office who in turn can set up an appointment for you with a Reach to Recovery volunteer.

➤ **Susan G. Komen Breast Cancer Foundation** at 1-800-IM-AWARE (1-800-462-9273) on Monday through Friday, 9:00 to 4:30 (Central time) connects you with an answering machine asking you to leave your name and number. A full-time staff person or a volunteer returns your call.

➤ **National Cancer Institute's Cancer Information Center** at 1-800-4-CANCER (1-800-422-6237) (in English or Spanish) connects you weekdays from 9:00 to 4:30 (local time) to a certified cancer information specialist who can send you free, up-to-date information about cancer, treatments, cancer research, current clinical trials and coping with cancer. Because they have 14 offices across the country serving different regions,

Take It from Us

Hotlines don't give medical advice and won't tell you what to do. But upon diagnosis, Helen called a hotline, asked to speak to a survivor, and talked to a total stranger for two hours. "She took away all my fears. She'd been there." Nine years out, Helen no longer remembers the woman's name, "But she got me through the toughest part. I'm so grateful to her."

Tales from the Trenches

Judy Perotti at Y-Me explains, "I'd been talking to a newly diagnosed survivor and we'd gone through a whole range of things. Finally she said, 'Thank you so much. You used all the words my doctor did but now I understand them better.' That really captures the essence of what we're about." Rest assured, someone there can help answer your questions, too.

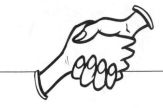

Helping Hand

Keep careful notes when it comes to calling hotlines. If you're calling a national hotline, lots of different folks answer the phones, so it's the luck of the draw who takes your call. As a result, if you call back, it's unlikely you'll get the same volunteer who'll know your particular concerns. So have your notes ready.

your call is usually answered fairly promptly. They can also provide referrals for information from other agencies.

➤ **Y-Me Breast Cancer Hotline** at 1-800-221-2141 provides information 24 hours, seven days a week, from trained peer breast cancer survivors, including help for partners and men survivors. (For Spanish, call 312-968-9505.) No matter when you call, you'll get a live person: no answering machine, no menu. Or, you can e-mail questions from their Web site at www.y-me.org.

As you talk, take notes. Get names, dates, and times so you can remember later when and where you picked up information. When you get off the phone, go over your notes. Add details to help you remember what you've heard. Then add these pages to your notebook. After you've talked with someone, feel free to call back. Usually, once you've had time to think about what you've learned, or after you've talked to someone else, you have more questions. No one keeps track of how many times you call, so go for it.

Read All About It!

Maybe the hotline answered your most immediate questions, but you need more details than chitchat can deliver. Now it's time to hit the books. Before you think you can't go back to those school-day study binges, cheer up. You've started in the right place with this book. We'll give you a clear, accurate overview of what breast cancer is all about, help you get a handle on possible treatments and what to expect of each, and help you prepare for what comes after—after the surgery, after the chemo, after the radiation. And we'll do it in what we think—and hope you do, too—is a light, readable style.

But we're not medical people. So maybe you want more medical details, or maybe you just want another point of view. There's no shortage of information. In fact, you'll find more printed pages than you can read in a couple of years (and meanwhile more will hit the bookshelves), so how do you sort through all the volumes to find what you need?

Stacks and Stacks at the Library

Your doctor or clinic may offer a reading list. Or use Appendix B, "Further Readings," for a recommended reading list. Armed with your list, hit the local library. Check the computer or card catalog and search for the recommended titles. When you locate a book on the shelf, browse through nearby titles. You may find another treasure. And never forget to ask the librarian for help. Librarians are absolutely remarkable folks who have an amazing range of knowledge. Tap into it.

Tales from the Trenches

Culture instills in many of us a respect for doctors, so much so that we put them on pedestals as if they always know what to do for every human ill. We were taught to follow whatever they said. But they are human, too. Most doctors are well educated, trained, certified, and (for the most part) exceedingly well informed. But they must deal with hundreds of patients with hundreds of ailments. You have only one problem: a specific kind of breast cancer. You can devote 100 percent of your time to learning about that problem. Do it. The more knowledge, the less fear.

Keep in mind, however, that just because you read a "fact" in a book, doesn't make it true. Here are the problems:

➤ **On any date, out of date?** The library keeps books for years. Since information about breast cancer and its treatment changes daily, make sure what you're reading has a recent copyright date. (You'll find that date in the front pages.) If the book is more than two years old, leave it.

➤ **Authoritative author?** While no reputable publisher will knowingly publish inaccurate information, the author's background may better tell you what to expect. If you want a technically serious medical book, choose an author who is an oncology doctor or surgeon.

➤ **Topic or topical?** Rather than choosing books about cancer in general or some cancer treatment in general, go for those that deal with breast cancer specifically or that at least have substantive sections devoted to breast cancer. Otherwise, you're likely to waste hours of time.

Timely if You Have the Time

Magazines carry the most up-to-the-minute information, but you may spend hours searching before you find something worth reading. If you have the time, however, check your library's periodical index (it may be online, on CD-ROM, or in print), but

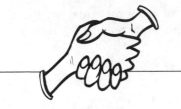

Helping Hand

Take the time to narrow your search. You can be overwhelmed by general information about cancer. Be sure to look for books or chapters that address just breast cancer. Use the tables of contents and indexes to make sure you're spending your reading hours most wisely.

consider the same advice we gave previously: Anything more than a couple of years old is probably too old to be meaningful. And anything really vital that is older than that will be in the newest books as well.

Bookstore Shelves

If your library lacks recent titles, your next stop should be your local bookstore. Usually, the books on women's health are categorized by type, so look for the section on breast cancer. If the section isn't obvious, ask.

Before you take home any book, browse through it. Study the table of contents. Check the index. Do you find there are topics about which you have questions? Then skim a chapter. Does it answer your questions? Does it footnote its sources so you can read more about a specific issue that interests you? Does it have a tone and style that you find easy to read, or at least accessible?

Books from Dot Com

If you don't find what you need in your local bookstore, or if you live in a community too small to offer adequate selections, turn to the Internet. Visit online bookstores like Amazon.com or Barnes and Noble at bn.com. Their online search engines will retrieve relevant titles.

Web Site Browsing

Another way to access current information is through the Internet. If you're afraid you'll get tangled in the Web, now's the time to overcome your fears. And before you cry that you don't have access to the Web, remember that most public libraries offer access, friends will likely let you browse, public schools sometimes let community members log on, and state universities usually allow community members access to their facilities (after all, you paid for it).

Yes, I know the Internet can be daunting. Your frustration level is fairly high right now anyway, and we don't want a Web search to reduce you to tears. So consider this advice:

First, check known Web sites. We've listed a bundle of them in Appendix E, but our top 20 are the following, arranged in alphabetical order. Most of them have links to other good sites as well.

➤ American Cancer Society offers information, outreach, and policy statements at www.cancer.org.

➤ American Cancer Society's Breast Cancer Network offers information and outreach at www.cancer.org/bcn/bcn.html.

➤ American Society of Plastic Surgeons offers information and resources at www.plasticsurgery.org.

➤ Association of Cancer Online Resources offers information at www.acor.org/.

➤ Breast Cancer Action offers information and support from a grassroots group at www.med.Stanford.edu/bca.

➤ Breast Cancer Answers offers information and details about clinical trials at www.medsch.wisc.edu/bca.

➤ Breast Cancer Information offers information at www.breastcancerinfo.com/.

➤ Cancer Care Inc. offers information, support, and outreach at www.cancercareinc.org/.

➤ Department of Defense Breast Cancer Decision Guide offers an online guide for making informed decisions at www.bcdg.com.

➤ Johns Hopkins Hospital offers information and resources at www.hopkins.med.jhu.edu.

➤ Susan G. Komen Breast Cancer Foundation offers information at www.komen.org.

➤ Mayo Clinic offers information at www.mayo.edu.

➤ MD Anderson Cancer Center offers information at www.mdanderson.org.

➤ Memorial Sloan-Kettering Cancer Center offers information at www.mskcc.org.

➤ National Alliance of Breast Cancer Organizations (NABCO) offers information at www.nabco.org.

➤ National Cancer Institute's CancerNet Information Service offers information specific to breast cancer at cancernet.nci.nih.gov/cancer_types/ breast_cancer.shtml.

➤ National Center for Complementary and Alternative Medicine details alternative treatments at nccam.nih.gov.

➤ National Library of Medicine's Medline Plus offers information and news at www.nlm.nih.gov/medlineplus/.

➤ Webmed offers detailed medical information, some of which is accessible by lay people, at webmed.org.

➤ Y-ME National Breast Cancer Organization offers information and support at www.y-me.org.

While you're browsing, keep your notebook handy. As you scroll and click your way through the sites, you'll eventually forget where you read something important. If you've taken notes on the Web site addresses, you'll be able to jump right back to that

Take It from Us

Exercise caution when browsing the Web! Since anyone can post anything out there, you may be exploring a site posted by a group of third-graders. Check the home page, see who's sponsoring the site, who wrote the material, and when it was last updated.

hot-topic page. Better yet, use a bookmark, the tool at the top of your Web browser screen to mark really good sites.

Of course, you can always print pages from the Web so that you can put the information directly into your notebook without the pain of writing lengthy, detailed notes. Before you hit the "Print" icon, however, you may want to check "Print Preview" in the "File" menu. You may be about to print something that runs hundreds of pages.

As you check out the Web, be alert to the reputation of the Web site you're browsing. Is it sponsored by a legitimate organization? Is the authorship valid? Has it been updated recently? Do reputable sites maintain links with it? And note what the Web site address tells you. If it ends in "org," the site is sponsored by an organization; if "edu," it's an educational institution; if "gov," it's government-sponsored. Always consider any possible hidden agenda of sites you browse.

And the Survivors Say ...

After you're brain dead from reading stacks of print and bleary-eyed from Web browsing, you'll probably want someone to talk to, to listen, to answer questions, to serve as a sounding board. Whatever the case, survivors are ready to help. (For more about connecting with other survivors, see Chapter 17, "Groupies: Yea or Nay?") How can you hook up with someone to talk with? Try some of these steps:

1. Call your local chapter of the American Cancer Society. The number is in the business White Pages. Tell them you need to talk, and they'll connect you with a volunteer.

2. Call one of the national support groups, like Reach to Recovery (part of the American Cancer Society) or Y-Me (phone numbers given previously), and ask about a local chapter. They'll connect you with survivors.

3. Ask at your doctor's office for someone to talk to. They may connect you with a survivor volunteer or one of the nurses. Nurses usually have more time than doctors do to answer questions and listen to concerns.

4. Call your local hospital and ask for Patient Services. Tell them you need someone to talk to. They'll help.

5. Call someone you know who's been through the battle, even if you don't know her (or him) well and especially if she's been through it recently. Treatments have changed dramatically over the last few years, so hook up with someone who's familiar with the how of now.

6. Finally, ask your healthcare professional to provide you with a password to CHESS (Comprehensive Health Enhancement Support System), a University of Wisconsin site that includes information, case studies, and a discussion group. The password ensures confidentiality and is available through any provider with a license to CHESS. (Call 1-800-361-5481 or 1-888-553-5036 for more information.)

Tales from the Trenches

Diedre, who had a mastectomy, chemo, radiation, and stem cell bone marrow transplant two years ago, says, "I don't know what I would have done without Carol Rogers, founder of Woman to Woman. She talked me through everything, asking questions, suggesting resources, and bolstering my spirits. She was wonderful. Never hesitate to call someone, even if you don't know the person whose number you've been given." Today, Diedre is working full speed ahead as an elementary school principal.

Armed with all the details from hotlines, books and magazines, and the information superhighway, and with your survivor's notebook as your log, you'll be an informed consumer confidently speaking an all-new vocabulary. As a result, you'll be far better prepared to join the new world of the battlefield and to march toward successful treatment.

The Least You Need to Know

➤ Knowledge is power, so it's important to be an informed consumer.

➤ Start your knowledge search with a thorough understanding of your diagnosis.

➤ Call on national hotlines, libraries, bookstores, Web sites, and local survivors for information.

➤ Keep a survivor's notebook in which you record all your questions and their answers and important information.

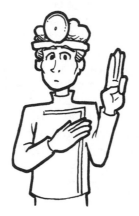

Chapter 4

Taking Their Word for It

In This Chapter

➤ Choosing your doctor and/or surgeon

➤ When—and *if*—to get another opinion

➤ What the survivors tell you

➤ What's right for you

One survivor put it bluntly: "It's important to find a doctor you really, really like and trust. He or she is going to lead you through some very unpleasant stuff, and attitude plays an important role in how well you tolerate it. It also plays a role in your willingness to follow through and be compliant."

Never forget this important tenet: You are the employer and the folks on your healthcare team are your employees. As an informed consumer, you make the decisions about your medical care. The overwhelming majority of healthcare folks are caring, compassionate, supportive men and women who entered their profession because they have a burning desire to help us get and stay healthy. But occasionally, the odd one out comes into your life. What do you do?

In this chapter, we'll show you some of the factors involved in creating a good patient-doctor partnership, getting a second or third opinion (even in a good relationship), and finding ways to make the partnership work.

Dr. Who?

To help you with your battle against breast cancer, you'll have a team of medical specialists, part of whom may already be in place. Your primary provider, family doctor, or gynecologist probably sent you for your mammogram. A radiologist read this x-ray, and when it showed something suspicious, a radiologist—perhaps the same one—did a biopsy. If the biopsy showed a pre-cancerous or cancerous condition, you were probably referred to a breast surgeon. Then there's the *medical oncologist,* the *radiation oncologist,* the *plastic surgeon,* and all their respective nursing and associated staff. It's quite a team.

Choosing a doctor/surgeon is a rather daunting task on a good day, but in the midst of the post-diagnosis chaos—well, it's plain overwhelming. And knowing that you'll have multiple decisions to make about a whole team of medical specialists may cause a moment of panic. Then, in the midst of that panic, you realize that you're about to meet a total stranger who, in the next few days or weeks, is probably going to do something fairly drastic to your body. But never fear! We have solid suggestions for making the right choices.

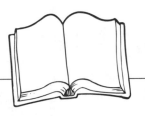

From the Book

A **medical oncologist** is a cancer doctor who specializes in the administration of drugs. A **radiation oncologist** is a cancer doctor who specializes in the administration of radiation therapy. A **plastic surgeon** does reconstructive surgery to rebuild a breast that has been surgically removed.

Tales from the Trenches

"I am still incensed by the first medical oncologist my surgeon sent me to," says Karla. "I was met by his receptionist, who put me in an examining room and told me to strip to my panties. No gown. It was July, and the air conditioning was set at 68 degrees. I waited 20 minutes for the great man. When he came in, he was wearing a three-piece suit with a white coat over it. He examined me and proceeded to tell me, still naked and shivering, what he was going to do for me. 'Just leave it all to me,' he said. 'I'll take care of everything.' I went home and called my doctor and asked if I had to put up with that. He sent me elsewhere."

Of course you want the best medical care you can get. Take the surgeon, for instance. It's a one-shot deal with this surgery, and it's your life lying there on the table under this person's knife. If he or she is going to take out part of your breast—or take off all of it—you need someone whom you can trust, someone with whom you can talk easily, and someone who has the time to listen to and answer your questions.

There are lots of surgeons, and all of them are trained to perform breast surgery. There are far fewer surgeons who specialize in breast surgery, but that's probably who you want for your surgeon. The specialists are the folks with the most experience and, in all likelihood, with the most up-to-date knowledge about breast cancer in its many forms. If they perform lots of breast surgeries, they will also be far more able to identify individual differences, namely yours. Just for a ballpark figure, try to find a surgeon who does at least 50 breast surgeries a year.

Take It from Us

Do background checks on your surgeons to make sure they have the experience you need and want! In 1996, almost 400 surgeons in Maryland performed only one or two breast surgeries. To find out a perspective surgeon's track record, call where he or she practices (maybe in more than one facility); ask about case volume. Or ask at his or her office. Or inquire at the state board of quality assurance. Aim for finding a surgeon who performs about 50 breast surgeries a year.

Say What? Trust and Tact

How do you find a good medical team? Where do you begin? One common practice is for your primary care provider to recommend a surgeon who in turn recommends the rest of the team. But your doctors may handle the process differently, and part of the procedure is dependent on your insurance carrier. Nevertheless, rest assured that you will have one or more recommendations readily available.

How do you know if you want to follow the recommendation? Three big issues tell the story: licensing, experience, and personality.

Certificates on the Wall

Your first concern, of course, is your doctor's or surgeon's credentials. Sure, they've graduated from some medical college and have a license to practice in your state.

What you don't know is whether they graduated at the top of the class or the bottom, and the diploma won't tell you. But there are other sources.

Generally, your best choice for a surgeon is one certified by the American Board of Surgery. You can check by calling The American Board of Medical Specialists at 847-491-9091 or by checking its Web site at www.abms.org. If your recommended surgeon has been practicing long enough, he or she may have earned credibility with other organizations as well, so ask about membership in the American College of Surgeons and the Society of Surgical Oncology, two organizations that work jointly to develop standards for breast cancer surgeries.

For other specialists, ask about board certification in their specialty (such as radiation oncology) and then in their subspecialty (breast cancer). And ask if they've earned the AMA Physician Recognition Award, an indication that they have attended a minimum of 150 hours of continuing education in the past three years. That means they have been keeping up with the research and new treatments that come out at warp speed these days.

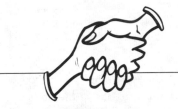

Helping Hand

Look beyond the surface. Experience is an important criterion when choosing a medical team. But there's a world of difference between twenty years' experience and one year's experience twenty times.

They've Seen It All

Ideally, you'd like an experienced medical team that's seen and done everything. You want to know that they have a broad range of experience, to be assured your treatment is not a first for them, that they know what to expect of your diagnosis, and exactly how to deal with it. Breast cancer specialists who work with the condition every day certainly have more experience than those who deal with only a few cases a year. Still, there's more to experience than simply the number of years they've been in practice. You'd like to know your medical team keeps up with the latest advances, the hottest news, the best treatments, and the finest procedures. You'd like to know that their equipment is state of the art and that their knowledge is, too. Since these are not certifiable details, you may discover them only by comparing what you've read and learned with what these folks tell you. Judge by the answers to your questions.

No Dale Carnegie Flunk-Outs

Some doctors show more patience and more compassion than others do. Some surely earned better grades than others in the course on bedside manners. Some carry an aura of arrogance, the "look-at-me-for-who-I-am" attitude. But then you'll meet some who are more gentle than others, those who remember that while they've explained a biopsy to hundreds of patients, this is the first time they've explained it to you. Those are the kind of medical professionals you're looking for: the professionals who seem to have had better training in communications or better upbringing with good manners than their less sensitive counterparts.

You should look for someone who is perfectly straightforward with you—not cold and impersonal, but honest and frank. You're into serious business here, so you can skip the sugar coating. You need—and have every right—to understand precisely your condition and your *prognosis*. Still, doctors are human, too. They may find it emotionally tough to give you bad news, especially if you're having a tearful time dealing with the news. Then, in spite of their best intentions, they may hold back a little, trying to regain composure themselves.

From the Book

A **prognosis** is the prediction for the course of the disease and your chances of recovery.

You want someone who will help educate you, to help you understand the technically complicated medical details they will be discussing with you. You want someone who will answer your questions—even the same ones over and over—until you fully understand. But watch out for medical folks who want you to leave it all up to them. You're a big part of the decision-making process, and any doctor who glosses over your role should get a glossy photo of you—as you walk out the door.

Take It from Us

Younger is not always better! One survivor said she thought younger doctors were almost always more compassionate, patient, and kind; but oncology nurse Christine Lammers says age has nothing to do with it. "It's personality, plain and simple. Doctors are just like the rest of us. Some are absolutely wonderful, warm, caring human beings. And some aren't."

Helen's doctor would probably win the personality contest hands down. He spent three hours with her and her hubby on the Friday afternoon before her scheduled Monday morning surgery. Then he gave her his home phone number in case she had questions over the weekend. That's compassion.

And the Winner Is ...

Before you make your final choice, check two more important details. First, does your insurance cover the services of the doctor and/or surgeon you want? If not, you may need to reconsider. Second, talk to survivors—particularly those whose doctor and/or surgeon is the one you're considering. Were they satisfied?

If worse comes to worse and you feel you need another choice, call your state or county medical societies or local hospital for referrals. Talk to survivors living in your area. Ask for their recommendations. They have nothing to lose by being perfectly blunt about their own care.

Finally, if you are willing to travel away from home, say so. Ask for referrals to area university hospitals or hospitals in nearby larger communities. Keep in mind, however, that you will continue to travel to and from your treatment center for about a year, and then follow-up visits continue afterward for as long as five years. If you choose to get treatment away from home, be prepared to commit to added burdens, including ...

➤ **Travel** (perhaps in poor weather conditions and frequently during very early or very late hours)

➤ **Time** (including hours on the road and nights away from home)

➤ **Effort** (even when you're nauseated, exhausted, and would rather be cuddled in your own bed)

➤ **Finances** (including cost of transportation, lodging, meals, and long-distance phone calls)

➤ **Loneliness** (being in strange surroundings away from close proximity of friends and family)

Still, this is your life at stake. Maybe travel, time, effort, finances, and loneliness aren't really big issues in your situation. In fact, the battle against breast cancer includes numerous little side skirmishes, and maybe travel-related hurdles are just that—inconvenient skirmishes. Our only job is to let you know your options so that you can make choices wisely, and with your eyes open. That way, you'll arrive on the battlefield fully prepared.

Second—and Third—Opinions

Let's assume now that you've settled on a doctor and/or surgeon. Does that mean that whatever he or she says is now the gospel? Hardly. Remember, you're an informed consumer. And doctors, like all the rest of us, think differently: some are more aggressive, others more conservative. Thus, you may need a second opinion. Or even a third.

So now you may worry, "Will I offend this doctor if I say I want a second opinion?" Do you worry about offending the car dealer when you decide you have a better deal down the street? This is a mega-bunch more important than a new car. And it will probably cost more.

You may want to begin by getting a second opinion of the pathologist's report. You have the right to the slides and lab reports and can take them (or have them sent) wherever you wish for another look-see. (Pathologists may be reluctant to let go of irreplaceable slides, but keep at it until you find a mutually agreeable means to the end.) After all, if the pathologist missed something, or misinterpreted something, everything else changes.

To check on the general quality of pathology work in your hospital, call the Joint Commission on Accreditation of Healthcare Organizations (JCAHO) at 630-792-5000 or check its Web site at www.jcaho.org. Ask for the hospital's inspection report. The reports have been available to the public since 1977.

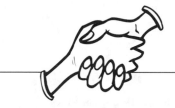

Helping Hand

Feel free to feel comfortable! If you want a second opinion and your doctor seems put out, so be it. Any doctor worth the diploma on the wall will welcome a second opinion. Don't trust doctors who try to play God.

When?

How do you know if you should get a second opinion? You should probably get a second opinion if …

➤ **You live in a rural area.** Of course you can get excellent treatment at small hospitals, but the medical folks there probably aren't breast cancer specialists and the hospital may not have the state-of-the-art equipment a large medical center will have. It's better to see the specialists. Ask your hometown doctor for a referral. He or she will understand.

➤ **There's something "borderline" about your condition.** For instance, you hear a statement like "We don't usually do chemo in a case like yours, but in this instance, I think we should." Or you hear the converse, like "We usually do a mastectomy in a case like this, but in your situation, I think we shouldn't." Better to check another opinion.

➤ **You're an HMO member.** While you can get superb care through an HMO, know that historically some HMO doctors have been prohibited from telling their patients about certain expensive treatments and/or those unavailable through the local HMO. Public outcry has severely reduced the so-called "gag rule," but who knows if and where it still exists. Better to find out, even if you have to pay for the second opinion yourself.

➤ **You've been given no hope and told there is no further treatment to help you.** Even if a doctor tells you your condition is inoperable or that the type of

Take It from Us

More opinions means more decisions to make. If you get a second or third opinion, be prepared to deal with the emotional impact of deciding who's right. One survivor had four opinions from four doctors—(her gynecologist, two surgeons, and a radiologist)—and ended up seeing a psychologist to help her sort it all out.

cancer you have is untreatable, get another opinion. There's a chance that a different doctor may give a different diagnosis, know of another treatment, or decide that your condition is, after all, operable. It may save your life.

➤ **You have a rare cancer.** We've talked about the importance of specialists already, and if you have a rare cancer, you really need a specialist in your kind of cancer. If the specialist is across the continent, then perhaps your doctor can at least consult with him or her via phone, e-mail, or fax.

You may have other reasons for seeking a second opinion, and they are probably valid. The most important issue is that you're comfortable that you've had the right diagnosis and the right advice about treatment. (More on making decisions about treatment in Chapter 5, "Decisions, Decisions, Decisions.")

Who?

If your condition (physical or emotional) warrants a second (or third) opinion, the next question, of course, is who do you call? If your doctor recommends someone for a second opinion, this new person probably works closely with your doctor, maybe thinks the same way, and perhaps even works in the same clinic, the same hospital, or with the same group of specialists. What you really want is an independent doctor, someone completely independent of your doctor. If you live in a small community, it may mean you have to go out of town, perhaps to a university or research hospital.

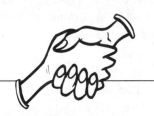

Helping Hand

Seek knowledge, constantly. Oncology nurse Judy Gianelos, herself a survivor, says, "I'm appalled at the number of people who aren't proactive about their treatment. The more you understand, the better able you are to deal with yourself and your condition."

To decide who to see for your second or third opinion, first call breast cancer survivor friends and medical folks for recommendations. For instance, surgical nurses have insights about surgeons that the rest of us don't. Or call a breast cancer hotline, the American Cancer Society, the National Cancer Institute, the American Society of Clinical Oncology, or your local medical society for a referral. (See Appendix E, "Informational Web Sites.") Call a hospital of your choice and request a referral to a breast cancer specialist, or call a local women's health center.

After you've made enough calls, you'll start hearing certain names pop up more frequently than dandelions in your lawn. When that happens, you're on your way to finding the right person for a second opinion.

After you make the appointment, get going with making your list of questions. And don't forget to take your notebook with you to the appointment. It's wise to take a friend or objective family member who can help take notes. You might even want to take a tape recorder. Always ask, but no responsible doctor or surgeon will object to your recording your consultation. Later, you'll be relieved that you're able to replay the conversation to make sure you didn't miss or misunderstand something. If your head is spinning anything like mine was, some details just spin off altogether. But not with the tape recorder. It just spins back the details, as many times as you want.

Tales from the Trenches

"My doctor came in, said I had a malignancy, that surgery was scheduled for Friday, and did I have any questions. Just like that," explained one survivor. "I was left breathless and had the impression that I had absolutely no time to consider other options or another opinion." In reality, of course, you do have time. Not months, but certainly days or a few weeks. The cancer has been in you for several years, maybe longer, so you can take the time to get the medical help you need. "The decision was made for me," she concluded, "so I wasn't part of the process."

Survivors' Advice

Karla, a survivor whose story you read at the beginning of this chapter, told me, "You have to like and trust your doctor." Her new doctor "actually calls me at home to see how I'm feeling when I haven't called him." Choosing your medical team is a bit like choosing your husband. It's a long-term relationship for better or worse, through sickness and health. So it's a crucial decision. Your medical team, however, unlike your husband, isn't much interested in granting you special wishes. Don't expect roses on your birthday. On the other hand, as in any marriage, you can put up with a few dirty socks on the floor or late nights at the office as long as the overall results work okay. Your medical team may have some quirks, too (don't we all?); but if you're happy with the overall results, you can probably live with the rest. Nobody's perfect.

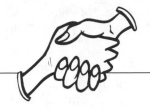

Helping Hand

Find the right doctor for you. Janelle, until she was widowed, lived on a farm and always had a few horses around. As an eight-and-a-half-year survivor, Janelle makes the comparison, "If the horse kicks, get rid of it. There are lots of good horses out there." Likewise, there are lots of truly wonderful, caring, compassionate doctors out there. You deserve one of them.

Take It from Us

Don't neglect your emotional needs when it comes to picking a surgeon. You may hear a comment like "He needs a better bedside manner, but he's a great surgeon." Maybe "great surgeon" is more important to you than personality. Choose what's most important to you or you'll be fighting more than breast cancer.

Not everyone seeks out doctors and surgeons on her own, and not everyone goes for a second opinion, much less a third. For example, my own surgeon is a prince of a guy. My primary care provider recommended him to me, and I liked him the minute I met him. He's young—30-something—so my only concern was that maybe he lacked experience. But my husband and I learned that he is a breast cancer specialist, works out of the local hospital–affiliated breast center, and is highly respected by others in the specialty. During appointments, he always gives my husband and me every minute we need; he answers lists of questions, sometimes more than once; he never talks down to us, never tries to sugarcoat the facts, never skirts an issue. He suggested I might be more comfortable with a second opinion; he recommended I see a radiation oncologist before surgery; and I followed his recommendations. Meanwhile, I talked to other survivors, read and checked everything he said against what I heard and read. It all fit. I felt comfortable. Who knows why he's so good at his job. Maybe it's learned behavior. His mother is a breast cancer survivor.

Some survivors have found unusual criteria by which to judge their medical teams. One woman is convinced that when the medical folks involved her in what was happening at the moment—what the new procedure was about, how it would be done, what would happen next—that she had just enough of a distraction that she experienced less pain.

Another woman blames her surgeon for literally promising her that her lump was benign. She had absolutely no preparation for the malignancy. If the surgeon had been more objective, she's convinced she would have experienced far less emotional turmoil.

Still another survivor complained about the lack of personal contact from her medical oncologist, that she was made to feel like just another body getting the medical recipe of the day. But another survivor shrugged off the whole idea. After all, she said, the doctors know more than she does.

Take It or Leave It

We've rattled on with advice about choosing your medical team and about second and third opinions, but the truth of the matter is, you must do whatever makes you comfortable. If you don't want to deal with second opinions and feel that your recommended surgeon is just fine, go with it. If you can't face up to checking out alternative medical folks, don't add further stress to your already catapulting world.

You have to do what makes you most comfortable.

The Least You Need to Know

➤ Choose a medical team that makes you comfortable.

➤ In some situations, you probably need a second opinion.

➤ Some survivors rely on whomever the primary care physician recommends; others don't.

➤ You have to weigh the alternatives and decide for yourself.

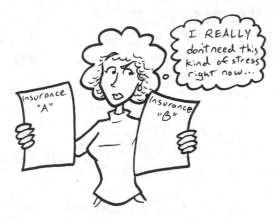

Chapter 5

Decisions, Decisions, Decisions

In This Chapter

➤ Decisions that are up to you

➤ When—and what—your insurance dictates

➤ Keeping the mind-body connection healthy

➤ Decision-making, the communication process, and your medical team

---

Some women take offense with the doctors who say, no questions asked, "Here's what we're going to do." Other women are scared out of their bras to hear the doctor or surgeon say, "Here are your options. Here are the percentages. Now, what do you want to do?" Most of us were taught to follow the doctor's orders. We break a leg, we go to the doctor, he puts on the right kind of cast, and tells us what we can and cannot do for the next six weeks. No decisions on our part. We do what we're told.

Breast cancer, however, doesn't have quite such an easy fix. In every case, you have the right to decide who's going to do what, when, and where. Sometimes, your insurance informs, or even controls, the decisions you make. Still, it's your decision, even if your doctor isn't one of those who asks you what you want to do.

In this chapter, we'll tell you what choices you can or must make, how to find out if and how much your insurance is going to pay, and what alternatives will help you feel more comfortable during treatment. By adding this advice into the mix, you'll be prepared—or at least better prepared—to choose from among your options.

Who, What, When, and Where

We've already talked about selecting your medical team (see Chapter 4, "Taking Their Word for It"). Now, assuming your surgeon and/or doctors are in place, your next decision is choosing what treatment is best for you. With breast cancer, "treatment" is usually plural, involving at least one kind of therapy and perhaps as many as three or four. Depending on the type of cancer you have and how advanced it is, you may have one or all of the following:

➤ **Local therapy** treats the tumor with surgery and/or radiation

➤ **Systemic therapy** uses chemicals or hormonal therapy traveling through the bloodstream to attack the tumor

➤ **Adjuvant therapy** is a systemic therapy used when your doctor suspects cancer cells may have escaped into other parts of the body even though no detectable cancer remains after surgery

The usual routine is for your surgeon to recommend a surgical treatment and, after the pathologist's report is in, send you on to oncology specialists who recommend the rest. In either case, though, you may be given two or even three choices. How do you think this through?

Recommendation, Please

Starting with first things first, let's consider the surgical decision. Refer to the notebook you began earlier (see Chapter 3, "Learning a New Vocabulary") and review what your biopsy showed:

➤ What type of breast cancer do I have?

➤ Is it in situ or infiltrating?

➤ Has it metastasized?

➤ What stage is my cancer?

These are the bare-bones facts on which you'll flesh out answers to lots of questions. Remember, breast cancer comes in many shapes and styles, and what was right for your sister or best friend may not be right for you. Know your diagnosis.

Until you've had some kind of surgery—a *surgical biopsy, lumpectomy,* or *mastectomy* (and we'll talk about these options in detail)—there are some unknowns. For instance, you won't know about lymph node involvement or the results of any *hormone receptor* tests (another topic we'll take up at some length later in the book). Without that information, no one can confidently recommend any local or systemic therapy. So your first decision may be whether to have a lumpectomy, mastectomy, or *bilateral mastectomy.* Without going into the details now (we will in Chapters 7, "Taking Your Lumps: Lumpectomy," and 8, "When They Take It All: Mastectomy"), we can still weigh the pros and cons.

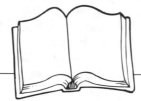

From the Book

A **surgical biopsy** removes a small lump of tissue for pathological examination. A **lump-ectomy** is the removal of a lump of malignant or pre-cancerous tissue along with a margin of tissue, said to be a **positive margin** if it contains malignant or pre-cancerous tissue and a **negative margin** if not. A **mastectomy** is the removal of the breast; a **bilateral mastectomy** is the removal of both breasts. Tissue that tests positive as a **hormone receptor** is sensitive to hormones and can thus be treated with hormonal therapy.

Ask your surgeon two questions:

➤ What is the usual surgical treatment for my kind of breast cancer at my stage?

➤ Is there anything about my case that would suggest something different from the usual?

Ask for explanations, and then compare the surgeon's recommendations with the chart later in this chapter, compiled from recommendations from the American Cancer Society (ACS) and the National Comprehensive Cancer Network (NCCN).

Standard or Not?

If your surgeon recommends something dramatically different from the so-called standard, ask for reasons behind his or her decision. At the same time, however, remember there's no such thing as "standard breast cancer," so "standard treatment" is only a set of averages. Every woman's case carries a unique set of details, and your surgeon and doctors have all these details in mind when they offer recommendations. My point? You won't be comfortable with any regimen unless you understand and accept it. So ask. Be an informed consumer. Then decide.

Take It from Us

Don't let time be the only factor in deciding which treatment you think is best for you! If one kind of treatment takes three months, another takes six months, or the whole regimen is going to take a year, focus on the fact that whatever treatment you take, it's just a temporary inconvenience. It will pass. Don't sacrifice the short term for the long term.

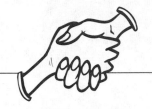

Helping Hand

Take advantage of the resources. You may want to use the Breast Cancer Decision Guide for Military and Civilian Families to help make decisions. The guide and detailed instructions are accessed online at www.bcdg.org/about_the_decision_guide.html. The site is sponsored by the Department of Defense as part of federal funding for breast cancer research.

What if your surgeon gives you a choice between a lumpectomy and a mastectomy? Or between a mastectomy and a bilateral mastectomy? How do you decide? By learning everything you can about your diagnosis, what it means, and what the options are. But you have to read—and you're on your way by reading this book—and then ask questions. Lots of them. Start by comparing the chart later in this chapter with your diagnosis, and then formulate a list of questions for your surgeon:

➤ What are the advantages of each kind of surgery?

➤ What are the disadvantages of each kind of surgery?

➤ Why would you recommend one over the other?

➤ What are my percentages for regaining full health with each procedure?

➤ What typical radiation and/or systemic and/or adjuvant therapies are recommended with each procedure?

Make note of the answers in your notebook. Then, to digest what you've been told, make a list. Put the advantages in one column and disadvantages in another. Then, call a hotline again. Read, check the Internet, and talk. Talk to survivors. Talk to family and friends. Keep track of their comments, suggestions, and observations, revising your advantages-disadvantages list as you go.

Finally, after you've done enough reading, studying, and talking, when you look at your list, the fog around your decision will lift. Take your list with you to your appointment with the surgeon to discuss your final decision. Then, if you have made a decision based on misinformation or misinterpretations, your surgeon can point out the error before you make a serious mistake.

Later, after you get the pathologist's report from whatever surgical procedure you have, you'll use the same process to make decisions about radiation, systemic, and/or adjuvant therapy. For instance, if your medical oncologist recommends a stem cell rescue (sometimes called a bone marrow transplant), you'll want to ask the informed-consumer questions to find out why. It's a fairly drastic measure used to treat advanced stages of breast cancer with such high doses of chemo that, without the rescue, would be fatal. A somewhat controversial treatment, it involves removing bone marrow prior to treatment and regenerating it through stem cell support or transplant. Still, it's saved lots of lives.

Standard Regimens for Breast Cancer Treatment

If You Have ...	The Usual Treatment Is ...
Stage 0	
Lobular carcinoma in situ (LCIS)	Observation OR in special circumstances with certain risk factors, bilateral mastectomy
Stage 0	
Ductal carcinoma in situ (DCIS)	
a. DCIS in 2 or more quadrants	**a.** total mastectomy (without lymph node dissection)
b. DCIS in 1 quadrant and negative margins	**b.** total mastectomy (without lymph node dissection) OR lumpectomy with radiation
c. DCIS in 1 quadrant with small, low-grade cancer and negative margins	**c.** lumpectomy with radiation OR lumpectomy without radiation OR total mastectomy (without lymph node dissection)
Stages I and II	
Invasive breast cancer	Lumpectomy and removal of underarm lymph nodes and radiation therapy OR modified radical mastectomy
Additional treatment dictated by tumor size and *nodal status*, as follows:	
a. Node negative and ...	
a-1. tumor smaller than .05 cm	**a-1.** no adjuvant therapy
a-2. cell type is tubular, colloid, or medullary and smaller than 1 cm	**a-2.** no adjuvant therapy
a-3. cell type is tubular, colloid, or medullary and larger than 1 cm but smaller than 3 cm	**a-3.** consider adjuvant therapy
a-4. cell type is tubular, colloid, or medullary and 3 cm or larger	**a-4.** adjuvant therapy recommended
a-5. cell type is invasive ductal or invasive lobular and tumor is less than 1 cm with no unfavorable features	**a-5.** no adjuvant therapy
a-6. cell type is invasive ductal or invasive lobular and tumor is less than 1 cm but with unfavorable features	**a-6.** consider adjuvant chemotherapy or hormonal therapy

continues

Standard Regimens for Breast Cancer Treatment (continued)

If You Have ...	The Usual Treatment Is ...
Stages I and II	
a-7. cell type is invasive ductal or invasive lobular and tumor larger than 1 cm that is hormone receptor-negative	**a-7.** adjuvant chemotherapy recommended
a-8. cell type is invasive ductal or invasive lobular and tumor larger than 1 cm that is hormone receptor-positive	**a-8.** Tamoxifen, with or without chemotherapy for tumors up to 3 cm and chemotherapy and Tamoxifen for tumors over 3 cm
b. Node positive and ...	
b-1. hormone receptor-negative	**b-1.** adjuvant chemotherapy recommended
b-2. hormone receptor-positive	**b-2.** adjuvant chemotherapy and Tamoxifen
Stage IIIA	
Invasive breast cancer, if operable	Modified radical mastectomy followed by chemotherapy and radiation (if hormone receptor-negative) OR chemotherapy, followed by modified radical mastectomy followed by additional chemotherapy, radiation, and (if hormone receptor-positive or uncertain) Tamoxifen, OR chemotherapy, followed by lumpectomy, underarm lymph node removal, and followed by additional chemotherapy and (if hormone receptor-positive or uncertain) Tamoxifen
Stage IIIB	
Invasive breast cancer, inoperable	Neoadjuvant chemotherapy, with or without Tamoxifen; if tumor shrinks enough to be operable, treatment follows treatments for Stage IIIA; otherwise, individualized therapy with no standard treatment
Stage IV	
Invasive breast cancer, if tumor is ...	
a. hormone receptor-positive and/or distant spread affects only bone or soft tissue	**a.** hormonal therapy followed in some cases by chemotherapy

If You Have ...	The Usual Treatment Is ...
Stage IV	
b. hormone receptor-negative and/or distant spread affects internal organs	**b.** chemotherapy and/or other chemotherapy protocol

Clinical Trials: Innocent or Guilty

One of the decisions you may face is your doctor's or surgeon's request that you participate in a *clinical trial*. Lest you think you've been asked to become a human guinea pig, know that prior to subjecting patients to this new treatment, the research protocol undergoes stringent review by a board of scientists, doctors, nurses, and laypersons. In most cases your risk is minimal, but you may have some real benefits.

Be assured that you cannot be placed in a clinical trial without your explicit permission, which includes your signature on a document called an Informed Consent Form. Sometimes quite lengthy and detailed, this form must ...

➤ Explain the rationale.

➤ Identify who is and is not eligible.

➤ Describe the procedure.

➤ Detail potential risks and benefits.

➤ Name the research participants (doctors, surgeons, etc.).

➤ Address concerns such as confidentiality, cost, and who to call if you have questions about your rights or the safety of this study.

Yes, there are justifiable cheers and jeers for participating in any clinical trial. The trials are so far-reaching in scope, however, that it's impossible to say here whether or not you should participate. You have to ask the usual informed-consumer questions of your doctor and of the research group involved. And, of course, you'll want to check with your insurance company to make sure you're still covered.

From the Book

A **clinical trial** is a research study conducted with patients to evaluate a new method of preventing, detecting, diagnosing, or treating a disease.

The advantage of a clinical trial is that you are getting state-of-the-art treatment that has shown promise of being better than the best treatment currently available. Be cautious, however, if your doctor is part of the study. Certain pressures—financial, professional, or personal—may (but not necessarily) influence his or her decision to want you on board. Be sure it's in your best interest.

Even if you sign on the dotted line, you can decide to leave the study at any time. Or your medical team can remove you from the study. Either way, your further treatment won't be jeopardized.

Tales from the Trenches

In 1998, Letta participated in the clinical trial for sentinel node biopsy procedure, now a fairly common practice. In the past, women may have had as many as 20 lymph nodes removed with perhaps only a few—or even none—testing positive. For Letta, as a result of the clinical trial, the only lymph nodes removed were those identified by the sentinel node biopsy procedure. That spared her undue removal of tissue and undue risk of lymphedema, always a risk with the removal of lymph nodes.

Insurance: Your Personal KGB

As soon as you have the slightest hint that breast cancer lurks in your future, call your insurance company. Get the name of a representative whom you can call on a regular basis. On the first page of your notebook, right below your doctors' names and numbers, write this person's name, direct phone number, and toll-free number. Explain your situation and ask for advice. Start a file (might as well make it a big one) in which you will keep track of every call, every question answered, every direction given—along with the date, time, and name of the person to whom you spoke.

Plan to keep five insurance-related files: bills, receipts, claims filed, claims pending, and claims paid. In another folder keep letters: those from your medical team explaining the necessity for a given procedure, requests for sick leave, and any correspondence about insurance. Better yet, since you are already stressed to the limit, turn this task over to someone you trust to keep detailed records—husband, adult son or daughter, or paid professional, such as an attorney or accountant.

Your primary concern, of course, is what your insurance will and will not pay. If you're past age 65 or have been permanently disabled for 30 months or more, Medicare will help pay your bills. It does not, however, pay all hospital expenses (you have a co-payment and an annual deductible), so call your Social Security office (1-800-772-1213) if you have questions. Even if you have Medicare, you probably have some kind of supplementary health insurance.

Whether you are dealing with your primary insurance, Medicare, or supplementary insurance, here are questions you need answered:

➤ Will my insurance pay for second opinions?

➤ Are second opinions required?

➤ Will it pay only if I am treated by certain doctors or surgeons, or treated in certain medical facilities?

➤ Does it require "evidence of medical necessity" before it will pay?

➤ Will it pay for any experimental treatments and/or off-label drugs?

➤ What is my co-payment?

➤ Is there a maximum payment?

➤ Are any treatments excluded from my policy?

➤ Do I need a pre-authorization number for each doctor's appointment, surgical procedure, or follow-up treatment?

➤ Do I need any special forms?

➤ Are there any deadlines, such as notice prior to surgery or filing deadlines?

Take It from Us

Don't forget to get it in writing! If you make any agreements about policy interpretation or coverage over the phone, be sure to get a follow-up in writing. When push comes to shove, verbal agreements don't count. Get that piece of paper.

When you get answers to these questions, add the details to your notebook. The answers will most likely influence your decisions about who, what, when, and where. Detailed records can eliminate major stress in the immediate and more distant future. I know families who, a year after treatment, are still trying to unravel insurance tangles.

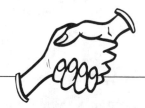

Helping Hand

Any time you talk to someone on the phone—about anything—be sure to record the essential information in your notebook: full name of the person with whom you spoke, his or her position, the date and time of your call, and exactly what the person said. If you're referred to someone else, get that person's full name, position, phone number, and/or e-mail address. Without this documentation, you'll face far more frustrations than necessary.

Be ready to fight if necessary. Let your medical team know about any battle with your insurance company, especially if your doctor/surgeon recommends a procedure or treatment and your insurance company reneges. Accustomed to dealing with the technical vocabulary and innumerable quirks of insurance policies, your medical team can often move boulders when you can only move pebbles. Sometimes insurance companies that have been reluctant to pay get a much-needed nudge by your telling them you're calling your lawyer. If that doesn't work, let your fingers do the walking, make the call, and get that letter from your lawyer; sometimes it's enough to start things rolling.

Medical assistance is available for people under a certain income level. Talk to your hospital social worker, hospital financial counselor, or cancer hotline. Organizations like the American Cancer Society also offer assistance. Don't hesitate to check them out.

Tales from the Trenches

While undergoing chemo, Beverly told me she felt trapped in an unhappy marriage. "I can't get a divorce because I don't work, and my health insurance is through my husband." To make matters worse, she now has a "preexisting condition" that may make it tough to get new medical insurance. Fortunately, some states have what they call "high-risk" insurance for folks like Beverly with a preexisting condition. It's pricey (so you'll need a source of income), but it's better than no insurance at all. In some instances, free medical service is available for those who can't pay. Inquire at your local cancer center.

Complementary Combos

Along with the treatment(s) you have decided on, you may want to consider certain complementary treatment. Some survivors report a resulting boost in their battle against breast cancer. We're talking about methods used along with, but *certainly not instead of,* treatments previously discussed. These are therapies that help manage stress and discomfort, ease side effects, or provide a nutritional boost. For additional details, check the National Center for Complementary and Alternative Medicine toll free at 1-888-644-6226 or on the Web at nccam.nih.gov/. Following are some methods you may want to investigate.

Mind over Matter

Several mind-over-matter therapies have worked wonders for survivors who talked with us. Visualization is one of these—a process by which you concentrate on seeing the healing process. Janelle reports that she listened to the "1812 Overture" during chemo and visualized with every crash of the cymbals the medicine blasting away the bad stuff. Carolyn reports getting "a clear picture of millions of tiny pink love hearts in my body. They were gooey and could slip into spots nothing else would fit. And every time they found something suspicious, they smothered it with love, digested it, and out it went." You can learn to use visualization by using readily available audio tapes or by contacting a therapist, either of which can help you come up with an image that works for you.

Take It from Us

Talk to your pharmacist if you take any complementary treatments. He or she is trained to keep track of your medications and what might interfere with them. Your pharmacist can also let you know if there are generic drug alternatives available if your insurance policy covers only certain classes of prescription drugs or if your policy doesn't cover drug costs at all.

Hypnosis also works for some. Seven-year survivor Susan Thomas, former oncology nurse and now founder and president of Susan's Special Needs in Detroit, said she used a hypnotist to help her through chemo. He went with her to every treatment, and, in her hypnotic state, suggested to her that the chemo was filling her with love. She never experienced nausea, never took anything for it, was never tired or sick, her blood count was always okay, and she took over 80 percent of the prescribed dosage. If you want, ask your medical team to help you find a trained hypnotist who can do the work for you or train you to hypnotize yourself.

Relaxation techniques rely on deep, even breathing and exercises to relieve stress. Variations include progressive muscle relaxation, tai chi, or yoga. Several survivors reported that using headphones and playing a new-age–type music tape during chemo (and, one woman reported, during her surgery!) helped them to relax. By extension, anything that helps distract you from immediate discomfort helps: a card game, a book you can't put down, a craft that requires your concentration.

Shown effective for reducing stress and managing discomfort, meditation is another mind-over-matter therapy. It is so well respected as a complementary method that hospitals, clinics, and community groups sponsor classes to help you get started. Ask your medical team.

Finally, remember that it's commonly accepted that the most important healing factor is your state of mind. It's the old I-can-do-this attitude. Sure, you need to know what you're up against, but then you need to deal with it. Whether that means you pound out your frustration on the jogging path or pound out your anger at the keyboard, whether you see a therapist every week or see your best friend over lunch every week—whatever you do, it's top priority that you maintain a positive attitude. You. Can. Do. This. What's more, if you need help, most hospitals can do psyche referrals, and the appointments may even be covered by insurance.

Take Your Vitamins (and Herbs), Dear

Medical folks often suggest that patients take a good multiple vitamin, minerals, and antioxidants. Always read labels, however, and know what they mean. Then ask your oncologist to make sure nothing you're taking will interfere in any way with other treatments. In addition, many survivors report using herbal teas and juices to help them feel better. Be aware, however, that there is no FDA supervision of the production, content, or safety of herbal remedies. For more on nutrition, see Chapter 23, "Life Goes On: Physical and Emotional Changes."

Tales from the Trenches

"I used an herbal tea, which I still drink," reports Letta. "It has four herbs in it that are also used in the making of Taxol, one of my chemo drugs. Everybody thought I went through chemo just great, and I often think that the tea was part of that."

Margie reports that she used fish oil capsules and flaxseed. "I grind the seed in a coffee grinder and mix it with applesauce. And it's great on ice cream!" But always check with the doc about anything you ingest, even vitamins.

Oldest Medicine of All

Acupuncture (with laser acupuncture a recent innovation) and acupressure are mainstays in Traditional Chinese Medicine (TCM). These methods, thousands of years old, now enhance many Western doctors' traditional practices. Acupuncture involves inserting thin needles into special places to relieve pain and treat illnesses, and some survivors have found it useful to relieve the side effects of chemo. Acupressure is a kind of massage in which the practitioner adds pressure to identifiable body pressure points. (Check the Yellow Pages under "Acupuncture.") Just remember that while TCM offers complimentary treatments for certain side effects resulting from medical cancer treatments, under no circumstances should you feel that any TCM can replace your medical regimen for cancer.

The Final Choice: Yours

By now you surely know that we're not here to tell you what to do. We can tell you about your options. We can tell you survivors' stories. We can tell you what to watch out for. We can suggest ways of thinking through your options. But the big decision, of course, is strictly yours. As you make these big decisions, however, keep the lines of communication open with your medical team. Consider the following suggestions.

The Question, Please

Ask good questions about your treatment, but avoid the confrontational "you" and replace it with the non-confrontational "I." For instance, replace "You said ..." with "I understood that ..." Ask good questions about your options, but ask parallel questions. For instance, if you ask, "What are the advantages of Option A?" be sure to also ask, "What are the advantages of Option B?" Same with disadvantages, side effects, and so on. (And remember to keep track of all the answers in your notebook.)

Learn the Lingo

Learn the technical medical language of your condition so you can communicate with your medical team. If someone uses a technical word you're not familiar with, ask. It's easy to say, "I don't know that word. What does it mean?" The technical medical language of your condition also lets you speak confidently and ask specific questions of insurance representatives. When you have questions about coverage, using the technical language will help your representative give a better answer.

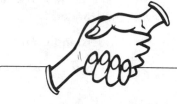

Helping Hand

Do unto others! You want to be treated as a person, not just a patient. Likewise, your medical team would like to be respected as people, not just doctors, surgeons, and nurses. It's a two-way street. Just as you expect your medical team to get to know you and your treatment, you have a responsibility to learn about what they do, the treatments, and their system.

The Envelope, Please

Don't seal details of your condition in the mayonnaise jar. Keep your medical team informed about what's going on in your life: your emotional state, family crises, financial stress, whatever. Since everything in your life affects your treatment, it's part of decision making. Your medical team can help. Likewise, keep your medical team informed about any complementary therapies you are using. Ask your doctor or nurse about any vitamins, herbs, teas, juices, or other oral complementary treatments you want to try. Make sure these won't interfere with your standard treatment.

As you struggle with the many decisions about treatments and get bleary-eyed from reading the fine print in your insurance policy, we hope you've found some lifelines here. And since this isn't a television game show, you can use every lifeline we and your fellow survivors have shared. After all, on the battlefield, every soldier looks out for his buddies, and, dear buddy, we're looking out for you.

The Least You Need to Know

➤ Make decisions about your treatment based on recommendations compared to the standard.

➤ Understand up front what your insurance will and will not cover.

➤ You may choose some complementary therapies to reduce stress and discomfort.

➤ Decisions are part of a good communication process between you and your medical team.

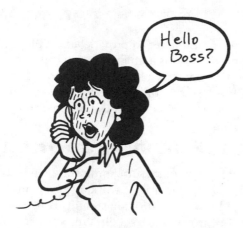

Call for a Working Plan

"And, what do you do for a living?" When you meet someone for the first time, do you often ask this question first? Whether we work inside or outside the home, volunteer our services or receive a paycheck, at least part of our self-esteem is attached to the work we do in our daily lives. For many people, work offers a sense of continuity and community; going to the office, setting up in front of a computer, or folding the laundry is part of a daily routine. But a diagnosis of breast cancer can—and probably will—disrupt this routine, at the very time when routine, structure, and continuity is what the doctor ordered! Indeed, more than 100 years ago, Freud said that the essence of life was "love and work." We need both.

In this chapter, we'll explore the challenges of working outside the home while at the same time coping with the physical and emotional demands of fighting breast cancer. Those challenges may include not only having the strength and stamina to keep up with the pace of work, it also may involve dealing with co-workers and superiors who may feel uncomfortable with, or resentful of, your condition and the extra demands on your time and attention it takes. We'll show you ways to meet those challenges, including what you'll need to do from a legal standpoint if you face discrimination in the workplace.

What the Law Says

Federal law and most state laws require an employer to provide an employee *reasonable accommodation*. Reasonable accommodation is a change in job duties to help you during the time you have breast cancer. It may be a change in actual job responsibilities or flexible working hours to allow for chemotherapy or radiation therapy treatments.

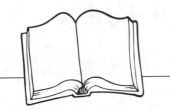

From the Book

Reasonable accommodation is a change in job duties to help you during your illness.

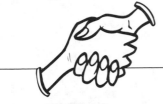

Helping Hand

The President's Committee on the Employment of People with Disabilities (1–800–526–7234) is a network that helps employers communicate with other employers and share ideas on what they have done to educate their staff about breast cancer. What a helping hand this is!

I Am Woman, I Am Strong!

For survivors, a routine or something close to normal is a great help. Staying at work, or returning after a medical leave, may provide stability and distraction for us, but it may create a difficult situation at work.

How your colleagues respond to your condition and the accommodations it requires may well depend on the lead your superiors—both your immediate boss and the management in general—take. If the office staff thinks you're contagious or under a death sentence, or assumes that you'll now be nonproductive and a burden, you're likely to feel quite uncomfortable at work.

If your boss or close co-workers avoid you or treat you as nonproductive, so will the other employees. However, if they are understanding and knowledgeable, your colleagues may well follow their lead. In addition, a boss who wants to educate his or her employees about breast cancer can do several things to increase everyone's understanding and to help you ease back into your job responsibilities.

First of all, he or she can talk with you about what "reasonable accommodations" would help. Reasonable accommodations are temporary changes in your job, such as flex time, time off, working from home, or job share, during and/or after your cancer diagnosis and treatment.

Second, he or she can bring in a healthcare professional to talk with the staff about breast cancer and the treatments. You can help find such a professional through your local support group or branch of the American Cancer Society.

Third, he or she can talk honestly and openly to you about what your capabilities are. You, in turn, may want to talk with your boss and close co-workers, openly and honestly, about things such as the reactions of more distant co-workers.

Knowledgeable and willing bosses also can act as a sounding board for employees who now feel uncomfortable with you and uncertain of what to say. He or she can offer them the right words—"I don't know how or what you are feeling, but I want you to know that I care and wonder if there is anything I can do to help?"—for instance. This is a major improvement over saying nothing at all and avoiding you completely.

Bosses can plan parties when you are finished with your treatments. They can suggest that co-workers treat you as naturally as possible, which will include asking you out to lunch (if they always did so in the past) or bringing you coffee when they go for their own. Remember, most people will want to help—they just may not know what to do. You can help educate and increase understanding.

We have heard so many stories of people who had such a good experience in going back to work. A woman who was getting ready to opt for early retirement decided to keep working. She was not prepared for two major changes at the same time, and her work helped her focus on something other than her illness. One woman decided to take unpaid leave time during her chemotherapy. All she could do was think about how badly she felt. She went back to work and felt better almost immediately.

No, you have not had a lobotomy and lost all of your intelligence with a lumpectomy or a mastectomy. No, all your job skills were not located in the breast tissue that was removed. Yes, you want to go back to work. Yes, you want to do, but do not *overdo*.

As frustrating as it may be, your boss and your co-workers may need you not only to guide them in their responses to your needs, but also to educate them in general about what having breast cancer means—to a woman and to an employee. Take a little extra time and make a bigger effort to ease their minds. It'll pay off in the long run!

Take It from Us

If you feel your job puts your health at risk, change it if you can. If you work around strong chemicals, hazardous material, or electromagnets, you may request a reassignment.

From the Book

Overdo is to do, use, or stress to excess. Doing is one thing, and overdoing is another. Do you need any more stress right now?

Working Through It

Although no hard-core data exists, it seems quite obvious to both survivors and their doctors that cancer patients who "have places to go and things to do" seem to live longer and enjoy the lives they are living more than those who withdraw from life. Keeping this in mind, you may want to keep working as much and for as long possible. To work most effectively and efficiently, keep these tips in mind:

➤ **Work in spurts.** Sometimes your energy comes in waves. Take advantage of the high points and make the most of the low points.

➤ **Don't call attention to what you "can't" do.** If there is something more difficult or time consuming than you can deal with, instead of saying you "can't" do it, see if someone will, covertly, trade responsibilities with you, even if it is for a short period of time.

➤ **Know the difference between doing and overdoing.** Do, but don't overdo. Overdoing could set you back. If you listen hard, your body will let you know the difference in no uncertain terms.

Do I Want to Stay Here?

Some cancer survivors panic at the thought of losing a job. Their job may be the love of their life, the reason for their existence, and they may fear that they will be fired or looked down upon because of their disease. They fear they may lose something they cherish and that gives them a reason to get up each morning. Even those who aren't passionate about the work they do may need the job to pay their bills or keep their precious health insurance. Indeed, for most people, work is not an issue of self-esteem alone, it is absolutely necessary for survival.

Tales from the Trenches

Carlene had the job of a lifetime—executive VP, corner office, triple-digit income, stock options, and recognition. She traveled 7 months out the year, worked at least 12 hours a day, and had no personal life. During her routine yearly physical, the doctor found a lump. Needless to say, Carlene was stunned. After her surgeries she called a headhunter to find her a new job.

Some people with breast cancer decide to leave their jobs because they assume that the daily stress that the job supplies is more than they can take at this time. In fact, if their jobs are particularly stressful, they may even blame their work for contributing to the development of breast cancer in the first place. Whether or not stress can actually cause disease remains a subject of some controversy. However, if you feel that the stress of your job wears you down, then getting rid of that stress may be helpful to your overall health, if you're able to do so without losing financial security.

Cancer survivors begin to ask themselves questions about their career. Are they there only for a paycheck and benefits? Do they stay there because, once diagnosed, they are afraid they won't be hired anywhere else or be able to get benefits anywhere else? Is there too much stress with the job? Are they satisfied with the job? Depending on how they answer these questions, they could be out the door tomorrow.

Regardless of how you see yourself in your workplace there is some place to turn for help.

The Sick Day Option

Can your company establish an attendance policy? Yes. Are you allowed sick days? Yes, in most cases. What are the guidelines in this situation?

The Family and Medical Leave Act of 1993 requires employers with more than 50 employees to provide a certain term of unpaid leave time for serious illness of self, child, spouse, or parent. Here are some of the specifics of this act:

➤ During a year, employees are allowed 12 weeks of unpaid leave.

➤ Employers must give employees the same or equivalent position when they return.

➤ Employees are allowed a reduced work schedule for the same time period if needed.

➤ Employers must continue to provide benefits during the unpaid leave.

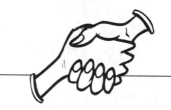

It's important that you treat your employer with as much consideration as possible. Try to give as much notice as you can, be available during specified times to answer calls from co-workers if you take sick days or an extended leave, or even go in to the office to check on things on your "good" days. By doing so, you'll help build a mutually respectful relationship with your employer and your colleagues.

Letting Others In

In addition to issues of job performance, you'll also need to deal with your colleagues on a personal

Helping Hand

Have the facts at hand. When it comes to asking your employer for medical leave, be prepared and get the facts in writing from your doctor beforehand. When you're trying to cope with breast cancer and treatment, the last thing you need is an extra run to the clinic or doctor's office to gather paperwork.

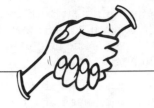

Helping Hand

Make a list of the people in your office you want to inform about your condition. Think about your relationship with each and decide how much information you want to provide him or her and when. Then consider how you think each person will respond to the news; that way you can prepare yourself for each encounter.

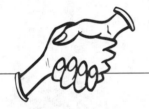

Helping Hand

Find out your rights as a breast cancer patient. Major cancer awareness groups such as the American Cancer Society, the National Cancer Institute, and the National Coalition of Cancer Survivorship have several pamphlets available at no charge that identify the legal rights of those with breast cancer. These groups are only a phone call away and will drop the information in the mail to you. It's a great place to start!

level as well, at least to some degree. And just as is true among your friends and family, you'll face a host of reactions when the news of your diagnosis spreads throughout the office (which it almost certainly will, no matter how discreet you try to be.) Some people will assume that you'll just pack up your tent and go home. Others will pity you. Others will offer just the right amounts of support and respect for your privacy.

Do remember that you have the right to keep your private affairs private at all times. But it probably makes sense to let certain people in on your condition, if only to allow them to support you when you're not feeling well or need time off.

When you talk to your colleagues, it's important to remain as professional as possible. Depending on the tone of the workplace, as well as your relationship to your co-workers, you could always try adding a little humor to the announcement. When people can laugh, they have distance from the problem and are able to cope with things. Humor also helps ease the pain, both emotionally and physically.

If there are others in your company who have had breast cancer, form a support group, or join any that they already offer. Since cancer, directly or indirectly affects about one in three women, it's very likely that you're not the only one in your company who has faced this disease.

Protecting Yourself at Work

What if you don't have workplace options? What if you don't feel you're being treated fairly because you have breast cancer?

If you feel that your cancer has caused others in your workplace to discriminate against you, take action. First, talk with someone in your human resources department, your boss (if your boss is not involved in the discrimination), or a support group. Find someone who is familiar with workplace discrimination to not only give you good advice and direction but also save you hours of researching, legal fees, and even hurt feelings.

You'll also want to know your legal rights. Fortunately, you have plenty of those, thanks in large part to the Federal Rehabilitation Act of 1973, which prohibits employers from discriminating against handicapped workers, including those women and men with breast cancer.

Although these federal guidelines apply to all 50 states, not every company in every state has to follow them. In fact, federal laws only apply to those who work for the federal government, employers who receive funding from the federal government, or private companies who have 25 or more employees. That means that if you work for a small firm with just six workers, you may have to turn to an applicable state law—if there is one—for help. Which also means you might have to get in the trenches and do some legal research yourself.

Becoming a Semi-Legal Eagle

Sometimes, the more you know, the more you need to know. That is the case with discrimination and breast cancer. Although no one expects you to become an expert—especially at this time when your top priority is your health—it's important that you understand your legal rights in the workplace as a person with breast cancer. Here are the basics: As of July 26, 1994, the Americans with Disabilities Act (ADA) banned discrimination by both public and private employers against employees who had disabilities. Although it doesn't specifically identify those with breast cancer as part of that class, past court rulings included those with cancer.

Tales from the Trenches

Although Teri had better qualifications and seniority, a co-worker received the promotion Teri was due—and the promotion took place when Teri was in the hospital for surgery. Not knowing where to turn, Teri talked to an administrator in her human resources department who took the information under advisement and began an investigation.

The Americans with Disabilities Act sets the following guidelines that all employers must follow:

➤ You cannot treat an employee with disabilities differently than other workers.

➤ A potential employer can ask you medical questions, but only after you have been offered employment and only if the questions involve a condition that would relate specifically to your ability to perform the job in question.

➤ A potential employer cannot ask you to take a pre-employment exam used to screen out those with cancer.

➤ An employee cannot be punished for filing a discrimination complaint.

Take It from Us

Don't delay! Discrimination suits must be filed within 180 days of the date of the actual act of discrimination. If you feel your employer has discriminated against you because of your medical condition and you want to file suit, talk to a lawyer as soon as possible. Keep your own accurate records of time, place, people involved, and what was said or done. The more detailed you are and the more facts you have, the less is left up to supposition and a "he said or she said" situation. Trying to mentally recall very specific information is difficult for most of us.

For your information, section 504 of the Federal Rehabilitation Act of 1973 demands that you file any complaint of discrimination within 180 days from the time the act of discrimination occurred. If you're a federal employee, the deadline is within 30 days. For more information, you can contact the Civil Rights Division of the U.S. Department of Justice in Washington, D.C., or your nearest EEOC (Equal Employment Opportunity Commission) office, or call 1-800-USA-EEOC.

The Least You Need to Know

➤ Continuing with work, for most people, is a good idea whether they are a paid or nonpaid professional.

➤ Determine if and how you will tell your co-workers.

➤ Do, but don't overdo.

➤ Talk with your boss and have him or her help educate co-workers.

➤ Be aware of your legal rights and know where to turn for help if you need it.

Part 2

Shock Waves: Dealing with Treatment

The initial shock that you have breast cancer turns into a rather long series of shock waves. Once diagnosed with breast cancer, you'll likely find yourself fully immersed in its treatment for most of the next year, maybe longer.

This part of the book takes you through the surgery (maybe more than one) and the likely follow-up with chemo, radiation, and/or hormone therapy. We'll detail each treatment and therapy, acknowledge their possible side effects, and suggest how you can best cope with them.

But the underlying message in this part of the book is plain and simple: The treatment—whatever it is—is only temporary. And it gives you the rest of your life.

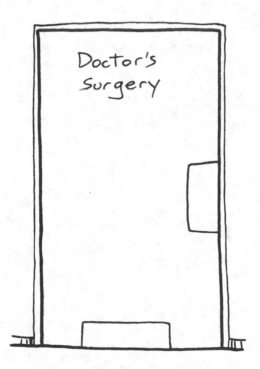

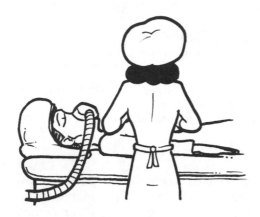

Chapter 7

Taking Your Lumps: Lumpectomy

> ## In This Chapter
>
> ➤ What "lumpectomy" means
>
> ➤ Anticipating the surgery
>
> ➤ What to expect during surgery
>
> ➤ The post-surgery forecast

When the surgeon says, "We'll take out a lump about the size of a golf ball," he may be describing your lumpectomy. Depending on the size and stage of your cancer and the size of you, a lumpectomy can refer to the removal of anything from 1 percent to 50 percent of your breast. Still, thousands of women who undergo a lumpectomy applaud the treatment for an obvious reason: it saves most of their breast tissue. Furthermore, today's research suggests that for a majority of women with breast cancer at Stage I or II, the combination of a lumpectomy and radiation therapy is preferable to a mastectomy.

Following a lumpectomy, most women never experience any change in appearance, apart from an inch-long scar along one side of the breast. If your surgeon recommends a lumpectomy (or if he recommends any of several other procedures that amount to the same thing), we're here to alleviate your fears and talk you through the experience. In this chapter, we'll tell you about the many terms used to describe the same surgical procedure and describe what you'll most likely experience before surgery, what the surgery itself is usually like, and what you can probably expect afterward—short- and long-term.

They're Gonna Do *What?*

A lumpectomy by any other name is still a lumpectomy, which is the removal of a lump or mass of tissue. For certain cancers, the lumpectomy combined with radiation therapy has proven equally as effective as a mastectomy, which is the removal of the entire breast. Your surgeon will use one of the following terms: surgical biopsy, (including perhaps a reference to excisional or incisional biopsy), partial mastectomy (maybe using terms like segmental mastectomy or quadrantectomy), or lumpectomy.

Surgical Biopsy

In Chapter 1, "It Ain't Gold in Them Hills," we talked about a core needle biopsy as a diagnostic procedure. A surgical biopsy serves the same purpose: to remove tissue in order for a pathologist to find out what's there. If your surgeon calls it an *excisional biopsy,* he plans to remove a suspicious mass as well as a rim of tissue in order for the pathologist to identify any malignancy.

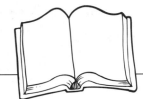

From the Book

An **excisional biopsy** is the removal of a suspicious lump along with a rim of tissue for pathological examination. An **incisional biopsy,** sometimes called a **wide excision** or **wedge excision,** is the removal of a wedge of tissue from a very large lump for pathological examination. A **segmental mastectomy** is the removal of a portion, or segment, of the breast. A **quadrantectomy** is the removal of a portion of the breast, although the term may not refer to the removal of a full quarter of the breast.

On the other hand, if it's called an *incisional biopsy,* you have a large tumor, and your surgeon plans to remove a wedge of the lump in order for the pathologist to determine what's there.

Since the surgery at this point is really diagnostic, typically neither kind of biopsy involves the removal of lymph nodes. Depending on what the surgeon and pathologist find, however, you may be in for more surgery.

Partial Mastectomy

Your surgeon may recommend a "partial mastectomy." The words sound scarier and more dramatic than "lumpectomy," as if somehow they're going to remove lots of tissue. In reality, "partial mastectomy" is often synonymous with "lumpectomy" and the term doesn't necessarily suggest how much tissue your surgeon plans to remove. In addition, a partial mastectomy may or may not involve the removal of lymph nodes, but your surgeon will tell you in advance what he plans to do. Otherwise, ask.

It's also possible your surgeon will recommend a *segmental mastectomy* or *quadrantectomy*. The terms may lead you to think you're in for the removal of at least a quarter of your breast, and you may be. However, some medical teams use the terms rather loosely—so again, ask if you're unsure.

Bottom line: these words—excisional biopsy, incisional biopsy, partial mastectomy, segmental mastectomy, quadrantectomy, and lumpectomy—can be synonymous.

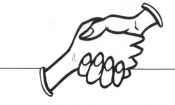

Helping Hand

A rose is a rose, but a lumpectomy is not a lumpectomy. Your case is different from your best friend's or your sister's because your case depends directly on the size and position of your lesion. No matter which term your surgeon uses—lumpectomy, partial mastectomy, segmental mastectomy, quadrantectomy, or incisional or excisional biopsy—you won't know from the words how much tissue they'll remove. Ask.

Lumpectomy

Given all the confusion about the terminology, it's comforting to know that the procedure for the lumpectomy itself is not nearly so confusing. In short, a lumpectomy is the removal of a mass of tissue that has been identified as suspicious either by mammogram, ultrasound, needle biopsy, or any or all of the above. The surgeon also removes what he—and you—hope is a rim of benign tissue all the way around the lump. In some cases, a lumpectomy may also be accompanied by another incision to remove underarm, or axillary, lymph nodes, a surgery technically called a lymphectomy. Typically, a lumpectomy is followed by radiation therapy, but that treatment is entirely dependent on the pathologist's report. More on that later.

Regardless of what it's called, a lumpectomy is fairly routine—not to you, certainly, but to your medical team. We're here to tell you what it's like.

From left: A lumpectomy removes a lump or wedge from the breast (wedge shown here), may or may not include lymph node removal, and you go home with a simple bandage.

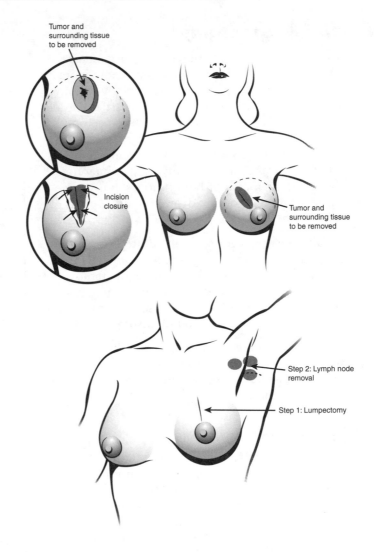

Tumor and surrounding tissue to be removed

Incision closure

Tumor and surrounding tissue to be removed

Step 2: Lymph node removal

Step 1: Lumpectomy

Minus One Golf Ball

Let's start with why your surgeon would recommend and why you would choose a lumpectomy over a mastectomy. The primary advantage of a lumpectomy over a mastectomy is fairly obvious: You still have two breasts when they're done. It's considered a breast-conserving measure, and for certain cancers, a lumpectomy combined with radiation has been proven to be as effective as a mastectomy. But there are some less obvious advantages, too. First, you'll recover much more quickly and easily after a lumpectomy (unless they took out lots of lymph nodes). Second, you'll retain most of the feeling in your breast and for some women at least, that sensation directly affects their sex lives. Third, there's minimal scarring.

But are there some situations in which a lumpectomy isn't an option? Yep. Aside from the fact that some malignancies are too far advanced for a lumpectomy (see Chapter 5, "Decisions, Decisions, Decisions"), there are times when an otherwise obvious choice of lumpectomy is the wrong choice:

1. You can't have radiation a second time in the same spot. So if you've already had radiation therapy on the affected breast, the typical lumpectomy–radiation combo won't work for you this time.

2. Maybe you have two or more suspicious areas in the same breast. If they're too far apart to be removed through one incision, a lumpectomy won't work.

3. If you've already had a lumpectomy but the margins weren't clear (i.e., cancerous tissue showed up in the rim around the lesion), your surgeon may try a second lumpectomy to get clear margins. After that, a mastectomy is your only choice.

4. If you have certain connective tissue diseases that make you particularly sensitive to radiation therapy, a lumpectomy won't work for you. Your doctor/surgeon will know and will pass the word along to you.

5. If you're pregnant and would require radiation before your baby is born, the lumpectomy–radiation combo won't work for you, either. Radiation can be harmful to the fetus.

Take It from Us

Don't insist on a surgical procedure that isn't right for you. And only if it's right for you will your surgeon recommend a specific type of lumpectomy. Whatever the recommendation, however, ask enough questions to understand why this surgery is the recommended route. Turn to your notebook, review your diagnosis, and make a list of questions. Record the answers in your notebook for future reference.

So, yes, sometimes a lumpectomy isn't an option. Talk it over with your doctor.

Recipe for the Routine

Again, it may not seem so to you, but lumpectomies are pretty routine. Just because thousands of women have been through the drill, however, doesn't make it any easier for you: This is your first go at it. So let's take it a step at a time.

First, it's same-day surgery. You're in and out in a few hours and may go right on with your business. Some folks go back to work in the afternoon after having a lumpectomy in the morning, but that really depends on two factors: whether you've had lymph node removal, and what you do at work. Still, you shouldn't miss work for more than a day, or maybe two, unless your job requires you to do lifting. Nix on that for about a week to 10 days.

First Things First

Before you leave home on the day of surgery, bathe with an anti-bacterial soap, skip the antiperspirant, and forget about food and water. You don't want to upchuck in the midst of it all. (Don't worry, your doctor will explain all of this to you as well.)

Wear loose clothing, something two-piece, and something that buttons or zips down the front. You're not going to like the way it feels to move your arm over your head, so a pullover shirt is really the wrong choice.

Getting Wired

Unless you have a palpable tumor, you'll first see the radiologist. That person's job is to insert a wire in your breast to mark the spot where the mammogram or ultrasound shows a suspicious area. I know that sounds a little crude, but we're not talking about coat hanger wire here; we're talking about a threadlike wire inside a needle. The wire has a tiny hook on the end so that when it's in place and the needle is removed, the wire stays in the lesion. (Of course, if your tumor is palpable, you don't need an additional flag to mark the spot.)

Sound painful? Strangely, it really isn't. It's more pressure than pain. The mammogram machine plates hold you firmly in place while they measure from the mammogram film: so many centimeters from the top; so many centimeters from the left; in we go. Your doctors verify the wire placement with another mammogram. The whole procedure takes less than an hour.

Why the wire? It's sort of like your personal antenna. When the surgeon cuts into your breast, the tissue all looks alike. There's nothing there that changes color or outlines a shape. So the wire guides him in, and *X* marks the spot.

Tales from the Trenches

One survivor told us, "After my lumpectomy, I remember getting up from the surgery table, walking across the sky bridge to an adjoining hospital building where my mother was a patient, feeding her lunch, and going from there to a business meeting that evening." So relax. It's not so terrible.

Getting Prepped

Wire in place, you're off to see the wizard. You'll strip to your panties, put on one of those fabulously chic surgical gowns, and get a pre-med shot to help you relax, make you drowsy, but probably not put you to sleep. If you want to sleep through it all, you'll probably have to make your wishes clear. Just remember that the anesthetic may be harder on you than the surgery, so be careful what you ask for.

If, on the other hand, the surgeon anticipates removing lymph nodes, the surgery takes longer and may cause more discomfort, so you'll be prepped accordingly. You may also encounter a slightly longer hospital stay, from a few hours longer to perhaps overnight.

Tales from the Trenches

Roberta explained, "After my pre-med shot, I walked down the hall, climbed up on the surgery table, asked questions while the medical team arranged the tools of their trade, and kept up a constant conversation with the surgeon during the whole process. Because of a tent-like affair above my head, I couldn't see what was going on, but it didn't take much imagination. There was no pain, only some discomfort and plenty of pressure. But nothing to bring tears to your eyes or make you want to yip and yowl."

Once in surgery, you'll lie on a narrow table with your arms straight out on little shelves perpendicular to the table (that gets your arms out of the way of the surgeon, makes it easy to maintain a constant check of your vitals, and makes the armpit area accessible if you're having any lymph nodes removed). Then you'll be scrubbed with an antiseptic, hooked up to all the appropriate meters and gauges (to check your heartbeat, blood pressure, oxygen levels, and so on), and have an intravenous line (an IV) inserted in a vein in your arm or hand. You'll feel them press to your skin—usually on your stomach or thigh—something that feels cold and a bit heavy. It's a grounding plate for the electrocautery, a gadget used to cauterize tiny blood vessels to stop bleeding. Finally, you'll be draped head to foot with green surgical sheets. And you're ready.

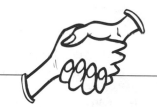

Helping Hand

Seeing is believing. During your follow-up visit after your lumpectomy, ask to see the x-ray of the tissue removed. You'll probably find it quite reassuring. If your follow-up appointment is at a location other than where you had surgery, call in advance to remind folks you'll want to see the evidence with your own eyes! They can then have the films available when you arrive.

Getting Exorcised

Now it's time for the surgeon to get the bad stuff out. You should feel no pain, but you probably will feel some pressure. If it really hurts, say so. Sometimes the surgeon has to go fairly deep, and the local anesthetic may be too local to get the job done. Speak up. The stuff works pretty fast, and there's no reason for you to be in agony.

In a surprisingly short time, usually a half-hour to an hour, you'll know that the surgery is done. Action stops, and you'll wonder what they're

81

waiting for. Answer: They're waiting on the x-ray picture of what the surgeon just removed. They want to make sure they got what they were after. The x-ray will show the wire, still in place, with this lump of tissue around it and the suspicious area surrounded by a rim of good tissue.

How Much Ouch?

With surgery finished, you'll be wheeled off to a quiet corner where you can finally get something to drink and hear the routine spiel for going home—instructions like these:

➤ You're bandaged well. You'll have to keep the bandage in place for two days (no showers until then).

➤ Keep an ice pack on the area for at least the next 24 hours. It lessens swelling.

➤ You'll wear your bra over the bandage for 48 hours—day and night.

➤ After two days, you can remove the bulky bandage. You probably won't have stitches, only some Steristrips—stout, waterproof tape—which stay in place until your next office visit.

➤ You'll do no heavy lifting with the arm on the side you had surgery on for at least a week. (You really won't have to be told; it hurts.)

➤ You can expect some bruising that usually disappears in about two weeks.

➤ You can drive unless you're taking pain medicine that makes you drowsy.

➤ You can eat whatever you want.

➤ If the pain medicine causes constipation (as it often does), your doctor may recommend a daily dose of two ounces of Milk of Magnesia.

In addition, you'll be given some warning signals: Call your doctor if you have …

➤ A temperature of over 101.5°.

➤ Chills.

➤ Redness of or drainage from the wound.

➤ Excessive pain from which you get no relief by proper pain medication.

If you've had lymph nodes removed, you'll have an additional two-inch incision at the bottom of your armpit, and you may have a drain that allows accumulated fluids to escape. For details about caring for a drain, see Chapter 8, "When They Take It All: Mastectomy."

You'll probably be really tired for a few days. Anesthesia can take the starch out of you, and you've had some rather dramatic emotional stress lately. Your body knows. So relax as much as you can, let someone else do the cooking and the dishes, and skip the housework for the next week. If you have to go to work, do so; but keep your energy output minimal. What about pain? They've cut a hunk out of you, maybe two. You'll be surprised how much muscle moves around in those areas when you raise your arm or pick up your coffee cup. So, yes, it's going to hurt a bit. You may feel a kind of burning sensation along the incision, maybe some numbness in the chest and upper arm, perhaps pins and needles, tingles, or short stabbing pains anywhere near tissue removal.

You'll have pain medicine, but if you're really sensitive to it, you might be groggy if you take it as prescribed. If so, you can cut the prescription in half. Some folks prefer a little discomfort to grogginess, so they may use nothing more than over-the-counter pain relievers, like Extra-Strength Tylenol or something similar. Someone on your medical team will probably warn you, however, to avoid aspirin since it functions as a blood thinner and could cause internal bleeding.

You might also find a sports bra (but *not* a pullover) to be far more comfortable than your usual bra. Because a sports bra holds equally firmly in all areas, it gives good support to the incision area. You'll likely find that more support feels better than less. Anything that stops jiggles stops ouch.

To get comfortable at night, haul out the extra pillows. Try sleeping on the side not operated on and propping a pillow under the affected breast. Even though you'll be wearing a firmly supporting bra, the pillow adds to the support. Anything that droops also pulls.

Take It from Us

Don't neglect exercise! There are simple exercises to help you regain full range of motion of your affected arm, and if you don't do them, you'll have restricted arm motion for the rest of your life. (See Chapter 9, "Between Surgery and the Rest," for more details about exercises to regain full range of motion.)

Within a week, you'll be really over the hump, and within two weeks, you'll have to stop and think about why a long reach is slightly uncomfortable. Meantime, you'll want to start exercising your arm—pain or no pain. Your medical team may refer you to a physical therapist if you continue to experience limited range of motion.

Going Topless: What's Ahead?

After two days or so when the bandage comes off, what will you see? For about the first two weeks, you'll probably have some fairly obvious bruising, depending on how easily you bruise. After that, the only obvious reminder is the incision scar, a short, straight line about an inch long. If you've had lymph nodes removed, you'll have another short incision under your arm, about where the top of your bra fits. It's a little unusual, but you may have some swelling. If it's extreme, your doctor may draw off the accumulated fluid to reduce the swelling as well as the discomfort.

Getting the Word

Within a week or 10 days, you'll have a follow-up appointment with your surgeon. At that point he or she will remove that really sticky tape and examine the incision and surrounding tissue. You'll also get a pathologist's report that tells you what's there—or more about what's there. (If this was a surgical biopsy, however, you'll probably know results sooner, probably within 48 hours.) Here's how the procedure works.

When the tissue was removed from your breast, it was—literally—dunked into a bucket of ink. The ink marks the edges. So the first thing the pathologist's report will tell you is whether the margins were *clear*. That is, was the malignant tissue surrounded completely by benign tissue? Second, you'll find out whether or not the cancer is *invasive*. That is, has it grown outside the milk ducts or milk lobules? Third, you'll learn whether the lymph nodes were *negative* or *positive*. If they are positive, the cancer has spread beyond the breast.

Answers to three questions determine your next steps: Are the margins clear? Is the condition still *in situ?* Are the lymph nodes negative? In a best-case scenario, you want to hear "yes" to all three questions. "No" to any one or combination of them automatically suggests a different regimen from here (see Chapter 9). In short, the pathology report guides the recommendations from here. Because this report is so important, you should get a copy and put it in your notebook. Then formulate questions about next steps based on that report and what we've talked about in Chapter 5.

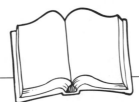

From the Book

Clear margins, also called **negative margins,** refer to benign tissue surrounding a malignant or pre-cancerous mass, showing that the malignancy has not spread. **Positive margins,** those that contain cancer, are not clear. **In situ** means that the malignancy or pre-cancerous condition is confined to the site, i.e., within the ducts or lobules. The opposite of in situ is **infiltrating** or **invasive. Negative lymph nodes** are those that tested benign, i.e., they show no sign of cancer; **positive lymph nodes** show malignancy.

The Long Haul

Over the long haul, you won't face anything serious from the aftereffects of a lumpectomy. Your fatigue should go away in a matter of a few days. You may experience tenderness for several months at the incision site, especially if your bra rubs the scar.

And you'll notice that the area from which the tissue was removed is hard and somewhat numb. In some folks, the numbness goes away in six months or so, but the hard lump may remain for a more than a year. In some cases, neither the lump nor the numbness ever goes away.

If you had lymph nodes removed, you may also experience some numbness in the back of your armpit. While this doesn't affect movement, it may be permanent. If so, you may have to use an electric razor. To nick yourself is to risk lymphedema (see Chapter 13, "The Big Arm: Lymphedema").

Finally, depending on how much tissue has been removed, you may find your breasts are now different sizes. And over the next five years or so, you may notice that the affected breast continues to shrink. Part of that may be the result of hormonal loss (especially if you take a follow-up hormone treatment), and part of it may be aging. At any rate, if that happens, you'll face the problem of finding a comfortable, properly fitting bra.

In the final analysis, a lumpectomy ranks way up there as part of the good news about breast cancer treatment these days. All the research says that a lumpectomy followed by radiation works as the perfect treatment combo for thousands of women. Sure, treatment depends on the kind of cancer you have, but given the right parameters, a lumpectomy (usually accompanied by radiation) is a remarkably wonderful tissue-saving approach to treating breast cancer. What a small price to pay for getting a new lease on life!

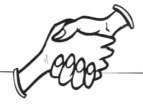

Helping Hand

If, after a lumpectomy, you find your breasts are different sizes, take a tip from survivors. Sports bras have solved the problem for many folks. But several were quick to point out that you can also use breast enhancers to create a perfect pair. (See Chapter 22, "Boob in a Box: Prostheses," for more details.) The enhancers fix you up for a better clothing fit. Other survivors who are large-breasted have chosen instead of an enhancer to have breast reduction on the healthy breast. Some have been thrilled that they can now wear clothing they could never fit into before. Consider all your options!

The Least You Need to Know

➤ Regardless of what it's called, a lumpectomy is a fairly routine breast-conserving procedure.

➤ A lumpectomy may or may not include the removal of underarm lymph nodes.

➤ As a same-day surgery, a lumpectomy has a short recovery period with only minimal long-term aftereffects.

➤ For certain cancers, a lumpectomy followed by radiation therapy has proven as effective as a mastectomy.

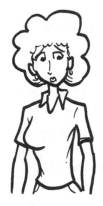

When They Take It All: Mastectomy

Some years ago, the only treatment for breast cancer was a mastectomy, the surgical removal of the entire breast. In many cases, then as now, some kind of adjuvant therapy, such as radiation or chemotherapy, followed. Although many women with breast cancer today have other options, for some this surgical procedure is the treatment most likely to provide the best prognosis.

So how do you know if and when a mastectomy is the best treatment for you? We talked about the "standard" treatments in Chapter 5, "Decisions, Decisions, Decisions." But we also said that in spite of recommended "standard" treatments, there is no such thing as "standard" breast cancer. So the bottom line is that your doctor/surgeon will look at all the facts and make a recommendation based on your particular diagnosis and situation. Simple factors like the location or size of the lesion or the size of your breast may affect the doc's recommendation for breast removal. And even if the doc's recommendation is for a mastectomy, you may not have the same kind of mastectomy as your neighbor or colleague. In this chapter, we'll tell you about a half-dozen different kinds of mastectomies, each involving a different amount of tissue removal. We'll tell you why and how they're done, why lymph nodes are removed, and what to expect after surgery. Above all, however, rest assured that your doctor/surgeon will consider breast-conserving measures before he or she recommends a mastectomy.

Names and Their Faces

In certain cases, a mastectomy is the standard prescribed course.

Your doctor might recommend a mastectomy if you have the following types of cancer:

➤ **Ductal carcinoma in situ (DCIS) that is widespread.** Your mammogram or pathology report may show DCIS widespread enough to warrant a mastectomy.

➤ **Lobular carcinoma in situ (LCIS).** In special circumstances and after adequate biopsies, your doctor may feel that you require a bilateral mastectomy. These "special circumstances" include a wide range of risk factors (see Chapter 15, "Caution Flag: Risk Factors"), including extensive family history of breast cancer. You and your doctor must thoroughly discuss all the factors.

➤ **Stages I or II.** If you're in Stage I or II, you may hear a recommendation for a modified radical mastectomy for any one of several reasons, including if you've had prior radiation to the breast, if you have two or more lumps fairly far apart in the same breast, if a lumpectomy had positive (i.e., malignant) margins, if you have certain connective tissue diseases that make you super sensitive to radiation, or if you're pregnant and can't have radiation as a result of risk to the fetus.

➤ **Inoperable stage IIIA invasive breast cancer.** If this is your diagnosis, you will most likely face a modified radical mastectomy.

If your surgeon recommends a mastectomy, you may get the recommendation in any one of several terms:

➤ **Radical mastectomy.** Removal of the breast along with both chest muscles and all axillary lymph nodes on that side; now considered an outdated treatment.

Take It from Us

Don't be misled! A bilateral mastectomy doesn't eliminate your chances of ever facing breast cancer again. No mastectomy can remove all breast tissue; it runs from your collarbone to the bottom of your rib cage and from your breastbone to under your arm. Remaining tissue can host breast cancer—against the chest wall or even in the incision itself, both common sites for recurrence.

➤ **Modified radical mastectomy.** Removal of the breast and nodes but leaving the chest muscle; usually now replaces the radical mastectomy (see the accompanying figure).

➤ **Subcutaneous mastectomy.** Removal of most of the breast tissue; keeps nipple and outer skin; fills space with an implant; controversial because of the amount of breast tissue remaining.

➤ **Simple (or total) mastectomy.** Similar to the modified radical, but without the removal of axillary lymph nodes.

➤ **Bilateral mastectomy.** Removal of both breasts; may be modified radical, simple, or any other form of mastectomy, and may use the same or different surgeries on each breast.

➤ **Prophylactic mastectomy.** Removal of an apparently healthy breast in high-risk women in whom cancer has been diagnosed in one breast but not the other.

➤ **Contralateral mastectomy.** Removal of a healthy breast for symmetry; considered cosmetic surgery.

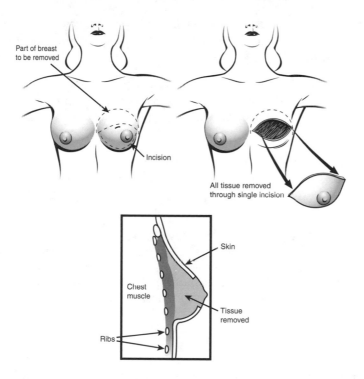

A modified radical mastectomy removes breast tissue, skin, and lymph nodes but leaves chest muscle intact.

While you're discussing surgical options, ask if anyone at your facility is trained to do *sentinel node biopsies* (or sentinel node mapping). It's a fairly new procedure but saves the removal of lots of lymph nodes at random. Here's how it works: In military lingo, a sentinel is the first to see the enemy creeping in. With breast cancer, the first lymph node to get drainage from a breast tumor is called the sentinel node. To locate that node, trained medical folks inject the tiniest bit of radioactive substance around the tumor, followed by a blue dye. Then they track where dye goes, thus identifying the sentinel lymph node. By biopsying the sentinel node, your pathologist can determine whether or not the cancer has spread. Meanwhile, if it hasn't spread, you've been spared the loss of all the other lymph node tissue, will recover much more quickly, and reduce your chances of getting lymphedema, a condition 10 to 20 percent of survivors face (see Chapter 13, "The Big Arm: Lymphedema").

Tales from the Trenches

Some survivors told us they chose a mastectomy, bilateral, or prophylactic mastectomy because they could then avoid the six weeks of daily radiation therapy typical after a lumpectomy. They felt it would disrupt their work.

Others said that the long-term routine wasn't an issue because they were concerned about family history and the likelihood of recurrence. They called it "peace of mind." As one astute lady put it, "It's like double-bolting a door: It can't prevent you from being robbed, but it makes you feel safer."

Still, don't choose a mastectomy for the wrong reasons. While a mastectomy significantly reduces your chances of recurrence, it's not a 100 percent guarantee.

It's All Procedure: Yours

If you and your medical team agree that a mastectomy is your best treatment option, you'll want to get prepared. Before you hit the hospital halls, make some plans, both medical and personal. Get your notebook and make a checklist. Let's start with the medical.

Pass Your Tests

You'll undergo certain medical tests prior to surgery, and your doctor and his or her staff will ask you many questions about your medical history, including your regular meds (name everything you take—including herbs, vitamins, and aspirin—since some may interfere with surgery), allergies, and previous surgeries. Then they'll put you through a battery of tests, usually including chest x-ray, blood tests, and an electrocardiogram (EKG) that checks your heart and circulation. Mostly the medical folks are making sure you have no problems that could complicate what should be a relatively routine surgery.

In addition to the tests, before surgery you ought to attend to two other medical details. First, get a *range of motion test* on the arm that will be affected by surgery. The results of the test will inform the physical or occupational therapist who will be working to help you regain the full use of your arm following surgery.

Second, get a *bone density test,* which is an x-ray that takes about 10 minutes and measures the sturdiness of your bones. Here's why the test is important now, as well as later. Hormones affect bone density. If you're pre-menopausal, your post-mastectomy adjuvant treatment (such as hormone therapy) may throw you into menopause and halt your usual hormone output. If you're post-menopausal, you've already stopped any hormone supplement. And if your follow-up treatment calls for an anti-estrogen drug (such as Tamoxifen), your body will be sapped of all estrogen hormones. These circumstances make you more likely to face *osteoporosis*. By getting a bone density test now, before your life is dramatically altered, your medical team can have a baseline measurement that will help them better evaluate any changes in your bones, especially over the long haul, and determine any necessary treatment.

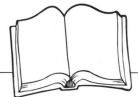

From the Book

A **sentinel node biopsy** identifies and tests the single lymph node that receives the first drainage from a tumor. A **range of motion test** records the amount of arm movement that is normal for you; then, after surgery your medical team will know when you've fully regained use of your arm. A **bone density test** measures how strong (dense) your bones are and recognizes, by comparison with future tests, bone density loss, a treatable condition if caught early. **Osteoporosis** is the deterioration of bone density leading to brittleness and an increased risk for broken bones.

Ask your doctor/surgeon if you'll need a blood transfusion. Chances are you won't, but if there is a strong possibility that you'll need blood (like maybe as a result of extensive reconstructive surgery), you may consider donating your own blood.

And as you check last-minute details with the doc, request a hormone receptor test on the tissue removed from your breast. If your lesion is hormone receptive positive, it means hormones are making it grow; if it's not, hormones will have no effect. It's a test the pathologist may or may not do without your request (sometimes it's routine; sometimes not), but the results will direct future treatment. (More on this in Chapter 9, "Between Surgery and the Rest.")

Finally, check in with your insurance company. Some companies demand prior notice of any surgical procedure. Get the *i*'s dotted and the *t*'s crossed.

The Personal File

When you've attended to the medical necessities, focus on the personal matters. Chances are, you'll feel exhausted, sore, and out of sorts when you come home from the hospital, so get your nest in order now. With the help of family and friends—don't try to do it alone!—make sure the house is clean and clutter-free. We're not talking wash-the-walls-and-windows cleaning; we're talking basics that annoy you when you sit down to rest but see all these things that need doing.

Cook up some soups or casseroles, package them in single-meal size, and put them in the freezer. Make sure the pantry and freezer are filled with easy-to-cook stuff: pastas, soups, veggies, stews. Prepare your family. Warn them they'll need to put meals on the table for a week or so.

You'll have three positive results if you do the nesting routine. First, after surgery, you'll be able to shut down and get the rest you need without feeling guilty about the clutter or worrying about nutritious meals. Second, you'll have something to keep your mind occupied at a time when you're likely to dwell on the unknown. Third, if you hustle-bustle all day, you'll sleep better at night—a real blessing as you prepare mind and body for the next battle.

If you're going to be in the hospital for a few days (and you will likely know this ahead of time), pack lightly but make sure to take your favorite bedclothes and your cosmetics (if you use them) as well. If you have one available, take along a tape player and headphones and music that you love or inspirational tapes that you enjoy. On the day before surgery, treat yourself to something special. One woman said she caught the train to a nearby large city, enjoyed the gorgeous department stores, had an elegant lunch, took a buggy ride through the park, and came home relaxed, refreshed, and ready. Maybe you'll choose a quiet lunch with friends or a visit to a museum. One survivor invited a dozen good friends over and had a bon voyage party for her breast. She said the laughter was an amazing emotional release for her. Do whatever works for you to keep your mind occupied with pleasantries.

Helping Hand

Be good to yourself during this time. As Janie put it, "Acknowledge your feelings. No matter what they are, they're yours, they're valid, and they need to be acknowledged. If you want to scream, cry, be mad as hell, feel scared or need a hug, just let it rip! You'll feel much better. Promise!"

Routine Rigors

Your doctor will give you instructions about preparing for the day of surgery. Every medical team requests a slightly different routine, but in general you'll probably be asked to …

➤ Bathe with anti-bacterial soap.

➤ Skip the antiperspirants.

➤ Eat or drink nothing after midnight (that means when you brush your teeth, you mustn't swallow any water).

➤ Take your regular medicines and bring them with you in their labeled bottles.

➤ Bring your glasses case or contact lens case.

➤ Leave valuables at home, including jewelry.

➤ Skip the makeup and nail polish.

➤ Consume no alcohol for 24 hours before surgery.

➤ Stop smoking at least 12 hours before surgery.

➤ Bring your insurance papers.

➤ Bring notebook and pen to note details and questions.

Wear really loose clothing, including a shirt that opens down the front: After surgery, it will be painful for you to raise your arm high enough to slip into a pullover. Go for comfortable low-heeled shoes, too. It's best, both emotionally and physically, for you to bring along a friend or spouse. For one thing, you won't be able to drive yourself home after surgery. For another, you may need the support of a loved one to get you through the strangeness of the hospital in general and the anxiety of the surgery in particular. When you hit the hospital doors, be prepared to sign all kinds of consent forms for surgery, anesthesia, blood transfusions, and so on—mostly routine stuff for any kind of surgery, but nevertheless somewhat disconcerting. They'll probably draw some more blood, and check your vitals. You'll strip to your panties (or maybe entirely) and don a lovely hospital gown. Then, the medical team will hook you up to an intravenous line (IV) through which you will get the anesthetic and/or any other meds necessary; they'll give you a shot of a mild tranquilizer, and after a short wait (unless somebody's running behind), they'll wheel you off to surgery.

Ten, Nine, Eight, Seven ...

You may find yourself wide awake when you get into surgery, but don't worry, you won't be awake long. The team will hook you up to various monitors to keep tabs of your vital signs, and then you'll get a general anesthetic that makes the lights go out like a switch. You won't know or feel a thing until hours later.

What's happening during the hour and a half or two hours you're in surgery? The routine varies

Take It from Us

Know your enemy. The more you understand about your treatment options—including surgery—the more free of regrets you'll be in later months and years. Once you know your strategy, focus on the battle to win the war.

from surgeon to surgeon, but basically here's the drill: The surgeon makes an oval-shaped incision with your nipple as the center of the oval. The incision may run five inches or so from tip to tip if you're a B cup, longer if you're bigger. The surgeon cuts out and discards an oval flap of skin and the nipple, and then removes the breast tissue. Next, the surgeon reaches under the skin to the armpit to take out lymph nodes. They're embedded in fatty tissue, and the number of nodes varies dramatically from person to person. You may have a half dozen or 30 or more.

The surgeon dips the breast tissue in a bucket of ink to clearly mark the edges, sends the whole mass to the pathologist, and closes you up. That oval opening now forms a neat, straight line, and you're fairly flat, but not entirely so. And actually, you probably won't see any stitches. Instead, you may have staples or, most likely, Steristrips, which are narrow but really tough strips of waterproof tape. You'll be well-bandaged with lots of padding and plenty of tape.

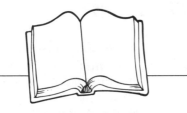

From the Book

A **drain** is a bulb-shaped apparatus attached to a tube through which fluids drain from the surgery area. The tube is inserted through a tiny incision and attached in place by a single stitch.

If you've chosen to have simultaneous reconstructive surgery, the plastic surgeon will work side by side with your surgeon, adding another hour and a half or two hours or more to the surgical process. (See Chapter 21, "Back to the Bikini: Reconstruction," for options and details.)

Finally, you'll get a *drain* (or perhaps two drains if your surgery was bilateral and maybe three or four if you choose to have simultaneous reconstruction). The doctor attaches the drain about halfway between the end of the mastectomy incision and the spot under your arm where lymph nodes were removed. Coming out from a tiny additional incision about a quarter-inch long, there'll be a plastic tube held in place with a single stitch. At the end of the tube is a transparent bulb-shaped container into which fluid drains.

Why a drain? Because anywhere the body finds a pocket-like area (like where the breast or lymph nodes used to be), it tends to fill the pocket with fluid, creating what's rather like a really big blister. Accumulated fluid causes swelling and that means a little pain! By draining the fluid the drain provides relief. At first, the fluid will look slightly bloody but, as time goes on, it's mostly clear to yellowish. You'll have the drain for anywhere from one week to as long as two.

When You Awake: What to Expect

Once the doctor finishes closing your incisions, you'll go from surgery to recovery and from there to a hospital room. You won't remember much about the recovery room, except that they keep asking you your name and you wonder why the devil they can't keep track of their patients. What they're doing, of course, is checking your vital signs and making sure you're coming out of the anesthetic okay.

Probably four to six hours after surgery, you'll finally wake up. Soon after, you'll be able to eat and, unless the anesthesia plays tricks on your tummy (and it does for some folks), you'll probably have a ravenous appetite. After all, it's been a while since you've had anything more than nibbles and sips. And don't worry about that slightly sore throat. You're not getting a cold; it's from the breathing tube you had while you were under the anesthesia.

You'll probably stay in the hospital overnight. If you've had reconstruction or if there were any complications, you may stay a day or two longer. In many communities, an American Cancer Society Reach to Recovery volunteer, a survivor herself, will call on you during that time (and in some communities, she may even visit you at home if you're willing). Because she's a survivor, she understands just how you feel. Don't hesitate to have a heart-to-heart. Of course, if you're in only overnight, you'll likely be out and gone before she can see you.

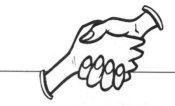

Helping Hand

Take advantage of the American Cancer Society Reach for Recovery program. Betty Slutsky, a 17-year survivor, is a volunteer. One woman she visited exclaimed, "I could ask questions of you that I wasn't comfortable asking the doctor." Another added, "With so many unknowns when you first hear the news, discussing this with someone who's been there lifts a weight off my shoulders."

The doc will be in to see you before you're sent home from the hospital. Assuming you have no fever (which could indicate infection) or other problems, you'll be out the door. The trip home won't feel particularly good. Every bump in the road is magnified at least 1,000 times in the site of in your incision. You won't like moving your arm, especially not upward. In fact, you must not lift anything for about a week.

On the Home Front

Once you're home and settled into your favorite recliner, you'll be more comfortable. Apply ice packs to the site of the incision and keep them in place for a day or so to reduce swelling. With any luck, your friends and family will offer to help around the house, but if they don't, just ask. Sometimes folks just plain don't know what you need. You'll soon see that they're eager to help; they're just not sure how.

You'll find that during this period you'll have limited energy. Even when you think you feel terrific, you'll find you tire easily, and it usually hits without warning. Pay attention to how you feel and take a break. On the other hand, except for avoiding lifting anything heavy, you should feel free to try to perform your daily routine. Unforunately, you probably will still feel pretty sore, even when it comes to the smallest things, like making the bed, picking up a pan from the stove, opening a window, brushing your hair, or pulling on panty hose. It will be more than a week before you'll be up to changing the sheets and even longer before you'll feel like using the vacuum cleaner.

Quite frankly, the drain is the most annoying part of the at-home post-surgery scene. It dangles from its tube, gets heavy as it fills, has to be pinned to something—your bra, your tee shirt, your panties—to keep it from pulling loose. That gets in the way, especially when you're trying to get comfortable in bed.

Take It from Us

Don't assume that a lumpectomy will necessarily be less painful than a mastectomy. After a mastectomy there is less tissue to jiggle around than with a lumpectomy. As a result, I found that there was actually less pain for a shorter time with my mastectomy than with my two lumpectomies.

In addition to the physical discomfort that comes with the drain, you'll also be asked to empty the drain several times a day and measure and keep a record of its contents. Most important, however, is the care you must take to be sanitary when emptying the accumulated fluid. Since the tube leads directly to the inside of your body, any germs touching the end of the tube have a direct link to your body fluids. Take your instructions seriously, for infection in the drain area is one of the most common problems associated with breast surgery.

Yes, your doctor will prescribe some pain medication and you'll probably need it for a few days. Take it as prescribed, unless of course you choose to take less. Frankly, most women say they have relatively little pain, some saying that they had more pain with their monthly periods than they did with their mastectomies. In any case, you'll probably be told to avoid aspirin because it may promote internal bleeding, but—with your doctor's permission—you may be able to take ibuprofen or acetaminophen.

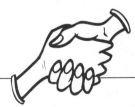

Helping Hand

Be prepared for a wide variety of responses to your surgery. You might hear from one friend, "Oh, yeah, mastectomies are same-day surgery now—it's nothing," while others may dash up to hug you only to stop short, not knowing which side hurts. And then there are those whose eyes meet your chest instead of your eyes. Solution? Make the first move by telling them what you need. They'll come around.

If you experience any unusual symptoms, like inflammation, undue tenderness, or fever, call your doctor—these are signs of infection. Also keep in mind that depression and anxiety may develop after such surgery. Try to keep your mind active and your body busy, but if you begin to feel persistently low or anxious, talk to your doctor.

The Great Unveiling

In about a week, you'll return to the doctor/surgeon's office. At that time, you'll probably get the pathologist's report (if you haven't had a call before then), and your doctor will remove the bandages and/or drain(s). The visit may throw you for another loop, so take someone with you. And take your notebook so that you—or whoever is with you—can jot down details and/or questions. Here's why the visit can be such a whirl:

➤ **The pathologist's report.** You'll need to listen carefully to details about the pathologist's report. Were the margins positive? Was the cancer invasive? Were the nodes positive? In a best-case scenario, you'll hear "No" in response to all three questions. No matter the answers, however, they determine every step from here on. Ask for a copy of the report and put it in your notebook. (More on the pathologist's report and what it means in Chapter 9.)

➤ **Removal of the drain.** It's a real milestone to get the drains out and at last be tubeless, but it's a bit uncomfortable as the doctor removes them.

➤ **Seeing the scar.** Most women see their scars for the first time at this appointment. For some folks, this is a highly emotional moment. Some women put off looking for weeks, but quite honestly the sooner you deal with your new look, the better off you'll be. Just understand that at first the scar will look really red and raw, but that goes away as it heals, and you'll be left with a pencil-line scar that continues to fade over the years.

Tales from the Trenches

A week after my mastectomy, my hubby was in the examining room with me when the nurse removed the bandages and took out the drain. After the doctor left, I turned bare-chested to him and asked, "Well, is it repulsive?" His answer came in the sweetest words I'd heard since he said "I do" almost 35 years ago: "No, it's not at all repulsive." It was all I needed to hear.

Because your breasts don't define who you are, you will come to see the new you as just that—a new you. It's a matter of getting used to the change, accepting it, and taking a positive attitude: If they hadn't taken the breast, the cancer would have eventually taken you. That's a no-brainer even on a bad day. As one daughter said after studying her mother's mastectomy scar, "Well, Mom, I think it's truly beautiful, so much better than seeing you in your coffin." It's all relative.

What should you expect over the long haul? You'll need to start exercising your arm immediately. Yes, it will hurt, but if you don't exercise, you'll pay the price for the rest of your life. (See Chapter 9 for details.)

You'll have some numbness around the scar, and it will likely be permanent. You may experience some *phantom feelings*, as do folks who have had a leg amputated but still feel pain in their toes. Yours may be stabs, throbs, burning, and itches; but if you do experience these feelings, they'll go away within a few months. The strangest sensation is cold. Drink a glass of ice water and you'll likely feel it in your scar. Weird, but it, too, goes away soon.

From the Book

Phantom feelings are real sensations that seem to come from a body part that has been removed, a result of remaining nerve endings sending messages to the brain.

Within a month or six weeks, you'll be completely healed, but long before that time, you should be able to get back to a fairly normal routine. A jogger told us that within a week, she was running three miles a day. Another woman said she took off work for two days and couldn't wait to get back. Four weeks after my mastectomy, three others and I left for a 17-day birding trip through Newfoundland and had an absolute blast. Getting back to routine is far more than chicken soup for the soul—it's champagne and caviar!

The Least You Need to Know

➤ Your doctor/surgeon may recommend one of several kinds of mastectomies, so you need to understand the terms.

➤ Get yourself ready for the surgery, both medically and personally.

➤ Mastectomies are rather routine, so unless you have reconstruction, you'll likely stay only overnight.

➤ At home after surgery, you need to rest, take careful precautions about your drain(s), and eat well.

Chapter 9

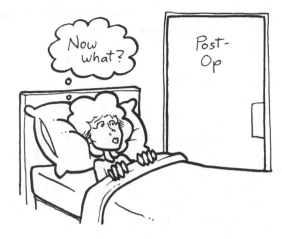

Between Surgery and the Rest

In This Chapter

➤ All about life after surgery

➤ The path pathology determines

➤ Aiding your recovery

➤ Preparing for follow-up treatments

Now it's intermission at the double feature. The first feature is over and ready for review. You've finished surgery, dealt with the lumpectomy or mastectomy and perhaps had reconstruction. Maybe you're up and about, back to at least part of your daily routine. Previews of the second feature, however, may have filled you with anxiety, even dread. Rest assured, dear friend, you'll do just fine, especially if you're prepared. And that's why we're here—to help you during intermission to prepare for the second feature.

So what do you do during intermission? Unfortunately, it's a bit more than getting up for more popcorn and Cokes. In this chapter, we'll bring you up to speed about what happens next, including showing you certain precautions that you must take—now and in the forever future. We'll also help you figure out what the pathology report means in terms of further treatment; and we'll help you get ready for whatever the second feature holds for you.

The Little Things That Count

Your medical dream team will probably give you a whole series of warnings, some written, some oral, about what might or might not happen next. Know that everything they warn you against won't necessarily happen and that it's more precautionary routine than information relating directly to your case. With that in mind, let's take a look at the kinds of challenges that may await you.

Non-Arm Arm: No Meds Here, Please

One of the most important things to remember is that if your surgeon removed any lymph nodes, you'll need to pay special attention to the care of that arm from now on. Here's the why and how: The body's *lymphatic system* serves to fight infection and to play a role in immunity to disease. Part of the lymphatic system circulates *lymph fluid* through your body, acting as a body-wide garbage disposal. The *lymph nodes,* located in little clusters throughout the body, filter out the garbage. Finally, in a complicated biological phenomenon, the lymphatic ducts dump all that filtered infection-fighting material into the bloodstream. And you know the rest: The bloodstream carries the good stuff everywhere in your body. Except not now. Not in your arm.

Here's what we mean: If you had underarm lymph nodes removed, or if you had radiation therapy in the underarm node area, that arm no longer has the full advantage of all its filters for those infection-fighting fluids—depending, of course, on how many nodes (or filters) were removed or scarred by radiation therapy. You now have somewhat less effective circulation in that arm, and you are also somewhat more susceptible to infection in that arm. As a result, you must now and forever take special precautions.

You'll read about this matter in detail in Chapter 13, "The Big Arm: Lymphedema," but we must emphasize here a crucial matter. Because circulation is somewhat restricted, you must follow three important guidelines now and forever in the future:

➤ No shots of any kind in that arm

➤ No blood drawn from that arm

➤ No blood pressure checks in that arm

Only you can keep track of these details. You'll have to tell the nurse who automatically takes blood pressures in the right arm to use the left arm now. Or you'll have to remind the nurse who always gives shots in the left arm to use the right arm now. A nurse

Take It from Us

Too many doctors and/or nurses neglect to emphasize the importance of some little things that in the long run really count, not just now, but for the rest of your life. To avoid complications even 10 or 20 years from now, take notice of the hints offered here.

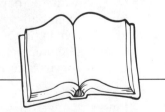

From the Book

The **lymphatic system** carries **lymph fluid** that circulates through the body fighting infection and providing immunity to disease. **Lymph nodes** serve as filters of the fluid.

won't likely check your record for lymph node removal or radiation therapy before she gives you a flu shot or antibiotics. For your own safety, you must take charge.

Yes, We Have No Razors

Because any kind of opening in the skin makes you susceptible to infection, you'll need to take other precautions as well. You'll want to be cautious about simple tasks that you never thought about before, like trimming your cuticles. In short, don't. Use a letter opener on envelopes to avoid paper cuts. Wear gloves if you're going to garden. Those rose thorns puncture and winter-dead stalks scrape and poke. Insect bites can be serious when they never were before. In addition, many folks who have lymph nodes removed find that they're now numb under the arm, sometimes in large areas. And some folks deal with a significantly sunken area where nodes were removed. So when you shave, you'll need to exercise caution. An electric razor may be the best bet for now; but survivors 10 years out tell us that after the sunken area fills out, you may be able to return to the safety razors.

These warnings apply now and always. The point is that early on you'll probably be overly cautious—and should be—until you learn what works for you. Better safe than sorry. We'll talk more about protecting your nonarm arm in Chapter 13.

Tales from the Trenches

One survivor told us she turned from throwaway safety razors to an electric razor. While she doesn't feel she gets as close a shave, she avoids nicking herself where she's numb. On the other hand, electric razors aren't foolproof, either. If not used cautiously, you can dig in with a corner or otherwise nick the skin. Be warned that any nick is serious—not just now but always.

The Path from Pathology

With those details out of the way, let's get on to what the second feature holds. We said in both Chapters 7, "Taking Your Lumps: Lumpectomy," and 8, "When They Take It All: Mastectomy," that the pathologist's report determines everything that happens from here on. That's why you'll want to get a copy of it, study it, and ask questions until you understand every word of it. Then keep it in your notebook.

While we hope your pathology report is filled with good news, that isn't always the case. Let's look at some of the broad categories of interest in the pathology report.

Positive Margins

If your pathology report says the mass removed contained *positive margins,* you have a clear indication that malignant tissue remains. For instance, you may have had a lumpectomy but the surgeon didn't remove enough tissue to capture the entire mass. (Remember, as the surgeon works, there may be nothing about the appearance of the tissue to tell him or her where the malignancy stops and starts. It's not like malignant tissue is green and everything else is pink. That's why the x-ray films are important to the surgeon.)

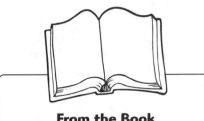

From the Book

Positive margins are those that contain malignant tissue; **negative margins** do not. Similarly, **positive lymph nodes** show malignancy; **negative nodes** do not.

What does it mean for your future if you have positive margins? It's hard to answer accurately, because cases vary dramatically; however, it may mean that you need further surgery. For instance, if you had a lumpectomy, you may now need re-excision or even a mastectomy. It's also possible, however, that surgery simply cannot remove all the malignant tissue. In that case, your doctor will discuss your options, including, perhaps, some super-duper chemo.

Positive Lymph Nodes

If your pathology report indicates *positive lymph nodes,* it may mean your cancer has spread from the breast into other parts of your body. You can have between 30 and 60 lymph nodes under your arm; we're all different. But the larger number of positive nodes, the more likely it is that your cancer has spread. Still, positive nodes are only a clue—not a fact—that microscopic cancer cells have spread elsewhere in your body. In about 30 percent of the cases, cancer has not spread. (But, then, some surgeons will point out that even with all negative nodes, in 20 to 30 percent of the cases, microscopic cells have spread elsewhere.)

So how do you know? Well, quite honestly, no one can know for sure either way. That's the sad truth about the battle with breast cancer. So if you have positive nodes, doctors make the assumption that the cancer has spread; thus, they treat with some kind of follow-up, like Tamoxifen, chemo, or radiation therapy. Better to err on the side of caution. Treatment is temporary. It gives you the rest of your life.

On the other hand, negative nodes are not always an all-clear sign. Your surgeon and pathologist will also look at the tumor removed. Depending on its kind, its size, and its aggressiveness, you may still be in for further treatment.

Tales from the Trenches

Diedre had a large tumor and 12 nodes. After chemo, doctors gave her a 28 percent chance of living 5 years. So, against her oncologist's recommendation, she investigated the benefits of stem cell transplant. She chose a hospital doing over 200 transplants annually.

After capturing her good stem cells, doctors administered 8 medications simultaneously 24 hours a day for 5 days. A day later, they replaced her stem cells. After 4 weeks, she resumed work, and took 37 radiation treatments, reporting for treatment every day after work. Doctors now project a 68 percent chance of her living 5 years. Three years out, she's a vibrant, active woman, who's a principal of a large elementary school.

In Situ, No; Invasive, Yes

Like positive lymph nodes, invasive cancer means more treatment, and maybe more surgery. As you study the pathologist's report, you want to learn to what extent your cancer is invasive. Has it just broken through the walls of the ducts? Has it invaded a major portion of the breast? Has it spread beyond the breast? In short, you want to know how far it's spread. The more invasive it is, the more dramatic the follow-up treatment. We've talked all along about the combination of a lumpectomy and radiation therapy being as effective in many situations as a mastectomy. When the pathology report for a lumpectomy shows invasive cancer, however, the situation changes. Almost certainly it will call for additional surgery, this time to remove lymph nodes. Then, depending on what they show, you may also be in for chemo.

Hormone Receptors Receiving?

The final broad category you'll be looking for in the pathology report pertains to the hormone receptor test. If your condition is hormone receptive positive (HR+), that means that hormones trigger the growth of the lesion. If your lesion is hormone receptive negative (HR–), hormones have no effect on it.

What does all this mean in terms of further treatment? First of all, most breast tissue is HR+. That's logical, considering that the breast responds to hormonal cycles (like tenderness during your monthly periods) and responds to pregnancy (by producing milk). All logic aside, however, if your malignancy (or even pre-cancerous lesion) is HR+, you must eliminate hormones to prevent—or at least retard—further growth.

That means no hormone replacement therapy when you approach menopause (and the immediate cessation of HRT if you're already on it). But it also means that you can use an anti-estrogen drug to eliminate whatever estrogen your body is producing, either before or after menopause. (For further details, see Chapter 12, "Hormone Therapy: The Pill.")

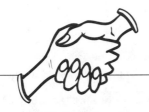

Helping Hand

Talk to your doc about your status. If your lesion is HR–, you may have a situation more difficult to treat. HR– tissue is foreign to the breast and thus complicates the medical follow-up. Discuss details with the doc.

Take It from Us

Don't rush into follow-up treatment. Usually, you'll have ample time to decide about your next steps. Before anything else happens, you have to heal. If you don't heal completely, the remainder of your treatment may be less effective or you may have other poor results.

Second Opinion?

After you and your medical team have studied and discussed the pathology report to your satisfaction, reconsider the so-called standard regimens set out in Chapter 5, "Decisions, Decisions, Decisions." Review your notes in your notebook. Take time to make another list of questions:

➤ What follow-up treatment do you recommend?

➤ What results should I expect from this treatment?

➤ What are the advantages of this treatment over a similar one?

➤ How long is each treatment?

➤ Do the treatments have to be taken in a specific order?

➤ What if I have to miss a treatment because of something like an infection or cold, or even a snowstorm?

➤ Is there a break between treatments?

➤ What short-term side effects can I expect?

➤ What long-term side effects can I expect?

➤ What are the disadvantages of this treatment?

➤ Are there other treatments equally or nearly equally effective?

➤ Why is the recommended treatment preferable?

➤ If this is a fairly new treatment, when was the latest study completed on this kind of treatment and what were the results?

➤ How will this treatment affect the healing of my surgical incisions?

➤ How many follow-up appointments are there for each treatment?

Make sure you understand your medical team's recommendation for treatments. Get your questions answered. Then, as before, if you feel it's necessary, get a second opinion.

Before More, Heal!

Depending on how much surgery you've had and whether or not you've elected to have reconstructive surgery, you may need anywhere from four weeks to two months to heal. Everyone wants to get on with whatever treatment is necessary if for no other reason than to get it over with; but until you heal, further treatment is out of the question. For instance, radiation destroys tissue, so what hasn't healed may not heal. And chemo isn't exactly a body builder.

So relax, rest, eat plenty of (low-fat) protein, and take good care of yourself. Do everything you can to help your body mend after surgery. Your body will better respond to the follow-up treatment if you do. This may also be a good time to find a support group to help you walk this walk. These women have been there, and you can get some real-life input on what to expect, when to expect it, and some do's and don'ts.

Exercise: Back to the Range

Meanwhile, you'll probably start feeling quite perky within a week or so of your surgery (depending on how much reconstructive surgery you had). So it's time to get back into the swing of things—literally. You may find now that the movement in your arm isn't what it used to be. To regain that movement, you'll need to exercise. The American Cancer Society's booklet *Exercises After Breast Surgery* includes an illustrated set of leveled exercises especially right for you. You may also want to consider initially seeing a physical or occupational therapist; then at home you can do the exercises prescribed for you. Meanwhile, let's look at a couple of easy exercises often recommended.

Probably the most frequently recommended exercise is the wall walk. Here's the routine: Stand facing a wall, your feet about six inches from the wall. Place your 10 fingers on the wall and let your fingers climb up—and then back down. Repeat several times, increasing repetitions each day. Gauge how far up you can walk the wall, striving to go just a little higher each day. If you had surgery on only one side, you'll be able to gauge the return of range of motion by comparing the affected side with the other side.

For the first week or so after surgery, your doctor may not want you to raise your arm more than 90 degrees, but later, you'll be ready to go for the rotation exercise. Simply stand in place, swing (gently!) your arms 360 degrees. You'll feel all the muscles pull. But keep at it several times a day. Rotate until both arms move with the same ease and the same range of motion.

In the hand wall-walk exercise, you'll face the wall and walk your 10 fingers as high as you can and then walk back down. In the shoulder flex exercise, you'll lie on the floor and reach both arms 180 degrees over your head.

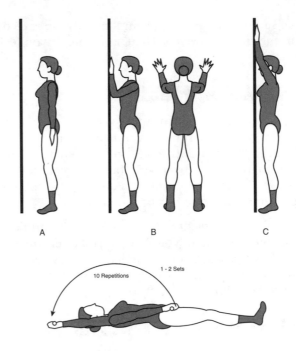

A third exercise starts by lying on the floor on your back with your arms parallel and down to your sides. Keeping your arms straight, raise them up and over your head, trying to touch the floor above your head (180 degrees). Repeat, building up to 10 repetitions. In this shoulder flex exercise, you'll notice that the unaffected side will touch the floor easily. Not so, the other. But keep working. You'll get there soon.

Tales from the Trenches

Janie, a 10-year survivor, found she could no longer reach back to fasten her bra as she had done only a few years ago. "I stopped doing the exercises," she explained. "I thought that was all behind me. Now I've discovered that if I stop exercising, I start losing range of motion. I've joined an aquatic therapy class, and that has made all the difference. We've also become a close-knit group of gals and go out to lunch once a month. Great therapy in more ways than one!"

Repeat these exercises as often as you feel comfortable. Try, daily, to extend the exercise time as well as your range of motion. This is truly a case of no pain, no gain. But wouldn't you like to be able to get into your jacket without help?

Port—or Starboard?

If after intermission you're facing chemo, you'll want to make a decision about whether or not to have a *portacath* (commonly called a *port*) implanted. Once in-serted, the port serves for every needle stick, from administering the chemo to drawing blood. Yes, your medical team will no doubt have a recommendation—one way or the other—but meanwhile, here's a heads-up about the whole picture:

Ports serve primarily to save your veins. The chemo does enough bad stuff to your veins without added abuse from lots of needle sticks. After you've had a few dozen injections (or even before the first dozen, if you don't have strong veins), the veins suffer severe damage and may even shut down.

To solve the problem, your doc can implant a port just under your skin in a rather minor but somewhat uncomfortable surgery. Different surgeons implant them in different parts of the body, but one common site is about two inches below the collarbone in line with your breast. It's about a 30- to 45-minute deal, but with that behind you, you'll have no more sticks in your veins. As we all know, just one stick of a needle is a whole lot better than two or more—and especially better than a few dozen more. Once the port is in place, the medical folks attach the chemo drip needle to the port or draw blood from the port for the many blood tests you'll likely have. Now the stick is only through the skin, not into a vein causing damage.

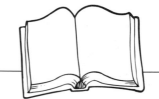

From the Book

A **port** (properly a **portacath**) is a small plastic tube with a rubber seal on top and metal on the bottom that is placed under the skin and attached to a catheter inside the body. Fluids enter and exit the body through the port with use of a special needle.

Why use a port? Consider the following:

➤ You don't have to endure stick after stick of a needle over the next many months.

➤ It requires little or no care on your part.

➤ It saves major wear and tear on your veins.

➤ It helps protect skin and muscle from accidental damage from very toxic chemo drugs.

➤ It's convenient and quick.

➤ It can remain in the body and be used for months and even years, especially for blood tests.

➤ You can feel it under your skin; but once in place, it doesn't hurt. (On treatment days, however, the area gets a bit tender, but it's okay in 24 hours or so.)

With all these advantages, why would you not use a port? Some folks cite these reasons:

➤ The biggest downside to the port is the surgery (rather minor but uncomfortable) and the three or four days of discomfort afterward; however, removal is much easier and may be done in the doc's office.

➤ Where the port is inserted and removed, you'll have a one-and-a-half- to two-inch scar.

➤ Some people worry that they might accidentally damage the port and thereby cause some harm to themselves. It's not likely, but the possibility may worry you.

➤ If not in use, the port must be cleaned monthly by medical folks.

➤ Some people worry about the port causing infections. That, too, is unlikely, but cleanliness is essential.

➤ Although it's quite rare, a blood clot can result from the surgery.

➤ Depending on its placement, you may need to wear a different style bra to avoid irritating the skin over the port.

For most folks, the advantages of a port far outweigh the disadvantages. If you hate being stuck with a needle and/or if you have less than perfect veins, you may want to discuss with the doc how a port might work for you.

Take It from Us

Investigate all options when it comes to injections and blood draws. You can have no needles of any kind ever in your affected arm. Thus, all blood work, chemo, IVs, even antibiotic or flu shots have to go into your unaffected arm. That's not just now. That's for the rest of your life. Taking care of your veins now may make a difference in the future.

Things Your Mother Never Told You

Just like your medical dream team, we've tried to be up-front about all the stumbling blocks you may face along the battle lines. And just like your dream team, we may have overlooked a few. So, during intermission, as you prepare for the second feature, reconsider some of the pointers from earlier chapters; check some of the resources in the appendixes; follow up with your insurance company about coverage. Granted, there comes a time when you need to quit reading and worrying and get on with life, but you're preparing now for whatever follow-up therapies your medical team—and you—deem necessary.

During this intermission, perhaps you'll find inspiration from Diedre. She went through what is probably the most difficult of any of the breast cancer treatments—stem cell transplant. Now, she says, lots of folks come to her really scared of whatever treatments lurk in their futures. "You know," she says, "treatment is only temporary. That's the operative word. Temporary. You have to think of it as an investment in the rest of your life. And the longer we survive, the better our chances for dramatic improvement in the treatments." This from a woman who raised her odds from 28 to 68 percent for living another five years. I'd say she's one tough cookie—and a tremendous inspiration. And yes, sister, you can do this, too! You really can!

The Least You Need to Know

➤ During this healing time, you can study and discuss the details in the pathologist's report.

➤ The pathologist's report determines future treatments, so understand the primary issues.

➤ While healing, you can resume exercise to regain range of motion in the affected arm.

➤ If chemo is in your future, seriously consider the advantages of a portacath.

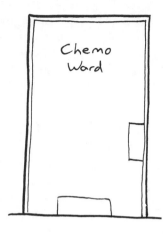

Chapter 10

Chemotherapy: Cruel to Be Kind

> **In This Chapter**
>
> ➤ Knowing how it works
>
> ➤ Learning your routine
>
> ➤ Dealing with the side effects
>
> ➤ Finding out how you might feel
>
> ➤ Discover how to cope

To most folks, anticipating *chemotherapy* is probably one of the most frightening parts of any kind of cancer treatment, including breast cancer. Unfortunately, however, many breast cancer survivors, in addition to having surgery, also require chemotherapy. In short, chemo involves the use of cell-killing chemicals to destroy cancer cells that may remain after your surgery. In this chapter, we'll discuss the uses of chemotherapy, as well as any risks and the side effects that may arise. And, above all, we'll reassure you that you can do this! In fact, some survivors never missed a day of work and kept up with their children's school and after-school activities all during chemo. Whatever your situation, however, remember that like all other breast cancer treatments, chemo and its common side effects are only temporary. And study after study shows that chemo will prolong your life.

The Why and Who of Chemotherapy

Doctors use chemotherapy to treat breast cancer in four ways, the most frequent being to kill any errant cancer cells that may have spread into the body and to treat a cancer that has metastasized. Sometimes if the tumor is quite large, however, the doctor will use chemo to shrink its size, usually in an effort to make the tumor more operable. Finally, infrequently, the doctor may administer chemo to watch how a tumor will react to a specific chemical or drug. But a fifth way comes along now and then. Given chemo's systemic approach, some survivors and their doctors agree to use chemo as a "chemical insurance policy" to lessen their chances of recurrence just in case the cancer might have spread.

In any case, chemotherapy is an adjuvant therapy, meaning it is only part of your treatment plan and used in conjunction with surgery and/or radiation therapy.

Pre-menopausal women who have been diagnosed with breast cancer with positive nodes are prime candidates for chemotherapy. Chemotherapy is necessary in such cases because positive nodes indicate that the cancer has probably metastasized (spread to other cells of the body) and pre-menopausal women are, by definition, still producing sex hormones, which affects the development of breast cancer in many women. If your doctor tells you that your breast cancer is "estrogen-receptor positive breast cancer," you are also a candidate for chemotherapy. This type of tumor has a protein attached to it that is receptive to or responds to hormones. As we have discussed before, most breast cancers feed and grow on hormones. (For more information, please refer to Chapter 12, "Hormone Therapy: The Pill.")

However, post-menopausal women, those who may be finished with or at the end of menopause and no longer produce sex hormones, may or may not receive chemotherapy. In studies involving post-menopausal women with breast cancer, chemotherapy did not necessarily improve the survival rate.

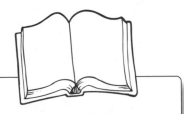

From the Book

Metastasis is the spread of cancer cells, by way of the lymph system or bloodstream, to areas of the body other than the tumor site. **Chemotherapy** is treatment of cancer with the use of cytotoxic (cell–killing) drugs.

Women who have node negative breast cancer (which means that the cancer hasn't spread outside of the breast) also usually do not require chemotherapy, although some opt to take chemotherapy as a "chemical insurance policy," just in case cancer cells have escaped detection. While chemotherapy may lessen your chances of *metastasis*, it is not an absolute guarantee that your cancer will not spread.

The decision to undergo chemotherapy is one that you must make with your doctor after hearing all of the facts about your particular type of cancer, your general prognosis, and what positive effects chemotherapy will have for you. Whether or not you had any positive nodes and whether your cancer tested hormone-receptor positive or negative all influence the decision. Once you've made the decision to go forward, however, it'll help you to know what to expect and why. First, let's take a look at how chemotherapy works within the body.

Doing the Chemo Dance: Who's Leading

The first thing you need to know about chemotherapy is that it kills healthy cells along with cancer cells, and that ability is what causes most of the side effects that patients experience. But we'll get to those later.

The second thing you need to know is why it works. Here goes. Cancer cells divide more quickly than normal cells. Cells that divide quickly are easily damaged or destroyed. Chemo works because even though it does affect some normal cells, it kills the quickly dividing cancer cells.

For now, let's look at how your doctor comes up with a chemotherapy protocol. You've heard that timing is everything? Well, that's certainly true when it comes to chemotherapy. Since chemo kills cancer cells and healthy cells as well, the treatments are given at intervals—typically about three weeks—allowing the body to generate new, healthy cells that the drugs have not affected.

The first step in developing a chemotherapy protocol is for your doctor to take a blood sample that determines the normal levels of certain of your body's cells. Then, he or she will test another blood sample to see if your body's ready for another dose.

The length and type of treatment differs with each person and diagnosis. Treatment schedules range from daily to monthly doses but the goal is to give the body time to recuperate and generate new healthy cells between each dose. The number of drips/shots given and/or pills taken vary, but a typical treatment protocol lasts from three to six months.

A typical routine is a three-week cycle over a six-month period. In other words, you get a treatment every three weeks, a schedule that allows the chemicals to do their job and for your body to adjust between treatments.

Which Cocktail Is Good for Me?

There are nearly 100 chemotherapy drugs currently in use. However, for the treatment of breast cancer, that list is narrowed to a baker's dozen.

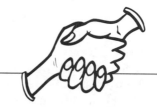

Helping Hand

Patients in chemotherapy treatment must be very careful of infections or other illnesses. The body's natural defense fighting cells are killed off in chemotherapy just like cancer cells and it takes time to rebuild immunity.

Tales from the Trenches

Karen knew that deciding to take chemotherapy was a difficult decision, so she read books, searched the Internet, and connected with others undergoing the same treatment. She asked lots of questions about the drugs, the benefits, and the side effects. Ultimately, she was happier with her decision to use chemotherapy because she had researched the alternatives.

The drugs fall into four basic categories:

➤ **Antimetabolites** are drugs that "starve" cancer cells while the cells are dividing.

➤ **Vinca alkaloids** impede cancer cells' division.

➤ **Antitumor antibiotics** work through your DNA, slowing down cancer growth.

➤ **Alkylating agents** also work through your DNA by binding with the cancer cell to stop it from dividing.

The chemicals or drugs are mixed much like a cocktail because some cancer cells can be resistant to one particular chemical or drug. Thus, bombarding them with more than one drug at a time may just do the trick. How your doctor mixes depends on the type of cancer you have and the stage it's in.

The following combinations of drugs are the most often used:

➤ **Cytoxin** (cyclophosphamide), **Methotrexate,** and **5-FU** (5-fluorouracil), usually called CMF for short.

➤ **Cytoxin** (cyclophosphamide), **Adriamycin** (doxorubicin), and **5-FU** (5-fluorouracil), usually called CAF for short.

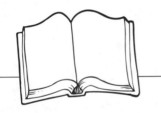

From the Book

Intravenous means "in a vein." In this case, intravenous means an injection in a vein directly from a syringe or from a bag containing a mixture of drugs. Most commonly, chemo is administered intravenously through a portacath, explained later.

➤ **Adriamycin** (doxorubicin) and **Cytoxin** (cyclophosphamide), usually referred to as AC, with or without **Taxol** (Paclitaxel) or **Taxotere** (docetaxel). Taxotere is substituted for folks who can't tolerate Taxol since it has fewer side effects compared to Taxol and can be administered faster.

➤ **Adriamycin** (doxorubicin) followed by **Cytoxin** (cyclophosphamide), **Methotrexate,** and **5-FU** (5-fluorouracil).

All of these chemo drugs frequently cause mouth sores, nausea, loss of appetite, low blood counts, menstrual irregularities (or even temporary or permanent cessation), hair loss, and sore throat. The CMF mix, as well as the Adriamycin followed by CMF, can also cause ulcers, rash, and conjunctivitis. And Adriamycin itself, while it's the strongest drug for metastasized cancer, can be toxic to the heart.

The Form of Medication

Chemo is usually given *intravenously;* however, rarely some is given orally in the form of a pill or liquid. If your chemo treatment is given orally, you can take your pills at home. If you receive the medication by injection, you'll visit a hospital or clinic for treatment. Depending on how you react to the drugs you take, you may have to stay briefly at a hospital for observation and monitoring.

At Home or in the Hospital

When it comes to receiving your chemotherapy, you'll most likely find yourself going to the hospital, a cancer center, or other such similar medical facility. Because— generally speaking—the more relaxed you are the better you'll be able to tolerate the treatment, consider bringing a tape or CD player with headphones and your favorite music to block noise, or ask friends to join you for conversation or a board or card game, or watch TV to help pass the time. You may want to apply fragrant hand lotion or perfume to mask chemical smells. In short, the more comfortable you feel, the better you'll be able to tolerate the treatment.

On some rare occasions, patients have taken their chemo at home, but most patients receive their treatments at a hospital, with a staff of medical professionals for support.

A Day in the Life of ...

Undergoing chemo certainly does change your life. It affects your health, both positively and negatively, and it alters your attitude and sense of well-being. The schedule of the protocol forces you to modify your daily routine. And, because all this is happening at once, it affects your relationships with your family, friends, and co-workers. It's hard to function at a normal level when you are anxious, depressed, angry, or so sick you can't get off the couch.

Once you've gone through the preliminary preparations, probably including the insertion of a portacath (see Chapter 9, "Between Surgery and the Rest"), you'll start to recognize a routine. Ask your doctor if you can schedule your chemo appointment in the morning (if you don't work or can take a whole day off), or in the afternoon (if you work or have other daily responsibilities and prefer to undergo treatment at the end of the day). You'll sign a consent form when you arrive at the hospital, and then a technician will draw your blood. The results of the blood test indicate if you can tolerate another dose or not. If your white blood cell count is not high enough, you'll go home for a couple of days and then try again.

If you're ready, you'll probably first talk to your doctor about any concerns you might have and tell him how you're feeling in general. Then, a technologist gets you ready. You get situated in

Helping Hand

Always stand firm when it comes to getting answers to any of your questions. If you decide to undergo chemotherapy, you deserve to know the facts and to receive those facts from a doctor you trust. If you even think you have a question, ask it. Medical folks can be intimidating but you have a right to know.

a comfortable chair and the tech inserts the drip needle into your vein or *port,* and the treatment begins. Depending on your regimen, you may be sitting for 10 minutes or several hours.

Today, most women do not suffer as severely from nausea as patients did years ago, thanks to drugs that help reduce severe side effects; however, some side effects are still a part of chemotherapy.

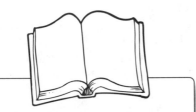

From the Book

Portacaths (usually called **ports**) are catheters that can stay in a vein for a prolonged period— months or even years. The port has a plastic piece attached to it outside the vein just under the skin where the needle is inserted. Ports are used to save your veins over prolonged periods of use, such as with the administration of chemotherapy.

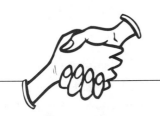

Helping Hand

Keep busy! If you work outside the home and can manage it, keep working. If you're at home, line up some projects that'll take your mind off of your treatment. That way, you'll be more able to shut out most anxiety and doubt.

When the chemicals hit your bloodstream, you may experience an odd taste in your mouth, your vision may blur, or you may just feel funny. Or, like some of the survivors we interviewed, you may have none of these exeriences. When the drip is finished, you're "unplugged," you schedule your next appointment, and you're free to go home. For several days after the injection, you may take pills that help relieve nausea. (Trust me, this is a blessing!)

Sounds simple, doesn't it? The procedure is; the side effects are not. To deal with the treatment and the side effects, you need a special cohesive ingredient: a good attitude.

The connection between the mind and the body is a crucial one, and that's especially true when it comes to tolerating the effects of chemotherapy. If you imagine that chemotherapy will be the worst thing you've ever experienced, your body might just cooperate and prove you right. If you focus on the healing power of the chemicals, on staying as healthy as possible throughout treatment, on coping day to day with the challenges you face, you'll fare much better.

The Side Effects: The Eyes of the Beholder

Other than the stick of the needle, receiving the chemotherapy is a painless procedure. However, many women experience rather nasty side effects. The on-cologist who establishes your chemotherapy protocol will meet with you and describe, as much as possible, what you can expect from the treatment. Depending on which drugs you take, and your own personal body chemistry, you may experience nausea, vomit-ing, hair loss, energy drain, weight loss, weight gain, or sleeplessness. Keep in mind that side effects vary from person to person: one gains weight; one loses weight. However, one universal side effect is anxiety: Because you don't know how the drugs will affect you (and neither does your doctor), you can't help but worry about what's to come. The bottom line: You must experience chemo before you know how you will react. It's walking a very long mile in your own shoes.

Menopause: A Change in "The" Change

Everyone knows the average age that most women experience menopause is about 50, but the changes that occur when your ovaries start to produce less of the sex hormones can begin as early as 40 to 45. Among the effects of menopause are dramatic changes in the menstrual cycle (culminating in the cessation of menstruation), hot flashes, dry skin, vaginal dryness, and mood swings. However, what most people may not know is that if you haven't yet begun or passed through menopause, chemotherapy may begin the process for you. Chemotherapy can stop the production of the sex hormones. If your breast cancer is called "hormone-receptor positive," it means that your cancer will grow and thrive in the presence of estrogen. Therefore, in order to stop the growth of the cancer, your body must stop producing the estrogen that feeds it. Certain chemotherapy chemicals can shut down the production of the sex hormones (estrogen and progesterone). This is why chemotherapy has the nickname of "chemical menopause."

While we cover this topic in depth in Chapter 12, it's important to mention menopause as a side effect. This is an incredibly difficult time for most. You are already fighting anxiety, anger, disbelief, and unnatural chemicals in your body—not to mention the chemotherapy side effects. Then you have mood swings and hot flashes to deal with, too. Wow!—talk about complications!

Sign, Everywhere a Sign

Some side effects can be serious and an indication that something is wrong. Keep track of these

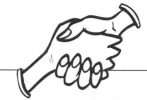

Helping Hand

Wait and see how you feel—don't let what your doctor or other patients say determine how you'll react to your treatment. Listen to what they say about potential side effects, but remain calm and think positive, life-affirming thoughts.

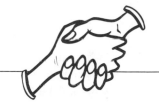

Helping Hand

Ask for help in gathering and organizing information about your treatment. When your doctor discusses your options and prognosis, it's a good idea to have a caregiver there—your husband or nurse—so they can understand some of the potential side effects, too. And take your notebook. Believe me, without notes, you'll never remember everything!

warning signs. The ACS guidelines list things you should take seriously and call your doctor if they occur:

➤ Fever of 101.5°+

➤ Bleeding or unexplained bruising

➤ A rash/allergic reaction, for example, swelling, severe itching, or wheezing

➤ Intense chills

➤ Pain/soreness at the chemotherapy/catheter injection site

➤ Unusual pain, including intense headaches

➤ Shortness of breath

➤ Prolonged diarrhea or vomiting

➤ Bloody stool or urine

Your body is trying to get your attention. If you experience any of these side effects, take them seriously and talk to your doctor as soon as possible.

Take It from Us

My warning sign was an allergic reaction. My treatment protocol called for six chemotherapy drips. After five normal sessions, my skin started to itch so badly I scratched myself raw. My tongue swelled. I had difficulty breathing. My allergist said I was having a reaction to the chemo. To me, my body was saying I had just had enough, and, in my mind, I thought I would die if I had the last injection. My choice was to have five treatments, not six.

Physical Reaction: Body Talk

As for side effects, be prepared for almost anything and question everything. You won't know until you have gone through round one, or sometimes through several rounds, how the ol' bod's gonna react. Remember, at your first visit with the oncologist, you were told what might happen. But "might" doesn't mean "will." In fact, the most often described symptoms are flu-like. And I mean a really bad case of the flu: aching muscles, nausea, fatigue, no appetite, headache, chills, fever, and all.

If you experience any flu-like symptoms, skip your usual flu remedies. Taking any other medication not prescribed by your doctor can complicate your chemotherapy treatment. Because chemo is pushing almost every organ and cell in your body to the limit, normal, "over-the-counter" drugs, as well as prescription drugs, may not function as they have done in the past. You already know that many drugs react adversely when taken together. The same goes for chemotherapy drugs. Combined with laxatives, pain medications, and, yes, even aspirin, common remedies can have adverse effects. Before you take your first drip/shot, consult with your doctor about "all" the medication you are taking, including vitamins and herbs. Mixing drugs can make a pretty potent cocktail.

Working Through It

With each drip/shot, you may feel more tired or drained. There will be days when you doubt if you can put one foot in front of the other; consequently, working while undergoing treatment may be an issue. Pace yourself with a part-time schedule or try working from home. Hopefully, you can create options for resting when you feel the need.

Some federal and state laws require employers to allow for flexible scheduling during treatment. Take a look at Chapter 6, "Call for a Working Plan," for more information, or contact the ACS in your area or call the national headquarters at 1-800-ACS-2345.

Tales from the Trenches

Millie was a cola-holic who drank six or seven colas daily. Several days after her first injection, she took a drink from a can of cola and immediately turned around and spit it in the sink. She could not stand what she perceived to be a strong chemical taste. She has not had a cola since that time.

Taster's Choice

Although this isn't a hard-and-fast rule, some survivors suggest you stop eating your favorite foods while going through chemo. Otherwise, you may never want to eat them again. You will be nauseous from the chemicals, and, further into the treatment, you will shed the top layer of cells of the lining of your mouth. That in turn, will change your sensitivity or tolerance for certain things or even your sense of taste. Something you once loved may suddenly taste terrible. It's like "guilt by association!"

However, there's a flip side to this coin: If you want to stop eating something (chocolate or pie, for example), try eating it during treatment. What a habit breaker!

Some foods, previously "so-so," will taste wonderful; some foods that you just love will gag you. For almost six months, the staples of my diet were cereal with really cold milk, iced tea, and potatoes. Talk to your doctor about vitamins or mineral supplements. It's more important that you keep eating than that you eat right.

In addition to these changes in appetite, further down the line you may also develop sores in your mouth, usually after the third or fourth drip. This condition is called stomatitis and is not only painful but also dangerous. The sores can become infected, and any infection is more difficult to fight during chemo. As a result, your doctor may prescribe ointments and gargles designed to coat and heal the sores. Although these medications generally taste terrible, the relief they provide is nearly instantaneous and long lasting. Ice chips also help numb the sores. Meanwhile, skip the potent spices, acidic foods, most mouthwashes, rigid toothbrushes, and dental floss. Now is the time to baby your mouth with cool, soft, mildly seasoned foods—even baby food—because they won't irritate a tender mouth.

Now's also the time to fight fire with fire. Almost the instant the chemicals enter your body, you'll receive a backwash of chemical taste in your mouth, one that will revisit you from time to time. You need a taste just as strong as the chemicals to counteract the taste. Prior to chemo, for instance, I never liked butterscotch because its flavor was too strong; however, after the first injection, I developed a love for butterscotch drops because they overpowered the chemical taste. During chemo, you will have different needs, new priorities, and unusual tastes when it comes to food. What you preferred before chemo, in the way of foods and taste, may not be what you prefer during or even after chemo. Listen to your body, experiment, and figure out what works for you.

Skinned!

Gray may be a popular color for fall fashions, but not as a skin color. Unfortunately, for many people who undergo chemotherapy, skin changes occur, and many of them are unpleasant (like having a gray undertone!). Your skin may suffer externally from acne, peeling, itching, rashes, and redness.

The skin is the largest organ of the body and needs special attention during chemo. Take quick baths with warm water, not long, hot showers, which can act to dry the skin. While still damp from the shower, pat the skin dry, but don't rub it. Then gently rub in moisturizers so the skin will absorb them quickly. Avoid perfumes and shaving creams that contain alcohol. If your skin becomes red and tender, a paste made of cornstarch or oatmeal is a blessing. And, last but not least, stay out of the sun.

Internally, the cytotoxic drugs are strong enough to kill cells. If for any reason these drugs escape the veins, cells in the near vicinity will die, also.

Asking for Immunity

Prior to chemo, the common cold would usually last 7 to 10 days. During and after chemo, the common cold seems to last forever. What has happened to your *immunity* and your *immune system?* What has happened is that chemotherapy has impacted your immune system and decreased your ability to fight against harmful foreign invaders like viruses and bacteria. Because some cancers attack your immune system or can be spread through the body by the immune system, chemotherapy also works through the immune system going after the cancer cells. While this major battle is going on in the immune system, it is hard for it to throw up defenses against any germs that are trying to attack your body.

Chemo has an effect on your red blood cells (oxygen carriers to the body), white blood cells (infection fighters), and platelets (helpers that stop blood clotting and, therefore, bleeding) because it directly affects the bone marrow where these three types of cells are produced. The drop in the production of these three separate types of cells can cause anemia, infection, and bleeding. Report any signs of anemia, infection, or bleeding to your doctor immediately.

From the Book

Immunity is an inherited, acquired, or induced ability to mount a defense to a specific disease-causing agent such as a specific bacterium or virus. Your **immune system** is a system designed to protect the body from invaders.

Most folks undergoing chemo fear infection above all. There are, however, some things that you can do for yourself to help avoid developing these side effects. Protect yourself.

➤ Avoid shaking hands with people.

➤ After contact with things, wash your hands.

➤ Avoid people with colds, measles, chickenpox, or the flu.

➤ Avoid crowds and gatherings.

➤ Avoid children who have been recently immunized.

➤ Do not receive any immunization shot unless you check with your physician.

➤ Pay special attention when using knives, razors, clippers, or scissors to avoid cutting your skin.

➤ If you do cut yourself, attend to the cut—now.

➤ For jobs requiring manual labor, wear gloves.

➤ Avoid "hard" toothbrushes.

➤ Get rest and talk to your doctor about vitamins and supplements.

➤ Pat wet skin dry; do not rub your skin.

➤ Use moisturizers to keep skin soft.

➤ Report unexpected bruising, changes in urine or bowel movements, bleeding in the nose or gums, headaches, dizziness, and pain in muscles/joints.

Bodily Functions

After several treatments, you'll know how you're reacting to the chemo, so this is the time to be on the alert for changes in your bodily functions.

What was "normal" for you as far as bowel movements before chemo may not be "normal" for you while going through chemo. Instead of struggling with either constipation or diarrhea, work with your doctor to find solutions to these uncomfortable problems. If you're constipated, drink fluids, have prescribed laxatives on hand, eat high-fiber foods and do some type of simple exercise. If you have diarrhea, avoid high-fiber foods, eat high potassium foods (bananas, potatoes, oranges, peaches, apricots) drink plenty of fluids, have prescribed anti-diarrheal medicine on hand, eat small amounts of food and eat more often, and avoid spicy or greasy foods and coffee, tea, alcohol, and sweets.

In addition to your gastrointestinal tract, other body systems are likely to be affected by chemotherapy. For one thing, you may notice that your energy level is lower than normal. You're not alone. In fact, most people experience fatigue as a side effect of treatment, the result of a low red blood cell count. Ask for help.

Furthermore, chemotherapy can also affect the nerves and muscles. Tingling, muscle weakness, or a burning sensation may occur. Not only should you see your doctor for help in coping with fatigue and muscle weakness, but you should also rest as often as you feel the need to do so.

Tales from the Trenches

Amelia was told her chemotherapy treatment could cause either constipation or diarrhea. After drip #1, she didn't have a bowel movement for three days. From then on, she avoided the misery by taking a laxative the day before the drip. This kept her system running smoothly.

Hair Loss: When Bald Ain't Beautiful

"Bald is beautiful" may be true for Yul Brynner or Telly Savalas, but not for most women. In fact, for some women, hair loss is the most difficult part of dealing with chemotherapy because it is so visible. And once you lose your hair, it seems to take forever for it to grow back.

Even if you don't lose your hair, it is likely to thin considerably. The one chemotherapy drug most often associated with almost complete hair loss is Adriamycin. The other drugs are more likely to merely make your hair thin. Your doctor can predict, with the drugs you're getting, how much hair you'll likely lose and when you can expect to lose it. (But sometimes women prove those predictions wrong!)

Some women decide to shave their heads and either wear turbans and wigs or simply do a Telly Savalas themselves. If you choose not to shave your head, some things you can do that may ease further hair loss are using satin pillowcases (because they do not tug on the hair like cotton does) and using mild shampoos and brushes. Consider getting a short haircut so you can let it air dry and avoid using rollers to set it. And for the time being, you should also avoid color treating your hair.

Creating a Calm During the Storm

Once you have information on how you *might* feel, begin to psyche yourself up to deal with the emotional and intellectual changes that are sure to follow. (See Chapter 23, "Life Goes On: Physical and Emotional Changes.") Now is also a good time to seek out women who have had or are going through chemo. Survivors speaking with the voice of experience offer wonderful suggestions and insight.

Take It from Us

Watch the wind if you wear a wig! Joan went to the mall on a breezy day. As she was getting out of the car, the wind blew her wig off. While people watched her chase it across the parking lot, she was so embarrassed that she went home crying.

Everybody's Waiting for the Weekend

With help from your doctor, you can choose when to have your chemotherapy sessions. For instance, if you're trying to keep your 9-to-5 job, you may want to ask that your treatments be administered on a Friday. You have three days to adjust, cope and overcome your immediate reaction. (What a way to spend the weekend!)

Put Your Hand in a Hand

Fear is part of this experience, from beginning to end, including chemotherapy. Until you go through this, you have no idea what to expect. Take someone with you to hold your hand, provide moral support, or just drive you home and help you get settled in. Doubt and discomfort are lessened by having the right person with you to reassure you.

Pamper Your Pantry

For the first few days you are not going to feel like running errands. Prepare your house and pantry in advance with comforting "goodies." Stay home; chill.

Keep the End in Mind

You have heard that you can face anything if you know there is an end to it. This is a great philosophy for dealing with chemo. Keep the timing in your mind and know the date and day it will end. After my first injection, I looked at my husband and said, "One down, five to go." Only diamonds are forever.

The Reed or the Oak

Because your family and friends are worried about you, one thing you will try to do is to prove, beyond a shadow of a doubt, that all is *okay*. Yes, there are times when you need to be the oak, but there are also times when you need to be the reed and bend with the wind. Don't try to overdo and show everyone you are a Samson. You are going through some pretty tough stuff. Be gentle with yourself.

Idle Hands ...

Idleness and loneliness help produce fear. Keep your mind focused on "other" things, not what you are going through. Read good books, rent funny videos, or work puzzles to help pass the time. Idle thoughts are your worst nightmare.

Your Secret Garden

Create and keep your surroundings pleasant and serene. Try not to argue with the people around you. Prepare your family so that they will give you an extra helping of kindness. Fill your house with pretty flowers and wonderful-smelling candles. This is the time to pamper yourself.

If the Shoe Fits ...

We all have different ways of relaxing; know what works for you. Your relaxation may come in the form of petting a lap dog, visualization, or even hypnosis. Whatever it takes!

It's possible to describe going through chemotherapy as a walk on the dark side. If you are prepared, emotionally as well as mentally, when the physical side effects come along, you are more able to deal with your chemotherapy treatments. But always keep in mind the guiding rule: Treatment is only temporary. Then you can go on with the rest of your life. Like over two million other women out there, you can do this. And you'll do just fine.

The Least You Need to Know

➤ Chemotherapy is a systemic drug that fights microscopic cancer cells that may have spread beyond your breast to other parts of your body.

➤ Know the chemo drugs you're taking and their possible side effects.

➤ Don't be afraid to question anything that is happening to you.

➤ Be patient and gentle with yourself. The emotional changes are just as dramatic and important as the physical changes.

➤ Others have walked this path before you and are more than happy to help. Please call and rely upon the medical professionals and the support groups to help get you through this trying time.

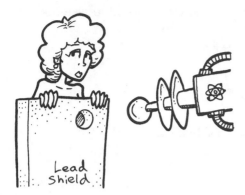

Lead shield

Chapter 11

Radiation Therapy: Getting Nuked

In This Chapter

➤ Radiation that helps, not harms

➤ Damaging and shrinking the tumors

➤ Understanding the process

➤ Feeling—and handling—the burn

In the past, the idea of radiation struck fear in the hearts of even the brave-hearted. Maybe we'd seen too many videos of atomic blasts and heard too much commentary on one of the resulting radiation. Is it any wonder we approach the recommendation for radiation therapy with concern? However, radiation has come a long way, baby. In the early years of radiation therapy, there were many unknowns, including what dosage, frequency, and direction were appropriate for each patient. Today, however, radiation is a proven, safe, and effective treatment helpful to many breast cancer survivors. In this chapter, we'll show you what you need to know if you face this treatment option.

Thirty Days Hath September

Nearly 50 percent of breast cancer patients undergo *radiation therapy,* and the number of those who achieve successful results through this treatment rises every day.

Radiation is usually used in conjunction with some other treatment, most commonly a lumpectomy and/or chemotherapy. Surgery removes the tumor; chemo tackles cancer cells that have traveled to other parts of the body. Chemo, however, is a systemic treatment and not the best ammunition at the tumor site. That's where radiation therapy comes in. It's the local treatment, the treatment at the cancer site.

Doctors use radiation in two instances: First, although it's unusual, they use it prior to surgery to help shrink the size of the tumor. Second, they most frequently use it following surgery, usually a lumpectomy, to "clean up the site" by killing or damaging any cancer cells that remain around the tumor. The reason is simple: Cancer cells that have been damaged do not grow, divide, or spread.

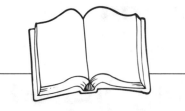

From the Book

Radiation therapy is the use of high-energy penetrating rays of subatomic particles to treat disease.

Treatment: Internal or External

With radiation therapy, timing for maximum benefit (killing the cancer) and minimum harm (keeping the patient healthy) is everything. The treatments must be scheduled on a daily basis for several (usually from two to five) weeks. Working this into your daily routine is often inconvenient; but because it's important, you'll find a way.

The first decision your radiation oncologist will make (in consultation with your medical oncologist) is how many and what dosage treatments you'll have. Fraction radiation therapy is the most common. It is administered daily in a five-day-on and two-day-off schedule by a machine called a linear accelerator. The doctor determines the amount of radiation that you should receive and divides it into a certain number of doses or fractions.

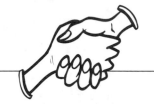

Helping Hand

Make sure you understand your radiation schedule. Although most radiation therapy is a daily occurrence for five to eight weeks, in special cases, radiation may be given twice a day for less than five weeks. This depends on you, your cancer, and your doctor's recommendations.

Near the end of your treatment, your doctor may decide to give what are commonly known as "boosts." Here's the difference: The regular radiation treatment covers a broader area and has deeper penetration than the boost. Because the boost, focused precisely on the surgical site, has a shorter penetration depth and a much-reduced coverage area, it helps destroy any remaining errant cancer cells and/or gives the rest of the radiation site some extra time to recover.

In a far, far less common approach, depending on your needs, your doctor may decide to use internal radiation, also known as brachytherapy. Brachytherapy involves the implantation of a radioactive material enclosed in a tube or capsule or bound by thin wires that the doctor puts in or close to the area needing treatment. Another type of internal radiation is given by injecting a radioactive solution into the bloodstream or ingested in a tablet form. Typically, your doctor will introduce internal radiation when you need a more intense or higher dosage in a shorter time frame than external radiation can provide.

The area surrounding the implant may be sore or sensitive. After all, you will have had at least two surgeries at the site. It is suggested that you get some extra sleep or rest, but then return to your normal activities as soon as you feel up to it.

Inquiring Minds

Yes, inquiring minds do want to know. And, you want to know why you are going through radiation therapy and what this means to you. Here are some questions you may want to ask your doctor, and you'll likely want to record the answers in your notebook:

1. What do you expect the radiation to do to my cancer?
2. Will I need treatment beyond radiation, and if so, what?
3. How will I likely feel while I'm getting radiation treatments?
4. Can I continue working?
5. What side effects will I likely experience and how long will they last?
6. What will happen if I decide against radiation?

The answers your doctor gives you should provide you with insight into what the radiation is going to do to and for you. It is important for you to know the answers to these questions so that you may decide if it is right for you. Keep these answers in your notebook, also.

If you decide to take radiation therapy, you're ready to work with your doctor to formulate a treatment plan. Let's take a look at how that planning usually occurs.

The Best-Laid Plans ...

The first day of treatment, you'll sign your informed consent papers, giving your permission to undergo radiation therapy and routine tests associated with it. In addition, the informed consent papers usually state that you have been informed of the benefits and risks of radiation therapy; so, please read them carefully and don't sign *anything* until you fully understand what it means.

Now, the planning can truly begin.

The doctor has a copy of your medical history and tests, and, additionally, he will do his own physical exam. Next, you begin your simulation. (And you probably thought that only astronauts went through high-tech simulation!) Simulation involves what looks like an x-ray machine, but this

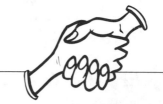

Helping Hand

Be prepared to relax! Creating your block is an hour-long process. To help pass the time, listen to music or talk with the medical personnel who are there to help you. If you feel chilly during the process (you'll be mostly naked!), feel free to ask the medical staff to raise the room temperature.

machine does not give off radiation. Its purpose is to allow the doctors and technicians to make exact measurements of your body in relationship to the available positions and motions of the real x-ray machine. You will usually lie on a table for about an hour, naked from the waist up with your arm above your head, so that the technicians can create your *alpha-cradle* and *block*.

There's one primary reason why you must take the time to undergo the simulation: You want the radiation to pinpoint only the immediate cancer site. To map your site, the technicians direct the machine over the entire chest area in order to make measurements that will avoid radiating your heart, lungs, or ribs. Your measurements are unique to you; hence the simulator.

From the Book

An **alpha-cradle** is a positioning device used to keep you in the correct position at all times while undergoing treatment. It is to provide accuracy for your treatment because the location and depth of your cancer site is different than almost everyone else's. Once you have been measured and tattooed while in the alpha-cradle, a block is made.

The **block** is the accurate measurements of your treatment area. Once this template is made, it is inserted into the x-ray machine (linear accelerator) each time you receive treatment so that only the affected area and not the vital organs are treated with radiation.

Lydia, the Tattooed Lady

Depending on your radiation oncologist's usual procedure, the next step may be the fulfillment of a secret desire: a tattoo! Unfortunately, your tattoo is not a lightning bolt or a rose or even a loved one's name. But it will be the most important set of dots you'll ever see. (Understand, however, that some radiation oncologists apply the tattoos only at the conclusion of your treatment and some may not use them at all.)

In order to get your set of tattooed dots (or marks, in the absence of tattoos), the technician locates the pinpointed lights beaming down from the block: wherever they hit your skin, you get a dot—tattooed or otherwise. Then, when you go in for your treatments, the technician can quickly line up the light from the block with the dots, virtually guaranteeing that you receive your radiation in just the right spot—every time!

During your office visit, your technician may use a dark marker to draw lines between the dots. The lines help him or her to align the block and x-ray. The lines are not permanent, and most technicians will ask you to use caution in order to avoid washing them off. Still, the marks will fade and/or rub off on your clothing (so old clothes are in order); and when they do, the technician will reapply them as necessary.

At the initial planning appointment, you and your doctor will set the time of each appointment. With rare exceptions, your appointment will be at the same time each day in a five-day-on and two-day-off schedule. The two days off, usually a weekend, allow the cells time to heal and regenerate. You'll also learn how many treatments you'll have, both full-blown and possible boosts. You are ready and set. Now, go!

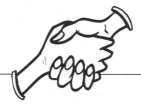

Helping Hand

Love your tattoos! The tattooed dots, called landmarks, can be removed with lasers after you have finished your radiation treatments. However, there is a word of caution here. Your radiation treatment is designed to give you the maximum dosage that is tolerable to your breast tissue. And, the dose remains there. Thus, tissue should not be radiated more than once. If, therefore, you require radiation later, either for a recurrence or new cancer, your doctor must know where you have been radiated before, either from your tattoos or from your medical records. Seen in that light, the tattoos are a lifetime safeguard.

A Day in the Life of ...

Do you know the saying, "you can't tell the players without a scorecard?" Here is a list—a medical scorecard, so to speak—of the staff members you will meet and interact with during your radiation treatments:

➤ **Dosimetrist.** One who calculates the number and length of your treatments

➤ **Radiation oncologist.** A doctor who specializes in using radiation to treat cancer

➤ **Radiation physicist.** A person who makes sure the linear accelerator is working properly

➤ **Radiation therapist.** A person who sets you up for treatment and runs the x-ray equipment

➤ **Radiation therapy nurse.** A person who provides care and helps you understand the treatments and side effects

➤ **Radiologist.** A person whose training is in reading and interpreting x-rays

Each person has a specific function, and each person will be more than willing to help you understand and cope with radiation therapy. Having your scorecard and knowing who to turn to for what information should be a source of comfort for you.

Beyond the cast of characters, you'll also have to learn the time frame. In addition to your travel time, plan for 30 to 45 minutes for the procedure. Also, think about what clothing you'll wear on treatment days. A two-piece outfit is best. You need to be naked from the waist up for your treatments, so wearing a two-piece outfit saves time and helps protect your modesty.

Every treatment day, you'll be escorted into a dressing room where you'll strip from the waist up, put on the hospital gown, and proceed into the treatment room.

Then, you'll take off the hospital gown and lie on the table. The radiation therapist will put you in the correct position. Generally, you'll place one arm above your head with a pillow under part of your back to elevate you to the correct position. Your special block will be inserted into the x-ray machine. The block and dots will be lined up, and you will be told to lie still, but you won't have to hold your breath. The therapist will go behind a radiation shield or step out of the room. From a panel and through a closed-circuit camera, the therapist is in contact with you and can operate the x-ray machine and monitor you throughout the brief treatment.

With you and the technologist in your respective places, you'll start to hear the x-ray machine making some strange noises that alternate between whirring and clicking, and the machine will move into the proper position for the treatment.

Usually in less than 10 minutes, you're done. The room is cool and dim. The procedure is totally painless. Take this "10" to heal and relax. Then you get dressed, and you're on your way. See you tomorrow. If, for any reason, you do experience pain or discomfort, tell the therapist or doctor immediately.

Once you have finished all of your treatments, you will need to have some type of follow-up to monitor your progress and to deal with any problem that may arise. The time and type of follow-up is something that you should discuss with your doctor. As with your treatment, your follow-up will vary from person to person. (See Chapter 14, "Again and Again: The Follow-Up," for more details.)

Helping Hand

If you have very large breasts, the breast may have to be netted to help keep it in place. Some women with extremely large breasts may have to use a special machine designed to handle tissue mass.

Cotton, Cornstarch, and Comfort

Because during radiation therapy your skin is subjected to direct rays from radiation, you need to be extra careful with it. There are some things to watch out for and some do's and don'ts to be aware of and practice.

Cotton, the Fabric of Your Life

Avoid tight, stiff, and starched clothing. It will irritate. Treatment will likely cause your skin to become red and maybe raw-feeling. Thus, any rough substance that comes in contact with it will irritate it. Even bras, because they are usually tight to help hold you in place, can be a problem. And, if you have large breasts and wear underwires, the wires can truly irritate your skin.

So what do survivors recommend? You may want to invest in all-cotton or cotton-blend sports bras. They are soft on your skin. They contain no wires, so they are not harsh or damaging, and they do hold you in place.

It is also a good idea to wear darker, heavier clothing. The dark lines the technologist applied can rub off on your clothing; or, if the blouse or top you wear is sheer, others can see the lines through your clothing.

Cornstarch for What Ails You

While going through radiation, avoid using deodorants. Most, if not all, deodorants contain some type of metal, usually aluminum. When radiation interacts with metals, it changes speed. If metal pieces are touching your skin during your radiation treatment, the potential is there for an unwarranted and unwanted skin reaction. Instead of deodorant, you might use cornstarch. Cornstarch holds the moisture and odor down. If you would like to use talcum or baby powder, please check the labels for metal ingredients and talk with your doctor.

You will also want to avoid fragrances and perfumes or products that contain them such as soaps, lotions, and cosmetics. These can also irritate the skin.

Tales from the Trenches

Marcia is part of the workout generation, so she's great friends with the StairMaster and treadmill. She kept up with a moderate exercise program while undergoing treatment. Because she perspired more than most while exercising, the cornstarch was not filling the bill. At a health food store, she found a natural deodorant that worked well for her.

The Big "C"—Comfort

Your number-one concern, right now, should be to baby your skin, especially in the treated area. Keep showers and baths a moderate temperature. Heat and cold can

133

cause discomfort to the treated area. After you shower, don't rub your skin; pat it dry. Do not use a straight razor, particularly under your arms. (Of course, if you've just come out of chemotherapy, hair under your arms may not be a problem. Chemo causes some folks to lose all body hair.) If you do have to shave, use an electric razor, but only after you have asked your physician if it is okay to do so. If it is not, you may, just for a while, have to adopt the European attitude about underarm hair and live with it.

From the Book

Acute refers to something that is short-term and occurs during the time of treatment. **Chronic** is considered long-term. They may take a long time to develop and can be permanent.

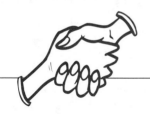

Helping Hand

Watch out for "dry mouth," a common side effect of radiation that causes a lack of saliva, that in turn can damage teeth and gums. Prescription medicines and over-the-counter fluoride rinses help. And since mint-flavored toothpaste can irritate, try using children's bubble gum–flavored toothpaste instead.

Try not to stick anything to the treated area, such as a bandage. Some types of adhesive tape are made of paper and they come off much easier than regular adhesive tape. Still, if you find it necessary to use a bandage, try putting the sticky part outside the treated area.

Protect the treated area from the sun. At this point, extra radiation, even from the sun, is not something you need. In fact, you'll need to protect the area from the sun for at least a year following treatment. Use a "sunblock" simply by staying out of the sun.

Possible Side Effects for a "Red Hot Mama"

With any treatment there are side effects. Naturally, radiation therapy is no exception! Because the side effects vary, you may have none at all or they may be very mild. All side effects fall into either the *acute* or *chronic* category.

The side effect survivors mention most often is fatigue. Yes, you're going to have to get yourself to the treatment center every day, and the journey itself may be tiresome. But you are also trying to heal yourself, and healing saps a great deal of energy from the body. Typically, your energy level will pick up after you have finished radiation. Pace yourself. Some people have no trouble; some stop working completely; some take a day off now and then. You do what you can and what works for you. Get as much rest as possible.

Another side effect is the change in skin tone. You already know that the treated area may be burned, sore, and dry. To help protect yourself, use very mild soap. Pat your skin dry. Your radiation oncologist and radiological nurse will keep a close eye on you and can prescribe or recommend special skin gels that help the skin heal. Radiation can also cause some hair loss, but usually only in or near the radiated area.

Your general health may be affected as well. For instance, if the white blood cell or platelet count is low as a result of the radiation, your doctor may decide to stop treatment for a brief time to give your reserves a chance to build back up. And if maintaining your general health requires your taking any additional medication, be sure to tell your doctor. You must make certain that one medication will not react negatively with another.

Your diet or food needs can also change. You may lose your appetite and begin to lose weight. While 99 percent of us want to lose weight, this is not a good time to do so. If you notice that you are losing your appetite, nibble, fix your very favorite foods, eat small meals and eat them often, or use a meal/vitamin/protein supplement (but only with your doctor's okay, of course).

Tales from the Trenches

I developed a radiation burn on my neck outside the designated treatment area. My doctor explained that as I raised my arm, a fold of skin developed around my collarbone at the base of my neck. Radiation gains speed when it hits the air as it did in the folded skin; and when it hit the skin a second time, it had speeded up and burned my skin. I changed to the boost to avoid the burn on my neck. It had time to heal and was fine in a couple of days.

Breast soreness is also an issue. Let's face it, your skin is getting burned. In the past, when you got a bad sunburn, you babied the burned area. You will have to do that now. You may want to sleep with extra pillows, on silk or satin fabrics, propped up in bed with an arm extended, or by yourself so that no one accidentally rolls into you. Do whatever it takes for your comfort.

Some side effects are signs of a severe problem. If you notice chronic pain, odd rashes, bruises or bleeding, lumps or swelling, unusual weight loss, persistent cough or fever, or vomiting, diarrhea or loss of appetite, please call your doctor immediately. In this case, safe is better than sorry.

Depression can be an aftereffect of radiation therapy. You are involved in the daily routine and counting down the days. You are active and occupied. When the radiation is complete, you come to a dead stop and don't know what to do next. Now's the time to focus inward on your own powers of healing.

Every person responds to radiation in his or her own way. You will, too. You'll probably want to discuss with the doc your own response and what it means in terms of participation in or return to sexual activity, sports, exercise, or work. If your radiation follows a mastectomy, the doc will also tell you when you can begin wearing a prosthesis or, if you chose to have delayed reconstructive surgery, when you can consider that option. (See also Chapters 21, "Back to the Bikini: Reconstruction," and 22, "Boob in a Box: Prostheses.")

The Least You Need to Know

➤ With rare exception, radiation therapy is a painless procedure.

➤ The planning stage is usually more complicated than the actual treatment.

➤ Be prepared for fatigue as the major side effect.

➤ Focus on pampering your skin during treatment.

➤ Arrange your schedule to make the daily radiation routine workable.

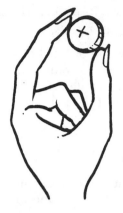

Chapter 12

Hormone Therapy: The Pill

In This Chapter

➤ Why, when, and how

➤ More side effects

➤ Benefits and side effects

➤ Real and chemical menopause

➤ Checking out your calcium levels

What's one thing that makes a woman a woman? Hormones, of course. As a matter of fact, they are so important to women that you get two for the price of one: estrogen and progesterone. But breast cancer treatment can play havoc with your hormones. As a result, you may well face at least one of three common situations:

First, if you were pre-menopausal at diagnosis and required chemotherapy, you may now find, as a result of the chemo, that you've been shoved unceremoniously into menopause and face all the side effects that go with it. Second, if you were already post-menopausal at diagnosis, you may have been taking hormone replacement therapy (HRT) to reduce the side effects of menopause, most notably hot flashes and bone deterioration. In virtually every case, a woman diagnosed with breast cancer must immediately cease HRT. That most likely means a return of the common symptoms. Third, after the completion of other breast cancer treatments, both local and systemic, you may find yourself taking a little pill called Tamoxifen. Referred to as "hormonal therapy," it is the most common follow-up treatment for hormone-receptor positive

(HR+) breast cancers. Because it is an anti-estrogen drug, it can cause hot flashes and, in rare cases, contribute to some more unusual side effects.

No matter which of these situations or combination of situations you face, your body will settle down after time. Meanwhile, though, you'll want to know how others have coped with the hormone havoc of breast cancer treatments. In this chapter, we will look at these hormone and hormonal treatments, their purposes, and their effects— good and bad.

Hormones: The Cycle of Life

Estrogen and *progesterone* are female sex hormones produced mainly by the ovaries. These two hormones are responsible for the development and maintenance of your sexual characteristics. The ovaries begin releasing these hormones when you're quite young; then, during your first menstrual period, you become more aware of your hormones because they may make your breasts feel sore or even lumpy.

While your body produces these hormones, you are fertile; that is, you can get pregnant. Evidence also suggests that estrogen may protect you against certain diseases, including heart disease and osteoporosis (bone loss), although research continues on that front. (Please refer to the last section of this chapter for more information.) When your body stops producing hormones, you go into *menopause*.

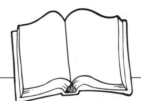

From the Book

Estrogen *is a female sex hormone produced mainly by the ovaries. It can also be produced by fat, the adrenal glands, and the placenta.* **Progesterone** *is another hormone produced by the ovaries and partly responsible for the menstrual cycle.* **Menopause** *occurs when the body stops producing these hormones (between ages 40 and 50), and you begin what is commonly known as "The Change." Once you have stopped having periods for a year, you have reached menopause.*

Menopause and the loss of these hormones have certain side effects, including some that are short-term (such as hot flashes, insomnia, and weight gain) and others that may be long-lasting (such as osteoporosis and heart disease). Because of your inability to produce these hormones as you age, many women begin taking medication known as hormone replacement therapy, or HRT.

Given all that background about how hormones have affected you your entire life, now there's yet another set of details about hormones as they relate to breast cancer treatment. For some women with hormone-receptor positive (HR+) breast cancer, hormonal therapy is the most common follow-up treatment. As of this writing, Tamoxifen is the most frequently prescribed. Although the common dosage is 20 mg a day every day for five years, your regimen many vary. Because hormonal therapy drugs like Tamoxifen are actually anti-estrogen drugs, they're quite different from hormone replacement therapy. These drugs, called SERMs (Selective Estrogen Receptor Modulators), help arrest the growth of those cancer cells that feed on estrogen. In this chapter, we will look at the benefits and side effects of the SERMs.

The Old "What For"?

To date, researchers aren't certain exactly what role hormones play in the development of breast cancer, but they do know it's a starring role. For most women, breast cancer is a disease affected by the circulation of female sex hormones. There are also hormone-related risk factors that further indicate that estrogen and progesterone may play roles in the development of cancer. Although you'll learn more about risk factors in Chapter 15, "Caution Flag: Risk Factors," we can tell you that the younger you are when you begin menstruating and the older you are when you enter menopause, the greater your chances of developing breast cancer. Menstruating for over 40 years, never being pregnant, and waiting until you are over 30 to have your first child puts you at higher risk. (As we'll discuss later, high-fat diets and high alcohol intake may also be risk factors.)

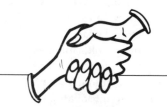

Helping Hand

Keep a detailed diary for your daughters and granddaughters that includes information about your condition but—even more important—about their own menstrual history, which could affect their risks of developing breast cancer later in life.

Needless to say, when fighting breast cancer or your risk for getting it, you're wise to reduce or eliminate as many risk factors as you possibly can. A few doctors have recommended hormonal therapy as a preventative for high-risk patients, but the treatment is unproven, and the jury's still out on that one.

Pill, Pills, and No Pills

Generally, women take hormones to lessen the discomfort of the side effects of menopause, including hot flashes and vaginal dryness. That's called hormone replacement therapy (HRT) because it's used to replace the hormones that the body, as a result of aging, has quit producing. In other words, HRT adds estrogen to the body.

Most women diagnosed with breast cancer can no longer take HRT. Instead, if their tumors are hormone receptive positive (HR+), they take hormonal therapy to keep the cancer from spreading, recurring, or taking their lives. These are anti-estrogen medications. Their purpose is not to add estrogen, but to remove estrogen from the body.

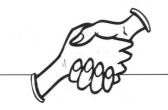

Helping Hand

Learn as much about the hormonal treatment as you can. Talk with your support groups. Ask who is taking what and what side effects they've experienced. Talk with medical professionals to see what they think. And carefully read the inserts that come from the manufacturer. You may think this is more information than you need, but, at this point in your life, the more information the better.

Research over the last 20 years (it usually takes 10 years to do a thorough study of a drug) has shown that Tamoxifen is very effective at helping alleviate breast cancer. If a tumor is HR+ (meaning that its growth is fed by hormones), then SERMs—those hormonal therapy drugs that adjust the reception of estrogen to the tumor—can block, starve, or neutralize the tumor. They can change the growth rate of the cancer cells as well.

Like chemotherapy, hormonal therapy is systemic, which means that the hormones must navigate throughout the body as well as to the site of the cancer. However, unlike chemotherapy, the side effects of hormonal therapy are relatively minimal, mainly because these "natural" substances lack the toxicity of chemo drugs. For instance, anti-estrogen drugs don't damage bone marrow, and thus don't affect your resistance to infection. Nor do they cause hair loss. However, hormonal therapy may increase your risk for uterine or colo-rectal cancer, so it is extremely important to do yearly physicals, be tested specifically for these two types of cancers, and report any abnormalities in these areas to your doctor immediately.

In Chapter 10, "Chemotherapy: Cruel to Be Kind," we referred to the drugs used as cytotoxic drugs, meaning that they kill cancer cells. In hormonal therapy, we refer to the drugs as cytostatic drugs, meaning to arrest cancer cells or hold them at bay. Although every case is different, most women who have had breast cancer require cytostatic hormonal therapy for about two to five years.

Today's Leaders

Currently, the only hormonal therapy drug commonly accepted to treat HR+ breast cancer is Tamoxifen (the generic name for Nolvadex). Basically, this drug is an estrogen blocker that is effective in fighting HR+ breast cancers, those that feed on and multiply in the presence of estrogen.

Since 1978, for post-menopausal women with HR+ breast cancer, Tamoxifen—either alone or combined with chemotherapy—has been approved for preventing tumor recurrence, additional tumors in the surrounding breast tissue, and contralateral breast cancer. Further, after a recent 20-year study, the FDA (Federal Drug Administration) has approved the use of Tamoxifen for reducing invasive breast cancer. It's become a household word among breast cancer survivors.

Raloxifene is a newer and in some ways similar drug. Currently, it has been approved by the FDA for the prevention of osteoporosis and is being studied as a second line of defense for reducing invasive breast cancer in HR+ women by working in ways similar to Tamoxifen. At this point, however, the jury's still out. (Currently, at least one major blind study is underway to compare the effectiveness of these two drugs.)

Take It from Us

Choose with care to become involved in a protocol study and be aware that there are certain criteria a person must fit to be part of a study. Before getting your hopes up about being part of any study, please call the organization sponsoring the study to see what the criteria are.

Two factors will determine whether you will or will not be asked to take hormonal therapy. First, when you had your surgery, your pathologist no doubt conducted a test to determine if your breast cancer tissue was HR+ or HR–. Only HR+ conditions are receptive to hormonal therapy. Second, you'll most likely need to be post-menopausal (although you may be post-menopausal only as a result of your chemo treatment). Statistically, post-menopausal women are more likely to be estrogen receptor positive than pre-menopausal women.

If you don't meet these two guidelines, you may or may not be a candidate for hormonal therapy. But there are other considerations as well. For instance, some women are actually allergic to hormonal therapy drugs and can't take them. If you are pregnant or nursing, you should not take them. Since blood clots in the legs or lungs are potential side effects of the SERMs, if you have a history of or a tendency toward blood clots or if you're taking blood thinners for the prevention of clots, you probably aren't a candidate for hormonal therapy, either. As always, talk with your medical team about every detail of your particular situation.

As you might expect, hormonal therapy drugs have their good effects and bad. The good we have discussed: For some women it's an award-winning cancer fighter. On the flip side, however, you must understand that many women commonly experience hot flashes, vaginal dryness, and, more rarely, vaginal discharge. And if for some reason you're taking hormonal therapy even though you aren't post-menopausal, you'll likely face irregular periods. While bothersome and anxiety-producing, these side effects aren't severe, especially taken in the light of the success of the drugs. On the other hand, some other side effects, while rare, can be more severe—including a higher risk of uterine cancer, blood clots, stroke, cataracts, and jaundice. For details about Tamoxifen studies, visit www.nolvadex.com.

Although there is some controversy about how long to take Tamoxifen, most medical folks as of this writing recommend taking it for five years. As research continues, the recommendations may change, so stay alert to current studies. And you'll also want to check out Chapter 14, "Again and Again: The Follow-Up," for suggestions for dealing with the long-term use of the drug.

Your personal reaction and interaction with hormonal therapy drugs is one of the main reasons for being diligent in your follow-up program.

Side Effects: What Can I Do?

When you undergo breast cancer treatments, you'll no doubt face one or more of a series of hormone upsets in your body. If variety is the spice of life, then side effects have to be the spice of hormonal therapy. And if there is one good thing that you can point out about these hormone upsets, it is that while they may be annoying, most of them are not debilitating.

Tales from the Trenches

Susan developed a red, itchy rash on her scalp while taking hormonal therapy treatments. Her allergist could find no cause, and she mentioned it in passing to her radiation oncologist. He said he had seen two other similar cases and took her off Tamoxifen. So, mention any questionable symptoms to each of your doctors. One of them may have an answer.

So let's take a look at some of the side effects and what you can do to help alleviate them. Keep in mind that you aren't likely to experience all of the side effects, and you may not experience any.

What's Typical … for Menopause

If you weren't post-menopausal before you were diagnosed with breast cancer, you may well be now—as the result of another of the not-so-wonderful side effects of chemotherapy. Or, if you were post-menopausal at the time of diagnosis but were taking HRT and have since stopped, you're probably facing some side effects similar to being newly menopausal. Or, finally, if you are now taking hormonal therapy, you may face some, but not all, of the same side effects. Let's sort them out.

You've probably heard about the common symptoms of menopause and some of them are also typical side effects of hormonal therapy:

➤ Hot flashes	➤ Heart disease
➤ Night sweats	➤ Loss of bladder control
➤ Fatigue	➤ Weight gain
➤ Headaches	➤ Loss of sexual drive
➤ Insomnia	➤ Vaginal dryness
➤ Depression	➤ Memory loss
➤ Osteoporosis	

Surely no one woman ever experiences all of these common symptoms of menopause; however, every woman experiences both natural and treatment-related menopause in her own way. Since you may be facing these side effects prematurely as a result of your cancer treatment, let's take a look now at the ones most likely to affect you, especially if you're taking hormonal therapy.

Hot Flashes

On a personal note, I think hot flashes are misnamed. To me, a flash is something that is momentary, like the blink of an eye or a camera snapshot. Hot flashes aren't momentary. You can feel your body temperature rising through your upper torso and then finally almost exploding out of the top of your head. Is this a "flash" to you?

Well, regardless of what you call them, many women experience them when they lose estrogen, either through natural menopause or through treatment. Some women have one hot flash a day and some women have four an hour. Worse, hot flashes wake you in the middle of the night, maybe several times a night, destroying much-needed and long-awaited sleep. You spend time throwing covers off and then pulling them back on, and some say that might make you irritable.

When it comes to reducing hot flashes, recent studies suggest that soy products help decrease the intensity of hot flashes. First let's look at why, and then we'll look at why not.

So first, why soy? Soy contains phytoestrogen, a weak form of estrogen found in estrogen receptor sites of a woman's body. Because hot flashes are related to a reduction of estrogen, many scientists believed that an extra dose of this plant estrogen would help lessen the intensity of hot flashes. Still, the studies aren't clear that soy can, indeed, reduce hot flashes. Having said all this, however, we need to add a warning: If your breast cancer is HR+, adding estrogen—even plant estrogen—may be a risk. It's another of those questions to which medical folks don't have the answer, so buyer beware.

Some survivors reported, in fact, that their oncologists told them to consume NO soy products in any form. As for other food-related matters connected with hot flashes, there's the issue of bioflavonoids. Foods containing bioflavonoids (a substance found in some plants useful in the maintenance of the walls of small blood vessels) such as broccoli, cabbage, and cauliflower seem to help lessen the intensity of hot flashes. In addition, some medical folks recommend taking a combination of vitamin B_6 and vitamin E (B_6 in the morning and E at night). Some folks find relief from additional vitamin C. Always check with your medical team, of course, before you take anything.

So what else can you do to find relief from hot flashes? Try dressing in cotton or natural fabrics, for they absorb perspiration. Dress in layers, keeping the bottom layer short-sleeved and of light fabric. For more suggestions, see Chapter 24, "Fashion Fling: New Clothing Priorities."

Vaginal Dryness/Itching

Typically, vaginal dryness is a part of menopause (as well as a side effect of hormonal therapy, but we'll get to that later). Most women can alleviate dryness by using creams, jellies, or suppositories specifically designed to help alleviate vaginal dryness on a temporary basis, usually for the purpose of sexual intercourse. For prolonged treatment of vaginal dryness, certain oral medications can be prescribed to work internally on vaginal tissue.

If you find that your vaginal area begins to itch, avoid perfumed soap, bubble bath, and perfumed toilet paper. Wear panties with cotton crotches and take warm, not hot, baths. If you want to use a douche product, be sure to check with your doctor about which would be the best to use.

Before you purchase any vaginal cream, lubricant, or douche, however, check the ingredients. Make sure they contain no estrogen, especially if your breast cancer is HR+. Your body can absorb estrogen through vaginal tissue. And if you can't understand all those long words on the ingredients label, ask your pharmacist to help.

From the Book

Quinine is a bitter, colorless crystalline alkaloid or powder made from South American tree bark initially used as a medicine to treat malaria.

Leg Cramps

Some days you'll think you've reverted to adolescence. You remember. You'd wake up at 2 A.M., screaming and cursing with those agonizing leg cramps. Well, they could be back.

One of the greatest remedies for leg cramps is so old it is as if it were out of the traveling medicine shows: *quinine* is usually a key ingredient in tonic water. In addition, make sure you're getting enough calcium in your diet (at least 1,500 mg a day by supplement if you're post-menopausal and taking hormonal therapy). And finally, make sure you get those eight glasses of water a day. One of the most common causes of leg cramps is insufficient water consumption.

Depression

To date, there has been no concrete proof that hormonal therapy causes depression, but this is a tough call. If you are dealing with depression, is it because of breast cancer, menopause, emotional situations with your family or co-workers, or hormonal therapy? It's probably impossible for you—or your doctor—to know for sure. You can, however, do some things to help relieve depression. Exercise helps release endorphins that boost your mood upward and helps aid in your getting a good night's sleep. Staying positive helps you focus on the good and your success. Relaxation and laughter with good friends or a good book can also help ease depression. Hobbies or other distractions keep your mind on the activity and not what "might" be happening to you.

However, if within two weeks or so your depression isn't relieved by some of the aforementioned activities, you may need help, perhaps in the form of antidepressant medication. At the very least, you need—and deserve—a proper diagnosis by a qualified professional. Tell him or her how you're feeling, emotionally and physically, and most likely you'll get some help to keep your depression at bay.

Odds and Ends

Other noted side effects of menopause, although not as common as the three aforementioned, are loss of bladder control, insomnia, weight loss, and night sweats. If any of these symptoms occur, don't spend time worrying about them. Adding more worry to what you already have is not a good idea. Consult your doctor. There are remedies. Monitoring fluids or taking a specific medicine may avert loss of bladder control. Insomnia can be more manageable with proper exercise, diet, or medication. Using a diet supplement can slow or reduce weight loss (but again, check with your doctor). And night sweats? They come and go, and with or without breast cancer, they seem to be a given of the aging process. Temperature control and layered clothing might make them more bearable.

Take It from Us

Don't worry alone! If you're like most survivors, every little ache and pain causes a scare. Is the cancer coming back? Is it advancing? Where has it spread now? With all you've been through, is it any wonder? Talk with someone—a doctor, a support group friend, or an expert from a national organization. Don't sit around and worry. That's the very last thing you need to be doing now!

145

Tales from the Trenches

"I can't stop gaining weight," cried Willie. She was following a new diet, walking her dogs two miles every day, and had a personal trainer, yet she still gained weight. She decided it must be the Tamoxifen. Even though she was not happy about the weight gain, when she compared adding 20 pounds to her weight or having a possible recurrence of breast cancer, she opted to buy larger-size clothes. A no-brainer for her.

The Serious Side of Side Effects

Although they are rare, some serious side effects can result from hormonal therapy. Indeed, they can be physically or emotionally distressing. They include …

➤ Shortness of breath.

➤ Blood clots.

➤ Inflammation in the throat.

➤ Painful joints and muscles.

➤ Stomach upset.

➤ Infections.

➤ Sinus trouble.

➤ Rashes.

➤ Changes in eyesight.

Remember these side effects are highly unusual, but it's better to be aware of the possibility rather than to let something serious slide by. If you have a serious reaction, the doc may take you off the hormonal therapy for a month or so, see what happens, put you back on, and see what happens again. This typical procedure helps you and the doc understand the relationship—or lack of it—between the hormonal therapy and your symptoms.

NOT!

You feel better when you know why you feel as you do. Yes, nausea could be a side effect of hormonal therapy, but you could also have the flu. Muscle aches could be a side effect, but perhaps you also started a new exercise program. Weight gain could be a side effect, or, as a result of recent stress, you could just have thrown your diet out the window and reached for "comfort" foods like cake, pudding, and pie.

Understand that all the changes you're going through may not be the result of breast cancer, hormonal therapy, or menopause. Something completely unrelated may be causing the problem. So before you panic or place blame, think of what may be happening in your life that could cause any of the changes you are experiencing. However, of course, "when in doubt, seek your doctor out!"

Dem Bones, Dem Bones: DEXA Scans

Because osteoporosis is a serious side effect of estrogen loss, checking your bone density should be on your list of "must do's." Osteoporosis is the gradual loss of bone density (softening as the result of a loss of calcium in the bones) as you age. Hormone replacement therapy, usually in the form of an oral medication, is a common recommendation for women wanting to avoid or delay this process; however, for breast cancer survivors with HR+ tissue, hormone replacement therapy is not an option. (Fortunately, however, Tamoxifen seems to help overcome the problem as well.) Nevertheless, you can do certain things to decrease your risk of osteoporosis, among them regular exercise (at least 30 minutes daily of weight-bearing activity, like walking or jogging, but not swimming) and taking calcium supplements (1,500 mg a day) along with vitamin D for absorption. In addition, some studies suggest that avoiding phosphates and cigarettes (probably including secondhand smoke) will certainly fall into the plus column.

Osteoporosis is evident in brittle bones and stooped posture—the so-called dowager's hump. Obviously, you'll want to eliminate or delay osteoporosis as long as possible. Because osteoporosis is associated with the reduced production of hormones, once you have been diagnosed with breast cancer and must deal with the loss of estrogen, your doctor will probably prescribe a bone density test called a *DEXA Scan,* a test designed to measure the calcium level in your bones. The part of the body they are checking is referred to as the "L-spine," which means "lumbar vertebrae." However,

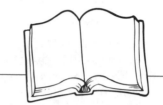

From the Book

A **DEXA (Dual Energy X-ray Absorptionometry) Scan** is a test designed to measure the calcium level in the bones.

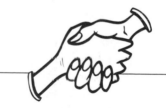

Helping Hand

Rest easy! Of all the tests you have taken, this is probably the simplest. You simply lie on a table that has an x-ray device built into the table underneath you. You lie still, and the x-ray moves. Compared to the rigors of all the surgeries, injections, and side effects you have gone through, on this test, just lie back and relax.

147

if there is any part of your scan that is in question, the hip and wrist will also be scanned. Your doctor, or referring physician, will determine what bones he wants scanned.

Here's the background: To determine the "normal" level of calcium in the bones, researchers scanned a cross section of women of different age groups (40s and 50s) and measured the calcium level, or bone density. The researchers found that as women age, they suffer from bone loss. The amount of calcium in the bones decreases, and when that occurs the bones become soft and can break easily. Thus, osteoporosis.

So what does this mean to you? If your calcium level is below the norm, depending on the kind of breast cancer you have, you may be put on a drug to prevent further calcium loss and the onset of osteoporosis. Because there are also medications available to aid bone density, the test can provide a warning to the doc to consider prescribing such a medicine. (For more information, see Chapter 14.)

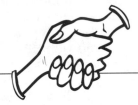

Helping Hand

Learn about your risk factors for osteoporosis as soon as you can, and help other family members understand their risks as well. Although until recently no one imagined it possible, your daughters can start to reduce their risks for osteoporosis in their 20s. So if you have daughters, sit down with them and tell them about the family history of osteoporosis and encourage them to exercise, eat right, and take vitamins. Forewarned is forearmed.

We now know more about calcium loss than we have ever known before, including some preventive measures every woman should take, preferably starting in their 20s. These steps include making sure you have a good supply of calcium in your diet, incorporating weight-bearing exercises into a fitness routine, and getting the daily recommended levels of vitamin D in your diet.

Our knowledge about hormones—both hormone replacement therapy and hormonal therapy for treating breast cancer—increases every day. Be part of it! Learn, be aware, help others, and pass it on. You'll help protect yourself, your daughters, and your granddaughters.

The Least You Need to Know

➤ As all women age, their estrogen and progesterone levels naturally decline.

➤ If you are not at high risk for breast cancer, you can take hormone replacement therapy (HRT) for three purposes: to help prevent heart disease and osteoporosis and to reduce the side effects of menopause.

➤ HRT should not be confused with hormonal therapy like Tamoxifen, an anti-estrogen drug used to ward off the recurrence of breast cancer in women with hormone-receptor positive (HR+) lesions.

➤ Hormonal therapy comes in the form of a pill taken once or twice a day for two to five years.

➤ Yes, there are side effects with hormonal therapy, but they are far milder than those of other therapies, and the benefits outweigh the side effects.

Part 3

After Shock: Dealing with the Tremors

The big shock waves are over. You've had your surgery—or even multiple surgeries. You've had the chemo and/or the radiation therapy. You may be on a five-year plan for hormone therapy. You may think you're home free.

Well, not quite. Unfortunately, the tremors from the big shock will follow you the rest of your life. Breast cancer is never in the past tense. As a chronic disease, it can—and does—recur. So how do you protect yourself physically? How do you deal with the emotional impact?

This part of the book shows you step by step how to take care of yourself by protecting yourself against lymphedema, by keeping regular follow-up appointments, by identifying your cancer risk factors, and by dealing with the emotional shake-ups from this series of tremors.

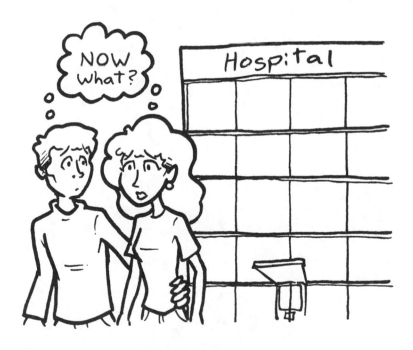

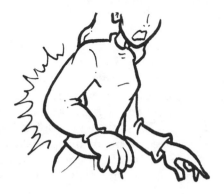

The Big Arm: Lymphedema

Walking behind her self-propelled lawn mower, about half finished with her task, Estelle felt the first signs of swelling on her left hand, from her knuckles to her wrist. When she finished mowing about a half-hour later, the tightness was creeping up her arm—the beginning of lymphedema, a condition resulting from her lymph node removal and a condition for which there is no cure. As she explained, "The lymphedema has altered my lifestyle far more dramatically than losing both breasts to cancer." Of course, unlike breast cancer, lymphedema doesn't threaten your life; and while it's manageable, it's certainly annoying and sometimes downright uncomfortable. The number of lymphedema cases among breast cancer survivors is hard to pin down simply because the problem can flare up months or many years after lymph node removal or radiation therapy. Certain preventative measures seem to help; but medical folks can't explain why 15 to 40 percent of survivors eventually face lymphedema but 60 to 85 percent do not. Some women claim the condition pops up even when they've taken extreme care and can point to no contributing factor. On the other hand, most folks who find themselves with a big arm can, in hindsight, say, "Yes, it was the push-pull of using the lawn mower for a couple of hours, getting really hot, and doing too much at one time."

In this chapter, we'll describe what lymphedema is, how you can best try to prevent it, what symptoms suggest a red flag, and, facing the condition, what treatments can help you manage it.

The Why in the Road

When it comes to lymphedema, there is bad news and good news. The bad news is that it can decrease your ability to move freely and do some of the things you've always done. And it's incurable. The good news is that if you learn what it's all about and take care, you can most likely avoid developing it. In short, you shouldn't have to give up everything you love doing for fear of getting lymphedema, so make decisions based on how much risk you're taking to gain the benefit you want. And if you do find yourself face to face with the condition, you can learn how to keep it under control. So let's get down to the nitty-gritty.

Lymph fluid is a clear, sticky fluid with the consistency of olive oil that floods the body, filling the spaces between the skin and everything else like water in a sponge. Remember scraping your knee just enough that it oozes but doesn't bleed? That oozing stuff is lymph fluid. It's not confined to vessels like blood is; nor is it pumped like blood pumped by the heart. As it flows through the body, it collects waste and works as a body-wide garbage disposal.

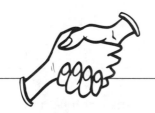

Helping Hand

Know your terms! Lymphedema isn't water retention, the condition that aggravates hypertension (high blood pressure). So don't confuse the swelling of lymphedema with the swelling from too much salt or too little activity. (Thus, so-called water pills won't help.) Rather, lymph fluid is a thick protein-rich fluid that gathers the body's garbage.

Lymph nodes are scattered throughout the body and serve as filters for the lymph fluid, filtering out bad stuff, including bacteria and viruses. The more active you are and the more you exert your arm, the greater the flow of lymph fluid into and out of your arm. Your body is running full blast. But the lymph fluid can't move through restricted (or missing) nodes, and so it accumulates and causes swelling—the big arm. But it's more than just swelling that's a problem. The impaired *lymphatic system* brings with it an increased risk of infections and slower healing of any injuries to that arm.

So where does all this fit in with the scheme of things in your life? First, the general picture: If your surgeon removed lymph nodes from under your arm when you had breast surgery, you lost part of your filtering system. Ditto if radiation therapy left scarring in the lymph node area. Your filtering system has been removed or disrupted. With the filtering system limping along, you're susceptible to lymphedema.

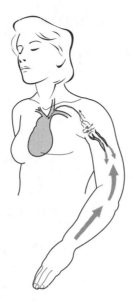

Removal of lymph nodes as well as scar tissue from radiation therapy can block lymph fluid flow from arm to heart.

Next, the specific picture. *Secondary lymphedema* (as opposed to *primary lymphedema,* which occurs from unknown causes) can develop after you've had surgery, radiation, infection, or trauma. Read between the lines here: We're not saying you'll necessarily get secondary lymphedema, because roughly 75 percent of breast cancer survivors never face the condition. For those survivors who do get it, however, surgery and radiation are the two major culprits, with infection or trauma as secondary causes.

And there's more. If the surgeon removed only your sentinal nodes, you have less risk of developing lymphedema than if he or she removed numerous nodes. But the risk remains. Generally, the greater the number of nodes removed, the greater your risk for developing lymphedema. And remember, it's the removal that counts, not whether the nodes were positive or negative.

Even if the surgeon didn't have to remove any nodes, you're still at risk for lymphedema if you had radiation therapy to the axillary node area. Radiation causes scar tissue to form around the lymph nodes, thus restricting the flow of lymphatic fluid. So if you've had both node removal and radiation, you have a double whammy. And if you get any kind of infection or trauma to the arm, the risk goes up even more.

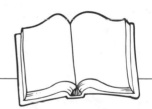

From the Book

Primary lymphedema results from unknown causes and can be present from birth. **Secondary lymphedema** is acquired as the result of surgery, radiation, infection, or trauma.

Okay, so that's who's at risk. But if you're at risk, when should you anticipate developing the condition? Unfortunately, there's no way to know. Lymphedema crops up in some folks within a month or so of surgery. Some get along just fine for 20 years or more and then suddenly wake up swollen. Some folks have only a mild condition that flares up and then recedes; others face more discomfort and require ongoing therapy. And, of course, lots of survivors never get it at all. Medical folks refer to the levels of severity by stages:

> ➤ **Stage 1: The "pitting" stage.** When you press your fingers into the flesh, you leave an indentation that stays there for several seconds. Usually at this stage, with therapy, the swelling is reversible.

> ➤ **Stage 2: The "spongy" stage.** When you press your fingers into the flesh, it bounces back and has a spongy feeling. At this point, the arm begins to "harden" and get noticeably larger.

> ➤ **Stage 3: The "hard" stage.** By now the swelling is irreversible, the arm is quite hard and quite large.

Take It from Us

Know your blood pressure history and fluid retention tendencies. While we've established that lymphedema is not the same as the fluid retention that aggravates high blood pressure, most experts believe that there is a connection. If you come into breast surgery with a tendency to retain fluids (your hands and feet swell regularly), you already have what's called a compromised circulation system. Thus, you're probably at a greater risk for lymphedema.

While all this may sound miserably uncomfortable, know that you can work diligently to try to avoid it. While medical folks really don't understand why some folks get lymphedema and others don't, they do agree that certain types of behavior seem to aggravate the condition. So, while there are no guarantees, following the guidelines does matter.

An Ounce of Prevention

Prevention begins even before surgery, first by your becoming well informed about lymphedema and what triggers it. Second, prior to surgery, you should measure both of your arms. Then you'll have a base for comparison if you suspect you're facing initial symptoms. However, if you didn't know about lymphedema before surgery and didn't measure your arms, don't despair. Just take that measurement as soon as you can.

After surgery, if other options are available, you'll want to follow some medical advice:

1. Never allow anyone to take your blood pressure in the affected arm.
2. Never allow anyone to draw blood from the affected arm.

3. Never allow anyone to put an intravenous line (IV) into that arm.

4. Never allow anyone to give you a shot in that arm.

It's up to you to make sure these things don't happen. Unfortunately, well-meaning nurses, therapists, and doctors may not know your complete medical history. You do. Speak up. And if you're worried about someone violating one of the medical no-no's while you sleep, consider these options: If you're hospitalized, tape a sign to the head of your bed that reads "No blood pressure, no needles in right/left arm." Better yet, for everyday protection, get a bracelet from the National Lymphedema Network with the same warning. For details, call 1-800-541-3259 or check www.lymphnet.org.

But what do you do if you've had bilateral mastectomies and lymph nodes removed from under both arms? You'll need to discuss your specific situation with the doc. Medical folks can give shots in your leg and draw blood from your foot. They can also take blood pressure in your leg, but it's sometimes difficult to get a good reading. So consider your options and make a decision. Maybe you'll choose one arm over the other because you've had fewer lymph nodes removed on that side. Or maybe you'll choose one over the other because you are right-handed.

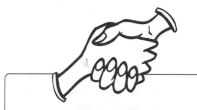

Helping Hand

Take care of yourself and you can reduce your risks of developing this unpleasant condition. We really don't know why some folks get lymphedema and others don't. Some survivors seem to have a predisposition for it. We have learned, however, that many women haven't been told that they must exercise special care with the affected arm. That lack of knowledge is probably the biggest contributing factor.

In addition to the medical alerts, following some other guidelines will help you protect yourself. (And if you're already dealing with lymphedema, these guidelines will help you control it.) Might as well get comfortable; it's a *loooooong* list.

➤ If you see any sign of swelling in your hand or arm or even your chest wall, or if you feel pain or discomfort in your arm, call your doctor. Now.

➤ Avoid wearing anything tight on that arm. No tight clothing, like tight sleeves, cuffs, sleeve bands, or anything with elastic. Avoid pushing those long sleeves halfway up to your elbows; that makes them tight. Likewise, no tight jewelry, like rings or expansion watchbands or bracelets. Wear them, but keep them loose.

➤ While exercise is beneficial, avoid strenuous and/or repetitious movement like rubbing, scrubbing, pushing, or pulling. So if you insist on washing windows, do only one or two windows a day. Skip lawn mowing all together—it's constant push-pull, even with a self-propelled mower and, yes, even with a riding mower.

Tales from the Trenches

Rachael faces regular bouts with lymphedema and admits that when she plays outdoor tennis in the summer, she can count on a flare-up. "It's the heat, plain and simple. All my life I've had some swelling in the summer—tight rings, that sort of thing. Now it's much worse." But she loves tennis. "You can't give up life, and that's a trade-off I'm willing to make."

After all, you don't steer the rascal with your fingertips! Likewise, depending on how much driving you do and if you can afford to, trade in any vehicle that doesn't have fingertip steering. And skip the stick shift.

➤ Skip hot: That means very hot water, as in washing you or anything else, including the dishes. Likewise, skip the hot tub and sauna. Avoid being out on hot summer days; getting overheated begs for trouble. And be careful with the sunbathing; you don't want a burn.

➤ Don't lift more than 15 pounds. *Ever.*

➤ Don't hurt the affected arm. No nicks, sticks, cuts, scratches, bites, burns, or hits or bruises. So skip cutting your cuticles. Watch out for paper cuts. Wear gloves and long sleeves when gardening to avoid pokes and scratches. Likewise for housework. Protect your arm from insect bites. Keep the hand and arm protected from the sun with fabric or strong sunscreen. And skip the bruising sports.

➤ Skip using a safety razor under the affected arm. Instead, go to an electric razor. Or consider having your underarms waxed (using warm wax, not hot). That will temporarily remove unwanted hair without nicking your skin and also will slow the growth of new hair.

➤ Keep on hand (and with you when you're away from home) antiseptic soap and antiseptic ointment such as Neosporin or Bacitracin. In the case of a scratch or bite, clean it immediately and keep it clean. It's okay to be obsessive about it.

➤ Keep the affected arm scrupulously clean. Pat dry; don't rub.

➤ Avoid anything heavy hanging from your shoulder. No heavy shoulder bag. No heavy prostheses (a significant issue if you're large-breasted). No tight bra straps.

➤ Wear properly fitting bras. No underwires. Not too tight. Add pads under narrow shoulder straps.

➤ Exercise is important, especially any that increases flexibility. Gentle stretching (but without lots of resistance and no weight lifting). Walking. Swimming (unless you insist on a fast crawl). Light aerobics. Biking (the easy kind). Whatever improves circulation. (Even erect posture and really deep breathing that squeezes the lymph nodes improves circulation.) However, the minute you feel the slightest ache in your arm, *stop*. Lie down and elevate it.

Tales from the Trenches

Marty told us that she mistakenly allowed her blood pressure to be taken in her affected arm. That same day she strained her thumb, carried in her groceries, and started wearing a heavy prosthesis. She woke up the next morning with lymphedema. A grandmother panicked when her grandchild ran into the street. She yanked him back and spanked him. That evening she had lymphedema. Another woman washed lots of windows during spring housecleaning. Bingo. Lymphedema. Another had a spider bite. Ditto.

On the other hand, Sue had a bad burn but kept it really clean and treated with antiseptic ointment. She had no aftereffects.

➤ Avoid anything that pounds your arm with constant jarring or vibration, like an intensive volleyball, tennis, or racketball game; a rototiller, chainsaw, or snow blower; a heavy-duty carpet cleaner, or a lawn mower—even the riding ones.

➤ Follow good health habits. Eat a high-fiber diet with adequate, easily digested protein, such as chicken, fish, or tofu. Skip smoking; avoid alcohol.

Okay, so we've given you such a *looooooong* list. But remember that you can't just sit on the couch and suck your thumb. Life goes on and you can't let the fear of lymphedema control your life. Armed with this information, you'll make decisions. If you love golf but playing in the heat is too much of a risk, hit the indoor air-conditioned courts. As one woman said, "I'd rather risk lymphedema than not have a life." In short, you'll make those risk-benefit decisions that parallel your personal priorities.

A special warning: In addition to the typical problems of lymphedema, watch for a significant rash or redness on your arm, perhaps accompanied by fever. If it happens, call the doctor immediately— or go to the emergency room. Any inflammation

Take It from Us

If you suffer from any itching, redness, or feverish sensations in your arm, go to a doctor immediately. Folks suffering from lymphedema are particularly susceptible to a condition called cellulitis, an inflammation of the connective tissue. If you have impaired lymph flow (from surgery or radiation therapy), your body can't effectively fight the infection, so it's serious business. Left unattended, it can be fatal.

159

or infection like this can signal a potentially dangerous condition. Ten minutes can make a dramatic difference. And without being an alarmist, I must tell you that infection in the affected arm, left untreated, can be fatal. Don't mess around. When in doubt, go.

Finally, if you travel, you'll want to consider some other pointers. First, ask your doctor for oral antibiotics to have with you in case of infection. If you're traveling by air, especially on a long flight, consider skipping the airline food and taking your own low-salt snacks, always drink lots of water, stand up and move around every hour or so during the flight, and consider wearing a compression garment (more on this later).

Diagnosis: And the Answer Is ...

The first symptoms of lymphedema are usually nothing more than a slight swelling in the fingers and/or hand. Your rings feel tight. Then maybe you'll notice your sleeve feels a little tighter than usual, at least tighter than the other one. As it worsens, most folks talk about a feeling of fullness, the same as you have from any swelling. The more the swelling, of course, the more uncomfortable it is, the more restricted your movement, and, according to some folks, the more painful. Of course, these symptoms all depend on whether you're coping with Stage 1 or Stage 3 lymphedema.

This woman's right arm (on your left) shows the swelling of lymphedema.

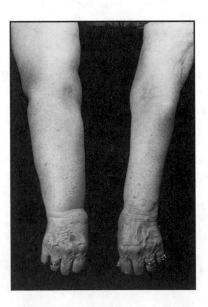

In its early stages, when lymphedema is more easily controlled, friends and family may not even notice the slight swelling. As the condition worsens, however, it will become fairly apparent, even though you may wear long sleeves to help conceal the hand-to-shoulder swelling. Ultimately, the affected arm can be significantly larger than the other. (See accompanying photograph.)

A Pound of Cure

Nobody should ever try to treat lymphedema herself. If any symptoms show up, see the doc immediately. And how do you find someone who treats lymphedema? First call your local health provider and ask, "Do you treat lymphedema? How do you treat it? Have you had special training, like continuing education courses, to prepare you to treat lymphedema?"

At present, we know of no state that offers special certification for treating lymphedema, so questioning is your only strategy for finding the right medical help. Even more unsettling is the fact that treatment for lymphedema has not been standardized. The National Lymphedema Network hopes that there will soon be some form of board certification to identify properly trained practitioners. Such a board would also help get insurance companies better aligned to pay for necessary treatments.

What kinds of treatment can you expect? If you have an infection, you'll get antibiotics, sometimes by IV if the problem is serious enough or aggressive enough. If, on the other hand, there is no infection but rather only swelling, you can expect a combination of treatments including all or some of the following: manual lymphatic drainage, bandaging, attention to skin care and diet, a compression sleeve, and remedial exercises. Here's what these typical treatments are all about.

Manual Lymphatic Drainage

In simple terms, the manual lymphatic drainage is a massage, but it takes special training on the part of a therapist to master the technique. It's unlike deep muscle massages you may have had in the past. Rather, this is a gentle pumping motion. In general, the massage helps decongest the tissue and get the lymph flow to move along alternate paths, thus reducing swelling. It's not magic: The swelling may go down, but it won't likely stay down forever. More important, however, the massage offers relief and aids in keeping the problem manageable. Be aware that most insurance companies pay for manual lymphatic drainage, but some don't. Check in advance.

Compression Bandaging

Compression bandaging, done properly, is quite helpful. It's a two-part process. There's a first layer of the bandaging that is a tight wrapping of cheesecloth-like gauze, beginning at your knuckles and winding up to your mid-arm or even to your shoulder. On top of the gauze is an Ace-like wrapping. You'll wear this combination bandage at night and any time you exercise. That means you'll have to learn to put the wrappings on yourself (or you'll have to have someone you live with devoted to your care). And in case you have any loving activities planned for bedtime, plan ahead. Once you're wrapped, you won't feel too frisky.

Compression Sleeve

If your condition warrants, you may be fitted with a compression sleeve. That eliminates the necessity for wrapping, but you'll wear it 24/7. (Well, of course, you can
take it off when you shower, or feel frisky, or go out to dinner in that gorgeous cocktail gown.) The sleeves come in many sizes, and you can even have one custom made
just for you. If you find you need a custom-made garment, make sure the fitter is certified and that you're being fitted when your swelling is down. Then you'll likely
have to wait a couple of weeks for its delivery. (And if it's custom-made and includes
compression chambers, it's pricey, probably in the neighborhood of $2,000 or
more, compared to $200 for the off-the-shelf models. As of this writing, many insur-
ance companies, including Medicare, will not pay, but check to make sure.)

Tales from the Trenches

As registered occupational therapist Trish Holcomb explains, "There is no cure for lymphedema. For breast cancer survivors who have lymphedema, it's a chronic condition that
can flare up and settle down. The bottom line is that survivors have to learn how to manage it. They'll learn that they can take the compression sleeve off to shower and go out
to dinner. But if they come home tired, go to bed, and then dash out first thing in the
morning to run errands—all without putting the sleeve back on—then the arm will begin
to swell again. Quickly."

The sleeves come in multiple flesh-colored tones, in a full-sleeve design or sleeve with
a separate glove, and come in a variety of fabrics, including cotton and poly blends,
all of which have elastic properties. But be prepared. In order to keep your lymphedema under control, you'll probably wear the compression sleeve the rest of your
life. Thus, you'll have to have regular replacements since they stretch and lose their
effectiveness after about six months. (And you'll need one to wear while you launder
the other.) Because it functions to help move the lymph fluid from your arm, however, it's an effective control for the condition.

Complex Decongestive Therapy

Complex decongestive therapy, or *CDT,* is the combined use of lymphatic drainage
and compression garments. Be aware that some insurance companies and HMOs are

beginning to pay for these treatments, but you'll need to be diagnosed and referred for treatment by a physician in order to qualify.

Also be aware that CDT may not be for everyone. For example, some lymphedema specialists take a dim view of the treatment for anyone with recurrent or metastatic cancer. They fear that the therapy may force the spread of the cancer. No scientific studies verify their fears either way, so be sure to talk with your medical team if you fit the description. (And if you suffer from congestive heart failure or a history of vascular disease, you may have further complications. Discuss these conditions with the doc.)

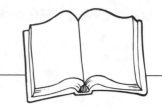

From the Book

Complex decongestive therapy (CDT) is a combination treatment consisting of manual lymphatic drainage and the use of compression garments, along with exercises and nutritional guidelines.

Proper Care and Diet

Proper skin care and diet remain important in the care of lymphedema. You'll have to keep the arm clean and moisturized by using a low-pH lotion to keep down bacteria growth under the wraps or compression sleeve. Remember that this arm is more susceptible to infection now, so you will likely become obsessive about cleanliness. In addition, skip the kinds of foods that might antagonize the condition, especially salt and high-fat, hard-to-digest proteins.

Finally, your therapist may prescribe a series of exercises, such as stretching and deep breathing, to improve your range of motion and to improve circulation. These exercises will help reduce the lymph fluid and make you more comfortable.

Tales from the Trenches

While your doctor and/or therapist are the experts in your treatment, there are some things you can do to make yourself feel better. None of these strategies has any proven benefit, but survivors who deal daily with lymphedema believe that these strategies help. First, most of them suggest that you try elevating your arm whenever you can; this seems to relieve the pressure a bit. Most folks recognized that it helps to cut out or at least cut way down on the salt. Reducing fluid retention gives the lymph fluids more room. And a few folks noticed that eating too much sugar worsened their condition.

Some Final Words

If, in the midst of your treatment for lymphedema, you notice a sudden significant increase in swelling, call your doctor immediately. It's possible that a recurrent cancer growth is further blocking the lymphatic flow. Always be alert to the possibility.

While all this may sound a little bleak, let's go back to where we began. The bad news—lymphedema can't be cured. But the good news is really good. You can do a great deal to prevent its occurrence. And if, in spite of your care, you find yourself with lymphedema anyhow, you can control it. You can go on with your life, pay your taxes, and hug those grandchildren. Just don't spank them.

The Least You Need to Know

➤ Lymphedema is an incurable condition brought on by either the removal of lymph nodes or radiation therapy to the node area.

➤ It can occur shortly after surgery or 20 years or more afterward.

➤ By minding certain cautions, you can most likely prevent the condition from haunting you.

➤ If you do find yourself with lymphedema, certain treatments can help alleviate and stabilize the condition.

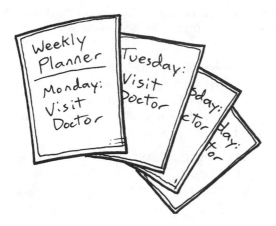

Chapter 14

Again and Again: The Follow-Up

In This Chapter

➤ Necessity of ongoing medical attention

➤ Kinds of exams and tests

➤ Importance of a plan

➤ Help for the tough days

There are two stories I've heard over and over again, and they both still make me cringe. The first story: "I've had breast cancer; I've had a mastectomy (or lumpectomy); I've had the treatment; it's over. There's no reason to have a mammogram now." This is a common misconception. Breast cancer can appear in remaining tissue, even if you've had a bilateral mastectomy. Sure, it's uncommon, but still possible. And possibilities cannot be ignored. The good news is that with each passing day, the breast that has been treated and had no recurrence has less and less chance of having a recurrence. But we can't ignore the rest of the story: Once you've had breast cancer in one breast, you're at an increased risk for developing breast cancer in the other breast. Or, to put it another way, once you've had breast cancer, your risk for getting breast cancer again is greater than the risk other women the same age face for getting breast cancer a first time. Among women who have had breast cancer, 1 in 100 will develop a new cancer in the other breast within a year.

The second story: "I'm past the five-year mark. I'm safe now; there's no need to worry." Also a common misconception. There is no five-year milestone with breast cancer. In fact, the older we get, the more likely we'll face either a recurrence or a new breast cancer. Breast cancers are often so slow growing that they can recur 20 years later. In short, breast cancer is never past tense. In fact, some medical folks are now suggesting it's wise to think of breast cancer as a chronic disease—one you'll live with all your life.

Of course, we all hope breast cancer never throws us into the line of battle again, but just like NATO members, we need to keep an active watch. No time now—now that you've fought and won the really big battles—to let down your guard and have the big bad guy slip back in during the dark of night. The solution: We keep a faithful watch ourselves, and we have professionals help us keep watch.

In this chapter, we'll tell you what and how to watch in the next several years and what to expect beyond that. We'll describe the kind of follow-up medical exams and tests you will most likely have. And we'll recommend a plan for your personal defense.

Parole Officer: Doctor's Visits

Surgery is over and the incision(s) have healed. You've had your umpteen rounds of chemo and/or radiation. The calendar has turned over lots of new pages, maybe 12 or more. Now, bingo! You've been turned loose. What happens next?

First and foremost, you'll continue to have follow-up medical appointments— probably lots of them. While every doctor handles cases somewhat differently and while every case is different, we can speak in generalities. So, in general, you'll most likely have a follow-up appointment every three to four months for the next year or so; then you'll go every six months for another year or so. After about five years, you'll be back to the typical routine: an annual clinical breast exam and mammogram. Most likely, you'll see only one doctor, perhaps your OB-GYN, your oncologist, or your family doctor—and it should be the doctor of your choice. If you had surgery and/or treatment at a breast center, you'll probably have your follow-up appointments there.

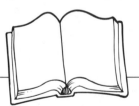

From the Book

Your **white blood-cell count** indicates how well your body is returning to normal. During chemo, the count drops dramatically; afterward it should return to normal levels, thus indicating your body can resume fighting most infections.

What happens during these frequent but routine follow-ups? You'll have a clinical breast exam and, if you've not had a mastectomy, a mammogram (probably every six months for a while). You'll likely have blood tests to check your *white blood-cell count* for signs of infection and blood cell production. And the doc will examine your breasts—or what's left of them—looking and feeling for new lumps, redness, and/or swelling. Finally, you'll probably be questioned about any other problems, especially if you're taking long-term medications, like Tamoxifen, or if you've had lasting side effects from chemo, like numbness in your hands or feet or irregularities in your heart.

To help you give your doctor an accurate report, you may want to keep a calendar of events. An ordinary wall or pocket calendar works just fine. There you can record joint or bone pain, headaches, tingling, numbness, blurred vision—whatever symptom presents itself. Why bother with the calendar? Well, you know how it is: The doc asks how long you've had this pain or that tingling. You think it's been a few weeks; in fact it's been two months—or vice-versa. So calendars help. They'll also help you pinpoint the frequency of any ongoing problems, a fact that will help the doc determine if the problems are side effects or otherwise related to your treatment, or the result of something else entirely (like, in my case, getting old—uh, I mean, more mature).

As long as you're getting any kind of follow-up treatment, you'll see the doc regularly. Some treatments, like Tamoxifen, may remain part of your regimen for five years or maybe more (although the studies are ongoing about precisely the most effective length of treatment). You'll need someone to help gauge the effectiveness of the regimen, and that's the doc's job.

Ongoing Going On

Once you've had breast cancer, the watch is ongoing. What's the recommended plan? It's the same three-point plan you read about in Chapter 1, "It Ain't Gold in Them Hills." Remember? Breast self-exam, clinical exam, and mammogram. All three. Always.

Your monthly breast self-exams (BSEs) are even more important now. Unfortunately, the breast on which you've had surgery will now be more difficult to examine. The skin thickens and you'll feel lots of scar tissue. Still, you'll need to do your BSEs religiously. You'll be watching for new lumps, redness, or any other changes. Just because you find a change, though, you needn't panic. It could very well be scar tissue. After all, you do have scarring—maybe lots of it—from whatever surgery you've been through; and in most cases, the scars inside are much bigger than the scars outside. On the other hand, if you feel changes in your breast, it could be the result of infection or—God forbid—recurrent cancer. So never ignore a change. Get it checked out. Now.

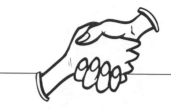

Helping Hand

We can't overstress the importance of regular follow-up exams. The bottom line: *Just do it.* Not just this year. Not just for five years. For the rest of your life.

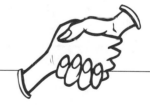

Helping Hand

The American Cancer Society recommends the three-point plan for everyone, before or after any battles with breast cancer. Do a monthly breast self-exam and have regular periodical clinical exams and mammograms. That holds for everyone, even (except for the mammograms) if you've had bilateral mastectomies.

If you've had a mastectomy, especially if you had a bilateral mastectomy, I know you think we're not talking to you. Wrong, dear friend. We are. I know what else you're thinking: How can I do a breast self-exam if my breast is gone? Well, although for all practical purposes your breast IS gone, breast tissue remains. Your BSE must examine all the remaining breast tissue, from the lower ribs to the *collarbone,* from the *breast bone* to back under the arm. Especially examine the incision site for lumps or any other changes. Ironically, the incision is one of the most common sites of recurrence. Ask your doctor to show you where and how to look.

And if you had a mastectomy (with or without reconstruction) you must also wonder about mammograms. If your breast is gone, there's certainly nothing left to take a mammogram of. And reconstructed breast tissue isn't susceptible to breast cancer. After all, a reconstructed breast isn't made of breast tissue. It's made of either muscle and skin from your tummy or back; or it's an implant; or it's a combination of muscle, skin, and implant. However (and this is an important "however"), breast tissue remaining under and/or around the reconstruction is most certainly susceptible to cancer. And yes, a reconstructed breast, even one with an implant, can and should be examined via mammogram. It's important, however, that your mammographer is trained in the special techniques necessary for dealing with implants and/or reconstructed tissue. In addition, of course, your doctor (and you) should check it regularly. (True, breast reconstruction complicates the exam for recurrence in the tissue remaining, but rest assured that your medical team knows how to cope with the difficulties.)

Assuming you have at least one remaining healthy breast, you need to have regular mammograms of it in case cancer shows up there. (Somehow I think the clinics should give a 50 percent discount to those of us who are now one-sided, but I haven't yet found a facility whose policy agrees with me.)

As you learned in the first several chapters of this book, keeping informed will help you avoid living in constant fear. So here's the scoop: Most cancers, like ductal carcinoma, do not spread from one breast to the other. However, as you age, your chances of getting a new ductal carcinoma in the second breast are greater than if you'd never had cancer in the first breast. Again, keep the watch. In fact, best advice: Never turn your back on breast cancer—even if you've never had it and you're reading this book just to be informed.

From the Book

The **collarbone** runs from your shoulder to the V at your throat. The **breast bone** lies at the center of your chest where your ribs attach.

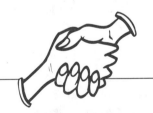

Helping Hand

Stay alert! The longer you go without a recurrence, the less likely you are to have one. However, as you age, having had cancer in one breast increases your risk of having a new cancer in the other breast.

If you're taking Tamoxifen, you'll also want to schedule an annual pelvic exam as a result of the increased risk of endometrial (the uterine lining) cancer. If, on the other hand, you've had a hysterectomy in which your uterus was removed, you're worry-free on this issue. Be assured, however, that endometrial cancer is relatively easily corrected, so it's not worth refusing Tamoxifen because of any fear you may have about endometrial cancer. (Besides, Tamoxifen fights cancer everywhere in your body, not just in the breast.)

If you're taking Tamoxifen, you'll also want to alert your eye doctor, whether you see an optometrist or an ophthalmologist. In a very small percentage of women, the drug leaves tiny white specks of residue on the eyes' blood vessels; however, the doc can easily detect any such specks and determine their seriousness. Then you can discuss whatever options remain. (For full details about risks and side effects of Tamoxifen, check out www.nolvadex.com.)

Finally, you should maintain your regular annual physical exams (or whatever is "regular" for you at your age), including all the usual tests and exams, and especially including blood work. Because blood tests can reveal lots of little secrets, your doctor may detect something otherwise overlooked.

Strike Two?

By now you've probably figured out whether or not you're a prime target for recurrence (see also Chapters 15, "Caution Flag: Risk Factors," and 25, "Recurrence: Safe to Go Back in the Water?"). If your medical team has admitted that you may face recurrence and/or if you're part of a clinical study, you may have more than the routine three-point program in your future.

Tales from the Trenches

Karla considers herself a poster child for follow-up exams. Unfortunately, she knows women who "stopped going for checkups because they didn't like the place they were going—hard to get an appointment, long wait, factory-like exams. I can only say that after 12 years of slogging to my doctor's every three months for blood tests, the blood tests finally picked up a cancer that wasn't palpable. Heaven knows when or how we would have found it otherwise, but it could have killed me by then."

While every doctor handles follow-up tests somewhat differently, and while every one of us fights a slightly different battle with slightly different victories, medical folks tend to use certain tests fairly regularly. For instance, you may have a *blood tumor marker study*. Its purpose is to check the so-called tumor count in your blood. It's a simple procedure from your standpoint in that someone will draw blood as they would for any other blood test. Since this test is somewhat complicated, however, it make take a bit longer for results—perhaps a week. Will you have this test at every follow-up visit? Maybe. Maybe not. Your situation will determine its necessity.

The results come back as a number, but when you see the number, don't panic. Some folks assume that if the cancer is gone, your tumor count should be zero. That's not the case. In fact, any tumor count between 0 and 38.6 is normal. Any future tests that give results within plus or minus five points of your original number are still well within the normal range. The test includes lots of variables far too complicated to explain here, but as a rule of thumb, if your tumor count jumps significantly (like by 50 or 100 points), you may be facing a recurrence. Still, tests can and do go wrong; so if your test shows a big jump in the tumor count, your medical team will probably retest within a week or so to verify the results. It's a tough week, with the waiting and not knowing. If the second test verifies the tumor count is still significantly higher, your medical team will start taking a much closer look at every nook and cranny of your body.

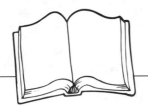

From the Book

A **blood tumor marker study** is a blood test that measures the tumor count in your blood, with a high count indicating a possible recurrence of cancer.

Take It from Us

Never drop your guard. While getting these regular follow-ups is, indeed, a constant reminder of your breast cancer, it is the key to maintaining optimal health. As one survivor wrote, "The devil you know is always better than the devil you don't know or don't want to know." With the new medical philosophy that breast cancer is a chronic disease, one with which we live all our lives, we're forewarned to be better armed.

Their investigation may include blood tests of liver function. They may do a bone scan, looking for any changes in your bones. Since breast cancer often spreads to either bones or lungs, those are logical, watchful steps. Ditto with chest x-rays. They may even do CAT scans of the brain, chest, or abdomen, ultrasounds of the liver, and a battery of blood tests. If these exams and tests suggest recurrence, then more treatment may be part of your future.

Keep in mind, however, that unless you have symptoms that suggest a problem, these tests have not proven useful. Big important point.

Know the Drill

Every doctor handles the follow-up drill differently. And your case is different from your sister's or your best friend's. So regardless of what is the right plan for you, above all, have a plan. And stick to it. Know what to expect; know what is irregular; be prepared with questions.

For instance, if you experience any of the following symptoms, be sure to report them to your doctor:

➤ Bone pain, especially if it gets worse over a few days (most commonly in the spine and hips)

➤ Cough

➤ Difficulty breathing

➤ Weight loss

➤ Lack of appetite

➤ Headaches

➤ Problems with balance

➤ New lumps

➤ New rashes or new allergies

➤ Bumps or redness in and around site of cancer

Likewise, report any other symptoms that are new to you or don't go away. Never hesitate to report a symptom, even if you think it's inconsequential. Sometimes the simplest indications give the doc a clear picture. (For more details about recurrence, see Chapter 25.) And never hesitate to ask your doctors to talk to one another—like asking your allergist to talk to your oncologist. Sometimes we can't use exactly the right terminology, so the doc shrugs off our concerns. Together, they may figure out the problem.

Take It from Us

Know the most common symptoms of possible recurrence so that you and your medical team can get the jump on whatever is happening in your body. Report those symptoms immediately, no matter how obsessive-compulsive it makes you feel to be monitoring every little ache and pain.

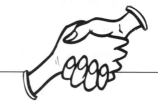

Helping Hand

Stay optimistic. Survivor Evonne recommends, "Expect a favorable outcome. Breast cancer is not as bad or as scary as many people seem to believe. Sure, get those regular checkups and follow the medical advice, but then put it out of your mind and get on with life."

Toolbox: Help Along the Way

Now that your treatments are over and you've been turned loose, what other help will you find along the way? First, don't turn your back on physical therapy. Whether you follow a prescribed exercise regimen at home or need a trained physical therapist to help you, you're apt to lose range of motion in the affected arm if you quit exercising. It's the old saw: If you don't use it, you'll lose it.

Certain alternative treatments may help you feel better, too. Some survivors found visualization and imaging helped them gain a toehold on positive thinking. Some report using vitamins, especially vitamin C (recommended by their plastic surgeon to aid healing) and vitamins E and B_6 (with B_6 in the morning and E at bedtime in an effort to reduce hot flashes). Some turned to herbal remedies and fruit juices. Still another turned to acupuncture, while others reported practicing yoga and various kinds of meditation. (See Chapters 5, "Decisions, Decisions, Decisions," and 18, "Mind and Body: Spiritual Support," for more details about these alternative treatments.)

Tales from the Trenches

One survivor asked her medical team on the last day of treatment what came next. The answer dumped her into a severe state of depression, for the nurse responded, "Well, we're all done. We just have to wait to see if it worked." Being an independent, take-charge sort of person, she investigated alternative treatments and ended up with a Chinese doctor who administered acupuncture, explaining that he was "helping the body get rid of the residuals from all the chemo." Years later, she feels terrific. While we're not medical people and cannot recommend treatments, if a regimen works for you, more power to you!

A few other details are worth considering:

➤ Thanks to its toxic effects on healthy cells, chemo has destroyed some of the immunities your body has built up since childhood. Thus, after chemo is over and you've regained some stability with the rest of the world, your doctor may recommend re-immunization—shots against those many childhood diseases you thought you'd never see again, such as chicken pox and mumps.

➤ Ditto with annual flu shots. You don't need the added risk of debilitating viruses.

➤ Ditto with those pneumonia shots, some of which are once a lifetime, others of which are once every five or ten years. You're more susceptible now to those bazillion germs drifting past your nose, so protect yourself any way you can.

➤ We suggested a baseline bone density test prior to chemo and/or hormonal treatment. If you didn't have one before, get one now. Some doctors claim that certain kinds of chemo will age your bones by 10 years, and we know what a lack of estrogen can do to the health of your bones. So if your bone density tests now show your bones significantly weakened, your doctor may recommend bone stimulator medications. There are several on the market—some quite new, including an implant.

➤ Take calcium. If you weren't post-menopausal before treatment, you may be now. As a result, your body's usual defense against osteoporosis has dropped. Daily calcium—1,500 mg a day by supplement plus what you get in your food—along with vitamin D for absorption will help you avoid becoming a stooped old lady.

Some folks like to say, "I'm through with cancer. I don't want to think about it, talk about it, or deal with it anymore. It's over." While the sentiment is certainly understandable, it's like saying you won't buy any more car insurance because you had an automobile accident and it's over and paid for. Well, if you're going to keep driving, that's not a bright move. And if you're going to keep living, it's not wise to ignore your past breast cancer and neglect the follow-up. To extend the metaphor one more step, let's look at it this way: You don't like paying those auto insurance premiums, but if you're going to drive, you'd better. It's the law. Likewise, you might not like keeping all those follow-up appointments, but if you're going to lead a long and happy life, you'd better. Plain and simple.

So, dear sister, here's to a long and happy life—yours!

Take It from Us

Don't second-guess your previous treatment plan. Now that the bulk of your treatment is behind you, you may read about new methods that cause you to think you should have done something different. Just remind yourself that what's past is past. Continue to get your checkups and follow your plan—but it's time to stop living only in terms of your cancer.

The Least You Need to Know

➤ Breast cancer is never past tense and thus necessitates regular periodic check-ups for the rest of your life.

➤ Monthly breast self-exams, regular clinical exams, and mammograms define the three-point plan for follow-up.

➤ While follow-up procedures vary from one doctor to another, you and your doctor should develop a plan and follow it.

➤ Certain symptoms may suggest a possible recurrence; never ignore them.

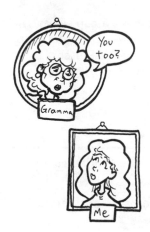

Chapter 15

Caution Flag: Risk Factors

In This Chapter

➤ Dispelling myths about breast cancer risks

➤ Known and suspected risk factors

➤ Risk factors among ethnic populations

➤ What to do now

A woman who is now president of her own manufacturing company told me that she spent her young adult life waiting to get breast cancer. Her mother and grandmother both died of the disease, and she figured it was just a matter of time before her number came up. She laughs at herself now, but it took some serious research before she realized her heritage was not her sentence.

Being female is the primary risk factor for developing breast cancer. And being female, even if you've fought one battle and won, you're at risk for recurrence. Those are the rotten facts, but fortunately, you can anticipate—and work at beating—the odds. In this chapter, we'll look at the risk factors for breast cancer—the real and imagined, the fact and the fiction about your chances for getting it or having a recurrence. Then we'll suggest a plan for you to get on with your life, whether you've already had a battle with breast cancer and fear another, or whether you're cancer-free and counting.

Once! Again?

Surely there's not a breast cancer survivor anywhere who hasn't at one time or another asked, "What caused my cancer?" Unfortunately, it's a question without an answer. And unlike the detection of cervical cancer via a pap smear, the detection of breast cancer has no easy test. There are, however, *risk factors* that help your health-care team know how and when to monitor you. While we discuss these factors in detail during the course of this chapter, the following chart gives you a quick preview of what's here.

Commonly Considered Risk Factors

Risk Factor	Significance of Risk Factor
Being female	Most important
Age	Second most important; older equals greater risk
Having had breast cancer	Very important
Family history	Very important, but 90 percent of women diagnosed have no family history
Ovarian cancer survivor	Very important
Diagnosed atypical hyperplasia	Very important
Population group	Important
Ethnic group	Important
Early menstruation	Slightly important
Late menopause	Slightly important
No children	Slightly important
Use of birth control pills	Uncertain
Hormone replacement therapy	Possible but uncertain
Smoking	Uncertain
Nutrition	Uncertain
Alcohol consumption	Uncertain
Diet pills	Possible
Environmental factors	Possible but uncertain

One risk factor is a history of having breast cancer. It's grossly unfair, but once you've fought the battle, you may face an increased risk of having to fight it again. But before you hit the panic button, talk to your doctor. Your risk is completely dependent on what kind of cancer you had before and how it was treated. You may be at risk for developing a new cancer in the other breast. You may be at risk for a recurrence of the first cancer. As strange as it sounds, you are never completely safe—even if you had a bilateral mastectomy. Here's the scoop.

Let's say you had a mastectomy on your left breast. Of course, it is still possible to get cancer in the right breast. And your risk is the same as anyone else's—even greater with some kinds of cancer. It is also possible (but less likely) to get cancer in the breast that was removed. Sound like double-talk? Not exactly. Some breast tissue remains after most mastectomies, and that tissue can develop cancer. (See Chapter 25, "Recurrence: Safe to Go Back in the Water?")

Since there's obviously not enough tissue to tuck between the plates of a mammogram machine, the only detection is through clinical and self-exams. So be aware of your risk factors. Ask your doctor if your cancer is likely to spread to the other breast or to recur in any remaining tissue. And keep up the monthly BSE and clinical exams.

Roots: Family History

We need to say up front that only 10 percent of women diagnosed with breast cancer have any family history of the disease. Nevertheless, family history does play a role in your risk factors. If you have a *first-degree relative* (mother, sister, or daughter) with breast cancer, your risk factor doubles. If you have two first-degree relatives with breast cancer, your risk factor multiplies by five. And if any of these relatives had breast cancer prior to menopause or if she had it in both breasts, your risk is even greater. So if your mother and your sister have had breast cancer, you are at a high risk, greater risk than if just your maternal—or paternal—grandmother had breast cancer.

Having first cousins and aunts, especially your mother's sisters, who have had breast cancer also seems to increase your risk, but so far the studies can't tell us by how much. If your father's side of the family has a history of breast cancer, your risk is also increased, but again, no one knows to what degree. Ditto for you if any male members of your family have had breast cancer.

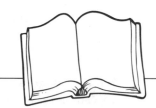

From the Book

A breast cancer **risk factor** is something—age, family history, lifestyle issues, menstrual history, etc.—that, if present, increases your chances of getting the disease.

Take It from Us

Don't forget to get the facts! When we talk about breast cancer, there are absolutely no guarantees. Even if both breasts have been removed, breast cancer can still occur—or recur.

Most hereditary factors involve something called gene *mutations,* or changes. Recent genetic research has identified two genes, BRCA1 and BRCA2, as the pivotal markers. Normally, these genes make proteins that keep cells from growing abnormally. But if they mutate, that protection is gone. Then, if you inherit a mutated gene from either parent, you have an increased risk for breast cancer. About 50 to 60 percent of women with mutated BRCA1 or BRCA2 will get breast cancer by age 70. (The mutated gene also increases the risk of ovarian cancer.)

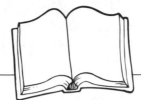

From the Book

Your **first-degree relative** is someone only one step away on the genealogy chart, like your mother, your daughter, or your sister. A genetic **mutation** is a change in gene structure that is abnormal. Some mutations contribute to various diseases, including breast cancer.

Another inherited abnormality comes in the form of the p53 tumor suppressor genes. As the name suggests, these genes naturally suppress tumors. If they mutate, however, the protection is reduced.

New genetic testing now available can analyze a blood sample and tell you if you're at risk. And if you are, you and your doctor can then decide if you need more careful monitoring, some kind of medication, or even a prophylactic mastectomy, a mastectomy to protect you against the risk of getting breast cancer. But serious issues surround testing to determine a mutated gene. First, the test is expensive, and some health plans don't pay. Second, many women worry that if their tests show genetic abnormalities they may not be able to get health insurance; however, a 1997 federal law prevents insurance companies from denying insurance on the basis of information from genetic testing. Of course, rates may become astronomical, but many states are working on laws affecting that area, too.

The real issue, however, may be emotional. If your tests show a genetic abnormality, you must understand that there is no known cure. How will you feel? Even if you don't worry about yourself, how will you feel about your daughters, your sisters, and your grandchildren?

Now, what if nobody in your family has had breast cancer? Think you're safe? Before you pat yourself on the back for having good genes, study the numbers. Only 5 to 10 percent of breast cancers are due to heredity. So just because you have no family history

Take It from Us

Don't jump into genetic testing before you know all the facts: get some counseling. There are complicated physical, emotional, and financial issues involved. For support, check FORCE: Facing Our Risk of Cancer Empowered, a Web site founded by a woman who carries the BRCA2 mutation and wanted to help women who have the gene, whether or not they've been diagnosed with breast cancer. Check it out at www.facingourrisk.org.

doesn't mean you're off the hook. Nobody in my family ever had breast cancer, but here I am, a full-fledged member of the sisterhood.

Identity Crisis?

The number-one risk factor (besides being female) is age. The older we get, the greater our chances of getting breast cancer. In fact, 75 to 85 percent of breast cancer is diagnosed in women aged 50 and older, with 64 being the median age for diagnosis. Women 20-something in age account for only 0.3 percent of the cases.

Here's the breakdown by age for your chances of being diagnosed with breast cancer:

➤ At age 20, chances are 1 in 2,500

➤ At age 30, chances are 1 in 250

➤ At age 40, chances are 1 in 67

➤ At age 50, chances are 1 in 39

➤ At age 60, chances are 1 in 29

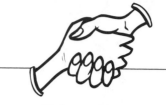

Helping Hand

Be aware that family history is only one small risk factor. Roughly 90 percent of survivors have no family history of breast cancer. Remember that all women are at risk. If you have been diagnosed, however, keep your notebook up to date detailing your diagnosis and treatment. It may be more important to your daughter or granddaughter than any other family album.

The numbers tell all. You're not safe at any age, but you're a lot less safe the older you are. In fact, many doctors don't do mammograms until age 40, when a baseline mammogram is usually in order and annual mammograms begin (see Chapter 1, "It Ain't Gold in Them Hills"). But if you're younger, don't let the averages give you a false sense of security. Younger women do get breast cancer, in rare cases even in their teens. And when they do, it tends to be more aggressive and more difficult to treat.

Age isn't the only risk factor relating to who you are. Depending on your ethnic group, you may have an increased risk of breast cancer. Where do you fit in the following?

➤ Caucasian women past age 50 surpass all population and ethnic groups, posting the highest incidence of breast cancer.

➤ For women under age 50, African-Americans face the highest risk of any group, including a greater risk of developing more aggressive forms of breast cancer.

➤ Hispanic women face a lesser risk than do either Caucasian or African-American women.

➤ Asian-American women who have been in the United States at least 10 years are at an 80 percent higher risk of breast cancer than are new arrivals. If you were born in the United States, your risk is about the same as that for Caucasian women.

Tales from the Trenches

Like a good girl, Letta went in at age 40 for a routine baseline mammogram. She felt great, her breast self-exams showed nothing, she had no family history of breast cancer, and neither she nor her doctor suspected a thing. But her baseline mammogram shocked everyone. Her cancer was already Stage II. After a mastectomy, heavy-duty chemo, and radiation, a year later she's back in the swing of things. What if she hadn't gone for the baseline mammogram?

➤ Among Asian-American women, Japanese are most at risk, with Filipino, Chinese, Vietnamese, and Korean following in that order, with Korean women less than half as likely to get breast cancer as are Japanese women.

➤ Inuit women have a higher incidence of breast cancer than do Native Americans or Hispanics.

➤ Native American women have the lowest risk of all, but in some areas of the United States, the incidence is rising.

To summarize the incidence of breast cancer by ethnicity, consider the following comparisons:

Rate of Breast Cancer Diagnosis per 100,000 Women

Caucasian	111.8
African-American	95.4
Hawaiian	105.6
Japanese	82.3
Inuit	78.9
Filipino	73.1
Hispanic	69.8
Chinese	55.0
Vietnamese	37.5
Native American	31.6
Korean	28.5

Your population group may cross some other lines as well. For instance, Jewish women of European heritage suffer from increased incidence. Researchers suspect the increased risk is genetic.

Women of higher socioeconomic classes have an increased risk. Researchers can't explain why, but the increased risk results in the study may be simply skewed results. Higher income women tend to be more conscientious about getting regular screenings resulting in higher rates of cancer detection. But some researchers are looking closely at diet and environmental factors as well (more on those issues later).

Pregnant women, especially those between 32 and 38, and of any ethnic group, face a greater risk for breast cancer than for any other cancer, occurring about one in 3,000 pregnancies. Researchers are reluctant at this point to say that late pregnancies cause breast cancer (there's really no solid evidence of that), but if a pregnant woman does get cancer, it's likely to be breast cancer.

Women partnered with women are at no greater risk than their personal history would suggest, since sexual orientation is not a risk factor.

And yes, men are at risk, too, but only in fairly rare instances, with about 1,300 diagnosed cases a year.

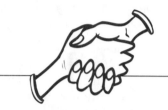

Helping Hand

Some population groups sponsor their own support groups, Web sites, and information centers. See Appendixes E, "Informational Web Sites," and C, "Support Groups," to find those most helpful to you.

Once Upon a Time: Personal History

After gathering detailed histories of women diagnosed with breast cancer, researchers have extrapolated the results into statements about who's most likely at risk. Only after a great deal more study may researchers eventually get at the why. So, here are some of the extrapolated personal history risk factors researchers have identified:

If you began menstruating before age 12, you probably are at a slightly increased risk for breast cancer. Ditto for late menopause, like age 50 or later. Whether or not you've had children also affects your risk factor. If you've never had children, or didn't have your first child until after age 30, you are at higher risk. If you breast-fed for at least a year and a half, you may have lowered your risk, at least by a little, but the jury is still out on that one. If you've had ovarian cancer, and/or you have

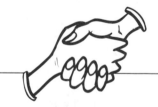

Helping Hand

In order to determine your own personal risk factor, call the National Cancer Institute at 1-800-4-CANCER for a computer program called The Breast Cancer Risk Assessment Tool that helps you estimate your chances of developing breast cancer—or developing a recurrence. It's free for the asking.

blood relatives who have had ovarian and/or breast cancer, you're a prime target. But removal of the ovaries before age 40 seems to reduce the risk of breast cancer.

Are you wondering about those birth control pills that are or were part of your life? Not a problem, report most studies, but the questions are numerous enough to merit your discussing your personal risk factors with the doc. Whatever slight risks birth control pills add are diminished within 10 years of stopping them.

Most studies that evaluated abortions and miscarriages as risk factors came back negative. Maybe they affect your risk very slightly, but probably not. And don't worry about ovulation-inducing fertility drugs. If you took them, they should not affect your risk of either breast cancer or ovarian cancer.

Hormone replacement therapy (*HRT,* sometimes called *estrogen replacement therapy* or *ERT*), however, may be a different story. It's the one risk factor women question most often. The answer is always the same: Nobody knows, at least not for sure. Nevertheless, most experts think that the risk, if it does exist, is minimal. Talk to your doctor to see if the advantages outweigh the disadvantages. If *osteoporosis* is bending your future, if you're at high risk for a heart attack or stroke, if the side effects of menopause make your glasses steam up, or if Alzheimer's disease runs in your family, you may decide to take the risk. See more about hormone therapy in Chapter 12, "Hormone Therapy: The Pill."

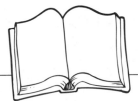

From the Book

Hormone replacement therapy is the oral administration of the hormone estrogen and, if used, usually begins with the onset of menopause. **Osteoporosis,** at one time called "dowager's hump," is bone deterioration resulting from the loss of bone mass density. **Fibrocystic breast,** sometimes still incorrectly referred to as fibrocystic disease, is not a disease at all, but a benign condition that occurs when fibrous breast tissue becomes dense; it often combines with the formation of small cysts. **Atypical hyperplasia** is excessive formation of tissue unlike that in the surrounding area.

Most women with *fibrocystic breasts* are not at any increased risk of breast cancer. If, however, you've had *atypical hyperplasia,* it does increase your risk. Unfortunately, no one can tell you which hyperplastic changes will turn into cancer and which won't. Do you puff the ol' cancer sticks? Smoking is directly linked to lung cancer, but how it affects breast cancer is an unknown. Likewise, studies are inconclusive regarding secondhand cigarette smoke and its effect on breast cancer. Some research shows, however, that smokers who get breast cancer have a much more difficult recovery, perhaps even a lesser chance for survival. Why add to the risk?

Some folks are convinced that we can reduce our risk of breast cancer with proper nutrition. The evidence is still inconclusive, but scientists do believe that a diet with lots of fruits, veggies, and grains is better than one high in any and all fats. Better to go low fat and high fiber than not; better to go olive oil and flaxseed oil than lard; better to go low salt than not—all known to be beneficial for warding off heart disease. For breast cancer, however, diet is not a guaranteed protector.

Even though some studies tout the importance of soy in protecting against breast cancer, the results are inconclusive. While it is a good protein substitute for meat, be careful how much you consume initially. If you suddenly begin eating lots of it, you'll probably suffer from gas. (And some folks worry that we really don't know whether or not plant estrogen, such as that found in soy products, feeds estrogen-receptor tumors the way animal estrogen does.) So many questions; so few answers.

In the end, we may find that food isn't a risk factor at all. Instead maybe it's the carcinogens (known cancer-causing substances) and hormones found in and on them—like the pesticides on veggies, the contaminants in fish, the artificial hormones in beef.

Tales from the Trenches

Anita says, "I tried to do everything right. I ate carefully, exercised regularly, didn't smoke, didn't drink. But my grandmother died from breast cancer, and my mother is a 20-year survivor. So when I got my diagnosis last year, I had to accept the fact that I'd fought it the best way I knew how. The early detection was my salvation. Now days go by without my even thinking about it. I had a mastectomy, chemo, and radiation. The cancer's gone. Sure, I go for my checkups regularly, but I'm going on with my life. There's so much to do!" And out the door she went, off to 18 holes of golf.

Some studies suggest that drinking those daiquiris and margaritas or other alcoholic treats, especially two or more a day, can increase your risk. Data are not clear. Another question.

We know for sure that too much of anything—margaritas or chocolate or dressing on the salad—adds calories; and while obesity is not a risk factor, some experts believe that weight gain, especially after menopause, is. Besides, we do know that fat consumption and being overweight are clearly related to heart disease risk, so why play with the numbers? Of course, exercise has been shown in some studies to help prevent breast cancer; it won't hurt to keep up the aerobics and daily walks.

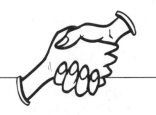

Helping Hand

Always follow your doctor's advice, no matter what the latest headline tells you. The confusion over what does and doesn't cause cancer—including breast cancer—makes great stories on the evening news. Follow a healthy regimen that your medical team recommends. It's the best you can do until further research gives us black and white answers instead of all these shades of gray.

And speaking of exercise and being overweight, do you look for miracles and try to lose weight with diet pills? Scientists are still studying the issue, but diet pills are a definite maybe as a contributing risk factor.

Periodic e-mail rumors have targeted antiperspirants and even underwire bras that supposedly cut off lymph circulation and contribute to breast cancer. No evidence for either. None. So buyer beware when it comes to understanding the truth about risk factors.

Is It the Water? The Environment

Let's say your parents gave you perfect genes. What could cause them to mutate and give you breast cancer? Could it be environmental carcinogens?

Unfortunately, certain geographical regions do have a higher incidence of breast cancer than do others. Research continues—some of it spearheaded and supported by survivors, others by the National Institute of Environmental Health Sciences, the National Cancer Institute, Centers for Disease Control, various governmental agencies, and numerous universities.

The springboard for research comes from a fairly straightforward fact: Scientists know that while some gene mutation is inherited, much of it occurs during a woman's life. The question is, of course, what causes it? Is it the water? Or the air we breathe? Something lurking behind the computer screen? The most current thought is that our genes interact somehow with the environment to finally result in breast cancer. Unfortunately, it's all shrouded in the deepest of mysteries.

Among the environmental factors under consideration are radiation, UV rays in sunlight, fumes (like those from household insecticides, cleaning solvents, paint), artificial sweeteners, pesticides, electromagnetic fields around high-tension lines and surrounding electronic devices like microwave ovens, cell phones, and artificial light. Other studies focus on environmental pollutants, such as pesticides used on lawns and golf courses. Even if you never walk in the grass, you're exposed. The residue never goes away; thus, rain washes the bad stuff into our drinking water. So you buy bottled water and take a leisurely hot shower. Hot water vaporizes the bad stuff and you suck it right into your lungs.

Other targets of investigation include PCBs (polychlorinated biphenyls, which are emissions from certain industrial processes) and other toxic chemicals as well as hazardous and municipal wastes. How any and all of these affect water and air quality is, of course, bottom line.

To date, studies have not identified any environmental elements as definite culprits. Research continues.

Forward March

What happens when you find yourself saddled with one or more of these risk factors? In a nutshell, everything! Knowledge is power. With the knowledge you have about your personal risk factors, you can work with your healthcare team to go for early detection, the key to everything—the best surgery options, the most effective treatment options, the best recovery path. The more risk factors you face, the more dramatic the monitoring— more frequent mammograms, perhaps even ultrasounds, and constant monthly breast self-exams and clinical exams.

Take It from Us

Take it easy on the news! If you dwell on every environmental threat that anyone suspects of causing cancer, you'll go bonkers. Try to avoid the obvious stuff—the pesticides and other known hazardous substances—but keep a level head. Of course, I'm one who washes all my fruits and veggies with soap! Go figure.

Tales from the Trenches

Because she had multiple risk factors, Gladys said, "I used to wake up every morning wondering if this would be the day I'd be diagnosed with breast cancer." Now, after counseling, she realizes how self-defeating her obsession was, and she's gone on to a healthy, happy life—of course, still getting those regular checkups.

On the other hand, Nancy felt a lump, figured she had no history of breast cancer in her family, and convinced herself it was just fibrous tissue. She didn't want to go for an exam for fear of what they might find. She waited too long. She was only 47.

Above all, get on with your life. Just because you're at risk doesn't mean you spend your waking hours waiting for the other shoe to fall. In spite of your knowledge of your risk factors, understand that there is little you can do to prevent breast cancer. Someday, we pray, we may have different advice.

Risk factors are just that. They're numbers. Averages. But it's best not to play the numbers game. Just know that if you're female, you're at risk. Take it from there. Take care of yourself.

The Least You Need to Know

➤ Every woman *is* at risk for breast cancer.

➤ The older you are, the greater your risk.

➤ Knowing your risk factors helps you and your healthcare team plan for more careful monitoring.

➤ Whatever your risk, get on with your life.

Chapter 16

Emotional Turmoil: Diamond in the Rough

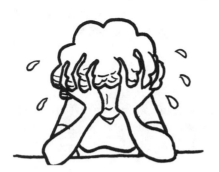

In This Chapter

➤ Fearsome foursome: shock, anger, fear, and guilt

➤ The pity party: You aren't alone

➤ Calling a halt to negative emotions

➤ Picking up the pieces and moving on

➤ Hope for tomorrow

How many of us have been driving down the road, minding our own business, when "BAM!"—someone slams into the side of our car! First, we are shocked that someone could hit our car while we're on the road in plain sight. Second, we are angry because someone *did* hit our car. Our insurance rates will probably go up, and it wasn't even our fault! Third, we sit in our seat "hiding out," waiting for them to get out of their car and come apologize to us. Fourth, we may feel a little guilty because our mind may have been on "auto-pilot." If we had been paying 100 percent attention, we might have been able to avoid the accident. Finally, we have hope when we know our car is repairable and still driveable, our insurance is up to date, we are not injured, and we know that while the car is being repaired, we will get all those extra little dings out of the body.

We go through all these emotions because of what someone else did to us. Having breast cancer really isn't much different. Most of us will experience this same range of emotions because cancer is that unexpected "BAM!" hitting us broadside. Were you *embarrassed* that you had a disease? Were you *angry* because it was happening to you?

Did you *envy* those who did not have breast cancer? Did you *fear* that you might lose a breast or only have a few months left to live? Did you feel *guilty* because you didn't get last year's mammogram? Did you *panic* about telling your family or how your co-workers would react to you? Were you *relieved* because you found out it was manageable? In this chapter, we'll look at those emotions and how to cope with them.

The Emotional Firing Range

Unlike many physical symptoms, emotional reactions to cancer, its treatment, and its aftermath are pretty unpredictable. You won't be able to pinpoint when you'll be feeling what emotion, or what circumstance or situation will trigger a laugh or a cry. In fact, you'll probably feel like you're on an emotional roller coaster taking you on the ride of your life.

Do keep in mind, though, no matter what you feel or when you feel it, your emotions are your own, for keeps. Please do not disown them; just learn to live with them and through them for a time. These emotions will be colored by what you've experienced in your life before cancer, what kind of support system you've set up, and your own unique personality. You should also keep in mind that, for most people, emotions are stronger than ideas or intellect, and an emotion can live with us for days at a time. That's good and bad news. Hope and happiness can replace sadness, worry, and guilt; consequently, worry and guilt will not last forever. Neither does hope nor happiness. We must work to rid ourselves of worry and maintain hope and happiness as much as possible.

From the Book

Shock has many definitions, and many of these can certainly apply to your reaction at being told you have breast cancer. "Heavy blow, impact, something that jars the mind or emotions, disturbance of function, surprise, agitation, and trauma," just to name a few.

Shock: No, Not Me!

Have you ever seen someone shocked with a mild jolt of electricity? They jump. Their jaw drops, and their eyes widen. They have a look of disbelief on their face. There's no doubt to any of us that they have been shocked. Wouldn't you have liked to see the look on your face when you were told you had breast cancer? Why, I bet the look on your face was one of *shock!*

The initial news is just like someone hitting us with a bucket of cold ice water. A million questions and thoughts will probably race through your mind, including …

➤ But breast cancer doesn't run in my family.

➤ Am I going to die or suffer?

➤ Will my insurance cover the expense?

➤ How will my family and friends react?

➤ I don't deserve this.

➤ This can't be happening to me.

➤ Can I keep working?

➤ I'm strong; I can deal with this!

➤ Will I be able to grow old with my partner and enjoy retirement?

The problem is, as your mind fills with these and other thoughts at the time of diagnosis and at odd moments throughout and after treatment, you're not hearing the words the doctors are speaking. You do not feel the gentle hand of your husband or your sister on your back, reassuring you. You don't register that someone has asked you a question and is waiting for you to reply. As a matter of fact, if breathing were not an autonomic reflex, you wouldn't even be sure you were still breathing.

Of all the emotions you'll experience, shock is probably the shortest lived. Getting over the shock will probably be the first step you'll take in dealing with breast cancer. It usually precedes the surgery and the treatment (although it can crop up at any time). The sooner we are able to get the shock of it all under control, the sooner we can get on with the treatment and recovery. It seems that getting the mind under control is just as important as keeping the body strong.

If you break the word "disease" into its parts, it becomes Dis-Ease. If we cannot move on, do we continue to be "not at ease" with ourselves, our life, or our cancer? The rest of our treatment may become easier once we recover from the emotional turmoil of shock. Once we pass shock (and, by the way, we do *not* get to collect $200; that money probably goes to the doctors), we can move on. Maybe that is why shock comes and goes rather quickly.

Even once you have passed shock, it will come to revisit you from time to time. Someone will say something that reminds you of your treatment, a good friend or family member will be diagnosed with cancer, or you will find a piece of clothing or a hat (thrown on the floor in the back of a closet) you wore to one of your therapy sessions. And, there is shock all over again. Your initial shock may be over, but—trust me—it will be replaced by other emotions, some of them much longer-lasting.

Tales from the Trenches

Pat chose not to have children, mainly because she remembered the horror stories her mother told of the pain and suffering during childbirth. In her late 40s, Pat was diagnosed with breast cancer and, after two surgeries, went through four months of chemo and a month and a half of radiation. All her "best-laid plans" of avoiding pain went down the drain. Sometimes, all we can do is cope.

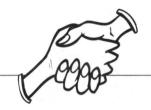

Anger: Why Me?

We stew in anger. We carry it with us. We relive what made us angry. We add fuel to the fire just to keep it and us going. Maybe we do this because anger is usually easier to deal with than fear. And, yes, we are afraid.

We are angry at our fate, our doctors, our cancer, and our "healthy" friends and family. We are angry we didn't deal with things when we had the chance and instead let them fester. We are angry because we allowed ourselves to be dis-tressed and dis-appointed, and we believe these have led to our dis-ease!

We wonder if all the frustration and inner conflict we have felt over a lifetime have been a partial cause of our breast cancer. Were all the "dis" emotions we felt accumulating over a lifetime helping produce our disease? Our frustration and inner conflict certainly seem to fuel our anger. Isn't anger referred to as "not a healthy emotion?" We can suspect, but we just don't know. And, we'd give worlds to know. Some of us have already given a breast, or at least part of one!

And, what's really funny is that we begin to wonder if all the anger we expressed helped cause our cancer. Now talk about a catch-22.

We will probably all go through some angry times and that's perfectly healthy. It's getting stuck in anger that's the real problem. Here are a few ways you, for yourself and for the people around you, can deal with your anger:

➤ Repressing it all the time doesn't seem to work well. You need to vent occasionally.

➤ When you need to vent, tell those around you that you are venting. Your mood and tone of voice are not directed at them, but to them. They may be just a sounding board.

➤ Now may not be a time to be too reasonable. Venting to release and reasonableness don't always go hand in hand. Sometimes, we need to be unreasonable, just for a moment or two.

➤ Think about the people you are expressing your anger to. Can you trust them not to repeat it or take you as 100 percent serious?

➤ Visualize your anger. Imagine, and I'm stressing imagine, yourself punching cancer cells and knockin' 'em dead!

➤ If you need to do something physical to release your anger, punch pillows, scream, run, cry, etc. Just don't do anything to damage yourself physically.

If you're the type of person who keeps things bottled up, you're likely to find that when your anger does finally burst through, it's over not just the issue at hand, but all of the problems you've tried to deal with inside. If you're able to express your emotions more openly and more regularly, then you might feel better all around—and you'll certainly be able to limit the sudden and extreme outbursts of anger.

Fear: Hiding Out

Fear may be a breast cancer survivor's meanest opponent. We are usually afraid of the unknown, and breast cancer involves many unknowns including how you'll deal with the challenges it will bring you, why you've been "chosen" by this illness, what effect it will have on your family and friends, and, of course, the spectre of death.

Fear may make us hide out or retreat from the world for a brief time. As with worry and guilt, a brief time spent alone and apart is understandable and perhaps even healing; a long time is not healthful. The greater our fear, and the deeper we bury ourselves into it, the harder it is for others to reach us. And, if we go too deep in fear, others may stop trying to reach us. At that point, our fear may lead us to loneliness and despair. Prolonged fear can also be an enormous waste of time because it drains you of physical and emotional energy.

If you feel yourself being overwhelmed by fear, try to break the cycle by becoming more actively involved in life. Force yourself to call a friend for company or to resume an almost forgotten hobby. Make sure you're not neglecting the needs of your family and friends; sometimes putting someone else first—even at this crucial time—can break the grip that fear has upon your life. Becoming well-informed about breast cancer in general and about your own unique case will also help reduce fear. Read, surf the Web, join and talk with members of a support group, get second opinions, and ask all of your healthcare providers questions. Once again, knowledge is power when it comes to fighting against fear!

Take It from Us

Don't try to hide the truth. Although many women try to be very secretive about their breast cancer, in most cases, when people know you well, they will see and hear subtle changes in your voice, facial expressions, or the look in your eyes. Others may not know exactly what is wrong, but they will know that something is up. Is it better to leave them guessing?

The other thing to keep in mind is that being afraid isn't the same as being fragile. You can use your fear as a weapon or as a tool of motivation. You can be strong and still be afraid. Your fear might make you withdraw from life temporarily, but it can also push you forward to face new challenges.

Guilt: Was It the Chocolate?

"I have been bad; that is why I have breast cancer." If that were true, everyone would have a bout of breast cancer since "to err is human," and no one on this planet hasn't been "bad" at least once in a while.

If you choose, you probably can make a long list of "mistakes" that your brain—in its uniquely undermining way—could potentially relate to the development of breast cancer. Remember the time you cancelled your yearly mammogram appointment? What about the fact that you resent that your friend has larger breasts than you do? And how can you rationalize away the cigarettes you smoked when you were a teen-ager? Unfortunately, unlike anger, guilt doesn't often motivate positive behavior. Most people who feel guilty simply sit around, stuck and feeling low, and certainly not getting much accomplished. If you wallow in guilt, you're bound to get depressed. And then we feel more guilty, then more depressed, and more and more helpless. This is a terrible merry-go-round to be on.

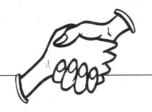

Helping Hand

Release your guilt. You were not given breast cancer as a punishment for past events and attitudes. It is *not* your fault!

Let's take a look at just a few of the reasons you might be feeling guilty at this moment:

➤ You forgot to get your mammogram.

➤ Your disease and its treatment is upsetting the lives of your family and friends.

➤ You resent the fact that others are healthy.

➤ You're envious that others are having a good time or have a normal life.

➤ You didn't exercise at least three times a week.

➤ You didn't watch your fat, sugar, alcohol, chocolate (you name the sinful food) intake.

Breast cancer is certainly bad enough by itself. You don't need to add dealing with a guilt complex on top of it! Watch the words you are using in your subconscious. Words in our head seem to filter into our lives and affect our ability to deal with things. Are you hearing your inner voice saying things like "It's my fault," "I didn't take enough care of myself," or "I'm a bad person"? None of us are perfect. We have all done bad or wrong things no matter how big or little the act may have been.

Try to give up all the bad things you did, and, most certainly do not make an itemized list of them. Bad and cancer are not synonymous; neither are good and health.

Forgiving ourselves is the first step in conquering our guilt. Breast cancer is not something that we contracted as punishment for the less than perfect life we have lived.

Hope: Light at the End of the Tunnel

At one point in the process, you'll be able to break free of all your anger, fear, and guilt, and this freedom will allow a return of joy, glee, and a sense of fun. There will come a time when you not only crack a smile, but you also just outright laugh at something funny. When you can do that, *hope* for a future has emerged.

How do you get past all of the other emotions to get to the happy glimmer of hope? First, you can look at the problem (breast cancer) and have a clear picture in your mind of what it is, which can help release the fear. Second, you can list your options. Basically, you have two: to live or to die. Third, you can make a plan. Fourth, list what you need to do to accomplish your plan. Finally, set your time line. I'm a firm believer that you can accomplish almost anything if you know how long it will take.

From the Book

Hope is a wish or desire supported by some confidence of its fulfillment; an expectation or trust.

Tales from the Trenches

After Carmen's mastectomy, she was talking with a golfing friend who was trying to cheer her up. Her friend remarked that since Carmen no longer had a breast in the way of her golf swing, her score should improve dramatically. Why, she could even call herself the "Amazon Golfer." (Amazons were women warriors who cut off their right breast to be great archers—hopefully not finding out later that they were left-handed.) Carmen started to smile and then just laughed out loud because she realized her friend was planning future golf games with her. Hope!

These steps seem simple, but they produce a wonderful result. You are planning on fighting this disease; you are planning on winning; and you have hope for a future? Yeah, you have arrived!

Others have lived through all the treatments, and so can most of us! Every day, scientists discover new ways to treat breast cancer. Every day, more and more people survive breast cancer. Every day, more companies initiate programs to help make people aware of the benefits of early detection of breast cancer and to contribute more money to fund the research.

No one can predict the when or the how, but every day we come closer to finding a cure for breast cancer. There is hope in that fact alone. In the meantime, you may not find a star to "hitch your wagon to," but you can certainly find a person who has gone through breast cancer, who has walked the path you are walking, and who shines just as bright as any star in the heavens for you. Attach yourself to someone whom you see as a person who is successful at living and surviving. They will not give you any fake cheerfulness. They will give you hope.

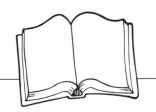

From the Book

Spirituality is the state of being spiritual. **Spiritual** is not tangible or material. It is concerned with the effects of the soul. A good spirit is the force within a living being that imparts courage. It is the essence or will of a person.

With your hope comes a new you. This new you is usually more mellow, and you may see a glow of this new inner spirit. Priorities have generally changed, and *spirituality* can be seen on your face.

With hope comes a new way of looking at yourself. You may be or have been scared, swollen, bald, tired, heavier, stinky, or disfigured. But you suddenly realize that the true you, your essence or spirit, wasn't housed entirely in just one breast! You may be slightly different on the outside, and maybe more than a little different on the inside as well, but you are whole and you are yourself.

The discomfort and pain you have felt will, in time, lessen. Your hair will grow back, and sometimes it grows back prettier than it was before you lost it. You may never be 110 percent satisfied with your body, but at least you're still alive and kicking, and as the days go by, you'll eventually learn to be comfortable with it.

Take It from Us

Don't lose your sense of self, even if others look at you differently. Instead, use the fight you know you have in you to provide yourself with a sense of peace and purpose.

You might want to think of the emotional healing process as a different kind of "reconstruction." Your internal reconstruction follows upon the shock, anger, fear, worry, and guilt of breast cancer. You've broken down, or deconstructed, for a while. Now you can begin to construct a new internal you—one that is stronger, more up to date, more tenacious. If you work at it, your new construction can be built on a strong framework that was shaken but has survived.

Your foundation is built on hope for tomorrow. Your framework has been treated and corrected for an indefinite period of time, and your façade glows with an inner peace. Hope.

The Least You Need to Know

➤ Don't bury or disown your feelings. They are a part of you. Living through them usually helps you recover faster.

➤ All the negative emotions of fear, anger, worry, guilt, and shock are the norm with breast cancer.

➤ Let others know how you are feeling emotionally as well as physically.

➤ One way or another, you will come out of breast cancer different than when you went in, and we are not just talking about physical changes!

Part 4
Shock Absorbers: Finding Support

While this bolt out of the blue called breast cancer certainly rocks the world of any woman diagnosed, certain shock absorbers cushion the blow. We're talking, of course, about those wonderful people whose soothing words, hugs, calls, cards, and carry-in dinners make you all teary-eyed with warm fuzzies. But other support is there for the taking, from the telephone to the bookstore to cyberspace to the spiritual world.

In this part of the book you'll learn how you can get the support you need by joining those women in the sisterhood who have survived the shocks and tremors and understand you as no one else can. You'll learn about more distant means of support as well as spiritual and professional support, for both you and yours.

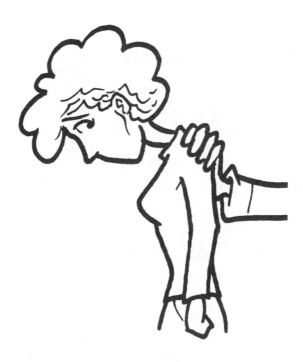

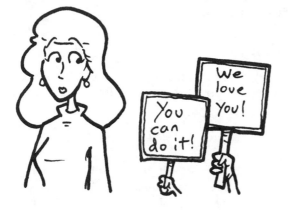

Chapter 17

Groupies: Yea or Nay?

In This Chapter

➤ Support groups' purpose and practicality

➤ Face-to-face and long-distance groups

➤ Great—or not so great—expectations

➤ When to steer clear

"No, I didn't join a support group," explained one survivor when we asked about it in a survey. And then in 10 pages of single-spaced typewritten detail, she poured out her heart.

While her story isn't unusual, it gives a poignancy to the benefit of sharing—and sharing sooner rather than later. A support group offers you the opportunity to share and can save you from the needless suffering from bottled-up anger, fear, frustration, grief, and who knows what other emotional drains that this woman endured. As another survivor told us, she attended her first support group meeting 20 years after surgery and finally found the emotional release she needed. Twenty years! After all that time, a small group of sincerely compassionate survivors listened to her sob out her story for the first time, shared her burden, and lessened her load. It's the amazing power of a support group!

Over 1.3 million breast cancer survivors are roaming the land of the free and home of the brave. Many of them recommend that you join a support group to share emotions, concerns, information, and broad shoulders. Still, groups aren't for everyone. In this chapter, we'll talk about what a support group can do for you, whether you might or might not find support groups a good thing, and what kinds of support groups you might encounter, from face-to-face to long-distance.

For That Let-Down Feeling

When you join this particular sisterhood, it's no cause for joy. Like others in the 'hood, you may seek out strength by osmosis. You'll most likely find your sisters and that strength at your local support group.

Schwarzkopf's Troops

A good support group does just what its name implies: It gives you the support you need to get through the battle. After all, not even General Norman Schwarzkopf fought alone. So, in what form does the support come? Usually the group is made up of breast cancer survivors who can say to you, "Yes, we've walked the mile in your shoes and we know how you feel." No one else—not even your medical dream team—can really understand the way a fellow survivor understands.

Tales from the Trenches

One survivor who, out of desperation, founded a local support group told us, "It's my dream that every woman diagnosed come to at least one support group meeting. It's so important to know that you're not alone, that you get the solid encouragement that others have survived and survived quite well."

A good support group can and does provide many avenues of support, including but not limited to the following:

➤ Offers a time and place for you to meet positive breast cancer survivor role models.

➤ Provides a group of caring listeners with whom you can talk freely about your feelings and concerns but who will also respect your choice to remain silent.

➤ Provides support before diagnosis (when you're worried about a lump or an irregular mammogram), after diagnosis (when you've been shocked out of your bra), before, during, and after treatment (when the rest of the world stands off and wonders what to say to you); and during post-recovery adjustments (when everyone else assumes you're just fine and that breast cancer in your life is past tense).

➤ Lends a sense of reversal for the sometimes overwhelming feelings of isolation.

➤ Offers a place to share helpful hints for fighting the battle—concerning treatment, the side effects, and relating to family and friends —not so much advice, but rather this-has-worked-for-me discussions.

➤ Allows survivors to share ways of coping as well as sources of information, perhaps in the form of speakers or literature or newly discovered Web sites on the subject of breast cancer.

➤ Instills a new level of strength and understanding that you can take home to your family.

Take It from Us

Take it slow and easy. Coping with breast cancer, according to one survivor, parallels tossing a stone into a pond. "At first the cancer was the center ring from the splash; everything revolved around it. As the phases of treatment passed, the cancer ring moved farther and farther from the center. Now, it's still visible but way out on the edge of my pond. Other beautiful rings are at the center."

Routinely Nonroutine

Most support groups meet in a comfortable, convenient location, once a week or once or twice a month, usually on a weekday evening. Some groups are open only to members of the sisterhood; others accept survivors and their relatives. Some groups are small—6 or 8—and others function with 30 or so. Critics say a larger group inhibits personal interaction, but my personal experience suggests otherwise. You do have to have a group, after all, to have group interaction. Some women like bigger groups because while they don't necessarily want to share their own experiences, they take comfort from hearing others'.

Usually folks sit in a conversational arrangement, begin with introductions (name, date of diagnosis, treatments to date), and proceed with whatever topics of discussion come up. The group is usually guided (not led or directed) by a facilitator (or two), an unobtrusive person who guides discussion but never makes speeches. That person might be a professional medical person, group counselor, or a peer leader, someone who herself is a survivor. She remains neutral and noncensoring (and, therefore, first-timers can be startled by the frankness of topics), creating a safe environment for all discussion. She strives for balance by gently quieting someone who tries to take over and by offering others an opening to speak out.

Some groups are short-term, offering support only from diagnosis through treatment. All members of the group fall somewhere along the continuum, and folks having completed their treatment are no longer encouraged to attend. Some short-term groups are also topical, i.e., they meet for a specified time, like six weeks, to address in depth a given topic, like nutrition.

On the other hand, some groups are long-term, ongoing forums that offer support to survivors at every stage, from the discovery of a lump or a suspicious mammogram through diagnosis and treatment to life beyond. Participants may be newly diagnosed or 20-year survivors, and those undergoing treatment may be dealing with a pre-cancerous condition or the late stages of an inoperable condition.

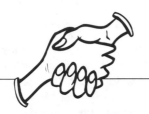

Helping Hand

If you feel guilty that your family needs your support but you don't have the strength to help them while you help yourself, then go for the strength in numbers and check out your local support group. Remember that you have to take care of yourself before you can take care of your family. Support group members know that and will help you find the way.

Some support groups meet annually for a week or a long weekend. Usually termed "retreats" at this point, they have tremendous potential for many undergoing the battle. One such retreat is housed on Madeline Island, the largest of the Apostle Islands in Lake Superior. Held in a condo-like setting, it's an annual affair for many survivors. You may want to ask about something similar in your neck of the woods.

Some groups have a set of bylaws, maintain membership rosters, collect dues, serve refreshments, have social functions, put out monthly or bimonthly newsletters, form committees, or any combination of the above. On the other hand, many groups do none of the above. So, what's the right answer? Any of the above. Because of their very wide range of definition, it's tough to say just what you'll find in your local support group. But let's make some guesses.

Finding a Bosom Buddy

How do you find out if your community has a support group? Ask your medical team. Nurses or other staffers will have names and phone numbers readily available. With the millions of other details on their minds, they may forget to offer those names and numbers, but I can guarantee you they'll be happy to get you the information if you ask.

If they have no suggestions or if for some reason you choose not to ask, you can call the American Cancer Society (1-800-ACS-2345), Y-Me (1-800-221-2141), or Sister's Network, Inc. (1-713-781-0255) for details about support groups in your area. Although the National Cancer Institute's Cancer Information Service (1-800-4-CANCER) doesn't have a list of support groups, it can refer you to certified mammography providers in your area. These folks, in turn, will probably have support group suggestions. Finally, also see Appendix C, "Support Groups," in the back of this book.

What will you find in your community? Depending on where you live, your support group may be different from or more successful than the one in the next town only because of the make-up of the group. Let's consider what you might find there.

If you live in a small community you may find a general cancer support group rather than a breast cancer support group. While certainly every kind of cancer differs from every other kind—in some cases dramatically so—still, cancer is cancer. You will find incredibly fine role models in these groups who fight the good fight all the while offering a broad shoulder for other battle-fatigued folks, perhaps including you.

In other communities, you may find breast cancer support groups connected with a specific medical facility. For instance, if there are three hospitals in your area, each may sponsor and/or affiliate with a support group. The advantage of facility-associated groups is that you and your sisters will be facing very similar treatments and follow-up regimes. The disadvantage is that you may not hear about the newest and best until you're way down the road. Sometimes competition is a good thing, even among medical facilities, because it keeps everybody on his toes—without stepping on yours.

Take It from Us

During a nearly 20-year study begun in 1976, Dr. David Spiegel at Stanford University discovered that women with metastatic cancer, Stage III or higher, who participated in a support group lived twice as long as those who opted not to. Studies also suggest support group participants enjoy a better quality of life. Surely that says something about human value in the long-term battle.

You may find that your local support group is affiliated with a national group, like the American Cancer Society, Y-Me, The Gathering Place, or Sisters Network, Inc. While there are obvious advantages with national affiliation (current information, readily available literature, visibility, and strength in numbers), there may be a disadvantage in your local situation. For instance, the group may necessarily become involved in fund-raising or may have a meeting format imposed on it. The bottom line is simple: You need to associate with a group that makes you comfortable.

Many support groups are not affiliated with any national organization or any medical facility. The group I participate in is of this form. The five survivors who organized it 11 years ago have kept the organizational plan simple and comfortable for all. We meet at a local library once a month and invite speakers (surgeons, oncologists, plastic surgeons, nutritionists, nurses, etc.) every other month. We begin promptly at 7:00 P.M. and end promptly at 9:00 P.M., and never have refreshments (so no one ever has to do any work). We wear name tags by way of introduction to first-timers (and there are always several present). We have no membership list or membership dues, no bylaws, no mailing lists, no committees, never release our names to the public or to any individual, and never permit anyone to attend our meetings unless they, too, are breast cancer survivors. We share stories and questions and the latest research. We share tears and fears and laughter and joy. We celebrate life, each other, and our dear sisters. The local founders named the group Woman to Woman because they felt that said it all.

Tales from the Trenches

DeeAnna, who works for an East Coast publishing company and spends much of her work week flying to and from major airports all over the country, couldn't fit a traditional support group into her hectic schedule. Instead, she said, "We had our own little informal support group at work. News travels fast in the office, so as soon as I was diagnosed, here came my new bosom buddies. I didn't even know until that moment that some had been through the battle. They were so vital, so wonderful, so inspirational. Unfortunately, a new sister joined our group last month; now I can offer her the same support the others have offered me."

Another group organizer told me, however, that their plan is quite different. They're in a small community, so the support group is open to anyone connected with any kind of cancer, including caregivers and partners as well as survivors. They meet in a church lounge that has a living-room-like setting and low lighting. In spite of the relaxed setting, because both men and women participate in the group, some first-timers hesitate to say the word "breast." Since the size of the community dictates the structure, however, folks soon get over any inhibitions.

The Long Reach

What if you don't find a support group in your hometown? Short of organizing your own group—and why not? You know you're not alone—you can find long-distance support. Okay, so it's not face to face, but maybe you'll even find it easier to talk to a total stranger about some of those really personal details you don't want to discuss with your own doctor, your dear husband, your sister (with whom you've shared absolutely everything over the years), or your best friend. If you know, in fact, you'll never meet this person in the grocery aisles or stand next to her in line at the bank or the post office, you may find it incredibly liberating, especially if you're one who tends not to share much of your personal life with anyone. Where do you find these long-distance support groups?

Earlier we talked about breast cancer hot lines (see Chapter 3, "Learning a New Vocabulary"). You may want to turn again to them.

In addition, however, you'll find chat groups and Web sites with both open and *closed discussion groups*. Here are some, listed in alphabetical order, that you may want to investigate:

➤ AMC Cancer Research Center's Cancer Information and Counseling Line at 1-800-525-3777 for easy-to-understand answers to questions about cancer; also equipped for deaf and hearing-impaired callers.

➤ Canadian Breast Cancer Network at www.cbcn.ca, a survivor-directed, national network of organizations and individuals.

➤ Celebrating Life at www.celebratinglife.org with information about breast cancer for African-American women and women of color.

➤ CHESS (Comprehensive Health Enhancement Support System), including a confidential discussion group and ask-the-experts, both protected by passwords; call 1-800-361-5481 or 1-888-553-5036 to find the provider nearest you that can give you access to chess.chsra.wisc.edu/bc.

➤ *Listserves* available free of charge by e-mail; subscribe by sending an e-mail message that reads only "Subscribe Breast Cancer" (minus the quotation marks) to LISTSERV@morgan.usc.mun.ca and see cure.medinfo.org/lists/cancer/bc-about.html for more information.

➤ SHARE (Self-Help for Women with Breast or Ovarian Cancer) at www.sharecancersupport.org for peer-led support groups with a hotline at 212-382-2111 where survivors answer the phone (for Spanish, 212-719-4454).

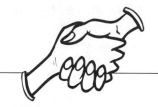

Helping Hand

Use caution on the Internet. If you subscribe to a computer listserve or post questions or responses to a bulletin board, remember that it's open to everyone, including, unfortunately, some kooks. You'll probably want to avoid sharing any highly personal details, always use a code name, and disguise your location.

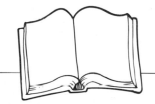

From the Book

A **listserve** is made up of a group of folks who share a common interest and who communicate by e-mail; every listserve subscriber receives all other subscribers' queries and posts, usually free. A **closed discussion group,** accessed at the sponsoring organization's Web site, requires a password for participation and thus protects privacy.

Surprisingly, in spite of the facelessness of phone, e-mail, and Internet support groups, many of the groups are highly personal. The CHESS site, to which the local breast center provided me access, is a perfect case in point. We all use code names; we're scattered across the country; we can—and do—talk about absolutely anything. We've asked one another about every imaginable experience: which books were most helpful, what happened with reconstruction, how the nipple tattoo went, how to deal with loss of libido, when to go back to work, whether you have sex with or without your wig, what to say when people ask how you're feeling, where to find great bras, what drugs helped best for nausea during chemo, which products best ease the radiation "sunburn," which vaginal estrogen-free lubricants are safe and successful, how to feel pretty when you otherwise feel ugly, and what to do when you're at your wit's end with the kids, the house, the husband, and the rest of the world.

I don't know a single woman personally, not even by full name, but I have learned from them and found their warm support nurturing and as comforting as my local support group. The big difference: I can access CHESS 24/7, but my local group meets only once a month. At 2:00 A.M. when I can't sleep, I can log on, read messages, moan and bitch to objective fellow survivors, and, the next day, get a whole raft of suggestions for getting to sleep the next night. It's like an all-night pajama party.

Tales from the Trenches

Positive attitude is essential in this battle. As two-year survivor Letta puts it, "The good days are great and the bad days are good because you're here to get through it and turn it into a great day again." She reminds us that we must "Find the good in things and make it positive. You have a limited amount of energy. Use it to get better, not to feel sorry for yourself." Letta turned to her extended family and church for her personal support group.

Skip the Pity Party

Historically, women talk, sharing over coffee, at PTA meetings, on the phone. We're storytellers—to our children and, culturally, to the world. We talk about how we feel, what we're thinking, what we're fretting about. Men don't do that. Thus, support groups tend to have a strong feminine appeal from the sharing/talking angle. On the other hand, we've been taught to be caregivers. To participate in a support group is contrary to giving, because it involves a great deal of taking. Many long-term participants, however, say they feel a tremendous sense of satisfaction in reaching out to others in the group. So while you may take more from the group than you give on the first few go-rounds, chances are you'll put back more than you took over the long haul. Nevertheless, a support group is only as strong as its individuals combined. While a great deal depends on the facilitator's expertise in guiding without stifling, some groups are less effective than others are.

Warning Signs

Certain support group actions might justifiably scare you away. Be cautious if you find any of the following:

➤ **Group members giving medical advice.** Even if some members are, indeed, licensed medical folks, they should never do more than suggest options or recommend appointments with specialists. The facilitator has the responsibility to get the group back on the right path.

➤ **Doctor bashing.** No human is perfect, of course, and doctors, like anyone else, can make mistakes. To undermine the skill and expertise of doctors in general, however, does no one any good.

➤ **Predominant woe-is-me attitude.** Everyone gets down once in a while, but one purpose of a support group is to help folks brush aside the pity and hit the positive. Thus, when a group member is down, others in the group should be offering a let-us-help-you attitude, not a can-you-top-this-sad-story attitude.

Tales from the Trenches

Some folks deal with the emotional crisis of breast cancer not by pouring out their emotions to a support group but by working them out with physical activity. When 10-year survivor Cordelia was diagnosed, "My five children came flying in all distraught, held serious discussions in the backyard, and looked like they had gathered for a wake. I threw myself into cooking massive amounts of food and had trouble putting down all the fuss." By choosing the physical activity route, however, Cordelia kept her emotions tucked away—away from her family as well as herself. If you choose the physical activity route, be sure you slow down enough to deal with your emotional well-being. Otherwise, as Cordelia ultimately did, you may well pay a big price later.

➤ **Advocating alternative medicine to the exclusion of traditional treatment.** While many complementary therapies are legitimate (you'll find some recommended in this book), it's a terrible risk to suggest they supplant rather that support traditional methods.

➤ **Cynical atmosphere.** Although cynicism is part of some people's personalities, you don't need to be subjected to it now.

➤ **Rude behavior.** A group provides support only if every participant's voice is heard and respected. Tact and courtesy are the order of the day even when the survivor reaching out is having a bad moment.

Stumbling Blocks

A good support group meeting leaves you feeling that you've been somehow enriched. No matter how wonderful a support group may be, however, some folks just aren't groupies. Maybe you're one. Still, maybe for the first time in your life, you'll actually find it advantageous to have a change of heart.

Stumbling blocks litter the way, however, and you may want to give a test kick or two to some of them. For instance, maybe you really fear any new or different situation. Perhaps because you don't know what to expect, you think the folks in support groups are sick, crying, and dying. Far from it. In fact, participants at most support group meetings share a great deal of zest for living and strive to help others feel the same way.

Tales from the Trenches

Sometimes support comes from individuals. "When I was diagnosed," one survivor wrote, "the surgeon gave me phone numbers of two women with similar diagnoses who were in the midst of treatments. I called both. The first, who had had a mastectomy three weeks earlier, was just heading out the door for her daily two-mile jog. The second, who was in the midst of chemo, wasn't home, but her husband said she'd be back in a couple of hours, that she'd gone to take her grandchildren to a soccer game and was going to stop off for burgers afterward. Wow! To hear that! Talk about coming out of isolation! Those two gals were wonderful support."

Maybe you're a bit insecure talking about anything so personal as breast cancer. True, before Happy Rockefeller and Betty Ford came out of the breast cancer closet, it was a hush-hush term that nobody spoke aloud outside family—and then not among the male members of the family. Well, folks, the times have changed. Women have learned that if we don't talk about breast cancer and talk about it plenty, the politicians (mostly male) will never allocate the necessary funds for breast cancer research. Still, I understand—it's your breast and your breast cancer you'll be talking about. That's really personal. But remember, you don't have to say a word. Nobody will push you to say anything, not even your name if that's the way you want it. Maybe after you listen to others for a meeting or two, you'll feel more comfortable. If not, stick to the mute mode.

For some folks, reaching out is a big challenge. Maybe you're one of them. Interestingly enough, however, some experts suggest that the women who participate in support groups tend to be take-charge people. While studies do prove that those who attend support groups live longer and enjoy a better quality of life, consider another angle to the same idea: Take-charge gals tend to recover faster than those who see themselves as victims. If a support group helps you change your perspective, then, aha! Look what you'll have done for yourself.

Some folks say that a support group lets them focus their concerns for a definite period each week or month. Whatever you're holding onto in the back of your mind can come to the forefront, get attention, perhaps reach resolution or even closure. That's not a bad result for a couple hours of your time.

Okay, it's true that not everyone needs a support group. Some survivors told us, "It's gone; treatment's over; I'm done with it. I don't want to think about it or talk about it. Ever again." As long as you're not bottling up feelings and hiding behind tough talk, go for it. But you can't know whether a support group works for you unless you check it out. Survivors who have walked in your combat boots have a keen understanding of your greatest fears.

Finally, understand that no matter the strength of the group and your relationship with it, it can never take the place of psychotherapy or counseling. When the scale starts tipping in the wrong direction, get the professional help you need.

Friendships formed in support groups sometimes continue for years. You're meeting folks with whom you share a very special part of your life; your only common thread may be breast cancer; but your battles together create a bond others will never understand. You'll hear them talk about feelings and concerns that you thought only you were experiencing. All in all, it's not really so different from the camaraderie military groups continue to experience years after the war has become a chapter in the history books.

May you have many happy victory parties with your comrades!

The Least You Need to Know

➤ Support groups help you step out of isolation and find broad shoulders among those who have gone through the fight before.

➤ By definition, local support groups vary dramatically, from size to philosophy to affiliation.

➤ In the absence of a local support group, you can find support by phone or Web.

➤ Some folks avoid any connection with support groups, formal or otherwise.

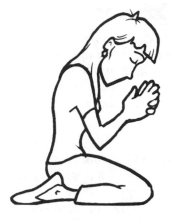

Chapter 18

Mind and Body: Spiritual Support

In This Chapter

➤ Connective healing—the mind and body

➤ What alternatives are available to you

➤ The "how to's" of alternative medicines

➤ Knowing what belief system works for you

➤ Calling upon your own strength

Have you ever seen the Hope Diamond? It's at the Smithsonian, but not simply resting on a velvet cloth inside an easily accessible glass case. Instead, it's set far back in a wall behind many panes of glass. To say the least, it's not easy to get an up-close and personal look at it, but people still stand in line just to view it from afar. Getting to see what lies within all the protective barriers seems to be worth the effort.

Isn't it the same with what's inside us? Aren't our hearts and souls buried behind layers and layers of protective covering? While we need these layers of protective covering, the bottom line is "it's what's inside that counts," and keeping what's inside whole, safe, and together gives the layers of protection a reason for being. It's a package deal!

In this chapter, we will discuss a few methods that may help you find some inner strength to get you through the challenges that lie ahead, including meditation, visualization, hypnosis, and faith and prayer. Even if you don't have an abiding belief in any or all of these methods, read on: You may find that one or more will work to help soothe your soul and focus your energy.

The Incredible Mind-Body Connection

In laboratories and psychiatrists' offices around the world, scientists are working to discover the intricacies of what's become known as the "mind-body connection" and, in particular, of how the emotions, faith, and attitude influence health among cancer survivors. Learning to focus your emotions is an important part of your recovery, working together with the medical treatments you'll undergo.

The mind-body connection appears to be located in the immune system. As you may remember from Chapter 10, "Chemotherapy: Cruel to Be Kind," the immune system works to protect us from viruses, bacteria, and internal abnormalities such as cancer cell development. Recent studies show that stress can affect the way the immune system functions. For instance, stress may affect the way the body metabolizes glucose, which can lead to depression, as well as destroy certain immune system cells, which reduces our ability to fight infection. Consequently, by combining both medial therapy and relaxation or meditative techniques, we'll have the best chance of success in fighting cancer or any other condition.

The spiritual techniques of meditation, visualization, hypnosis, therapeutic touch, yoga, and even laughter have been practiced in some cultures for centuries. While there is little documented proof that these methods lead directly to improved health, we do know that they cause us to relax and to focus, which helps to relieve pain, eliminate stress, and help give us just an overall better sense of well-being.

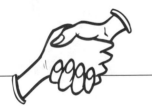

Helping Hand

Take an active part in the growth and maintenance of your inner being. Think, say, meditate, and pray. Give yourself the freedom to hope and offer other people hope as well. Hope heals.

Whether or not you believe that these techniques actually work, you'll probably find that using one or more of them will add to the quality of your life and bolster your ability to be proactive in your healing. You may even find that they help you conquer feelings of helplessness and give you a stronger sense of control.

After you've received your physical diagnosis and created a treatment plan with your doctor, it may behoove you to take the time to consider your inner, emotional self and what it will take to survive this ordeal.

Focusing on calming your mind and spirit through one or more of the techniques described in this chapter can help keep you optimistic and strong. Working with our own spirituality is a growth process that seldom has an end, and it is never too late to get started.

Meditation: A Pause That Refreshes

Meditation, quiet, silence, and calm are words that cause us to think of peace. To incorporate these methods into your therapy will hopefully help you beat fear, lessen suffering, and, most important, give you hope.

Tales from the Trenches

A woman I know got involved in meditation 20 years ago. As is true today, all patients were hospitalized during chemo, but mainly because the treatments almost always caused severe vomiting. This woman realized that the quieter she was, the less she vomited, but didn't realize she was learning to meditate. She believes that many people meditate without even knowing it. It may not be the "lotus position with ooming" type; it may just be something as simple as sitting still and focusing on one particular thought or issue.

Meditation is a technique that helps you to focus on something other than the here and now, the everyday world, in order to eliminate the chaos in your mind. Focusing on one thing, such as your breathing, helps eliminate some of the chaotic thoughts that are going through your head.

Dr. Mitchell Gaynor, in his book *Healing Essence,* says that meditation "requires you to be alert and aware of your thoughts and feelings without judgment or resistance; be free of your own criticism." Does this mean that meditation can cause you to be more accepting of yourself and learn to let go of what you cannot control? If this is true, meditation may be a way to heal your inner self by knowing the real you.

Meditation is a good way for anyone to begin and end a day. Quieting the mind and ridding ourselves of chaotic thoughts should heal the body and the soul. Begin practicing with a very simple meditation: Find a quiet place, free of distractions and noise. Find a position that is comfortable for you. Close your eyes and begin to focus on your breathing. Imagine a particular scene or say a word over and over again. Sit quietly for as long as you can; if a distraction interrupts you, begin again. Work up to about 20 minutes each session, once or twice a day.

Meditation is not a complicated activity. Here are a few tips to get you started:

➤ Pick a time of day when you have fewer interruptions than normal.

➤ Start by meditating for about 5 minutes at a time, then slowly work up to about 20 minutes or more a session.

➤ If you can meditate in two sessions—one at the beginning and one at the end of every day—you might find it enjoyable.

➤ Concentrate on your breathing.

➤ Think positive thoughts about health, love, healing, acceptance, success, happiness, wisdom, hope, and peace (to name just a few!).

➤ Remain as quiet and as focused for as long as you can.

Visualization: My Mind's Eye

Visualization involves creating a positive picture in your mind of an event or a process you want to accomplish. One successful visualization technique used by many cancer survivors involves the old Pac Man game: Survivors visualize these little creatures eating up their cancer cells as it runs through their bodies. You may want to see your antibodies duking it out with your cancer cells and winning the fight against your disease. You may want to see yourself 30 years in your future standing on the deck of a ship with your grandchildren. Or you may even want to see yourself with a full head of hair and a good color in your cheeks walking in some type of marathon.

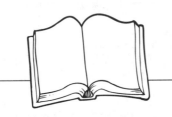

From the Book

An **image** is an optically (eye) formed duplicate or representation of an object, or something that closely resembles another. It is also defined as a mental picture of something not real or present.

Here are a few tips to help you learn to visualize:

➤ Relax, and let your mind go blank.

➤ Think about what you want to visualize.

➤ Begin to picture in as much detail as possible the image you are trying to create: the clothes, the surroundings, the people, the day, etc.

➤ Begin forming the words you want to hear—stating things in the positive, not the negative. Even eliminate the word *not*, i.e., "I am cancer-free," not "I do not have cancer." Sometimes negative words get a foothold we do not want them to have.

➤ Replay the vision or image in your head as many times as possible.

➤ In your mind and soul, believe it is true and not just a mind game.

In Napoleon Hill's book *Think and Grow Rich,* he states that "whatever a man can conceive and believe, he can achieve." I think that goes for us women, too. Remember, your purpose is to see, in as much detail and as clearly as possible, what you want to happen.

Tales from the Trenches

Between my diagnosis and my surgery, I spent a great deal of time visualizing. My *image* was cancer cells (in the form of crabs—like the zodiac sign for cancer) in a big net. They were trying to get out, but couldn't. My image was on keeping them contained. When my lymph node results came back clear, I figured I did a pretty good job of containing the cancer cells. Others visualize the antibodies as little boxers just beating the heck out of the cancer cells and finally killing them. Use an image that works for you. That way, it will seem more real to you.

Hypnosis: You're Getting Sleepy

Like meditation and visualization, hypnosis is not a new technique. As a matter of fact, hypnosis has been around for more than 200 years. Many patients, including those with cancer, take classes in self-*hypnosis* for pain control and to eliminate other unpleasant side effects. Hypnosis can also help alleviate stress.

Hypnosis involves the alteration of an individual's mental state by a suggestion provided by a trained therapist—although you can learn to do it yourself with training. When you're "hypnotized," you're actually in a state of deep relaxation; your mind is at rest, but alert. In this relaxed/alert state of mind your ability to respond to suggestions increases.

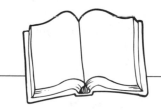

From the Book

A definition of **hypnosis** is "a sleeplike state resulting from a procedure of some type (you're getting sleepy) suggesting things that seem to be the result of the suggestion."

The hypnotherapist helps you become relaxed in any number of ways. Some use a metronome that makes a loud, repetitive, even ticking sound, others repeat certain words, still others have you focus on an object. After a time, you become transfixed, or so focused on the word, sound or object, that you do not recognize or respond to any other outside source. Then, in this trance-like state of mind, the hypnotherapist plants a suggestion in your mind. It could be something as simple as "I hate

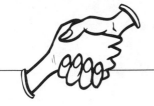

Helping Hand

Find strength wherever you can. Chemo was truly tough for Carolyn. After the first treatment, she knew she needed all the help she could get to get through it. During the rest of the treatments, she asked her church group to go to prayer for her at the exact time of her injection. "Injections two through six were much easier to handle. The prayers gave me strength."

cigarettes," if you're trying to quit smoking. Then, when you next encounter a cigarette or the craving for one, your mind will replay the suggestion to you. If the suggestion is strong enough, you'll believe it, and then be better able to break the bad habit.

In controlling pain or illness, your hypnotherapist may suggest "heal," "relax," or "alive." Again, a word that you can relate to or that is real for you. Or, in the case of self-hypnosis, you repeat the word over and over or listen to the repetitive sound. It is the focus that helps provide the benefits from hypnosis.

Hypnosis works for some but not for all. About 9 out of 10 people can be hypnotized, and some can even learn and practice self-hypnosis. If you'd like to try, ask your doctor to recommend qualified hypnotherapists in your area. To learn more about hypnosis in general, you can check out hypnosis.com for some basic information. And keep in mind that hypnotic suggestions seem to weaken over time; consequently, you may want to revisit your hypnotist to repeat and reinforce the suggestion.

Faith and Prayer

Faith is simply a "confident belief in a truth, value, or trustworthiness of a person, idea, or thing." You can rest your faith in medicine, in a higher power, in your own ability to fight and to heal, or in a combination of these things. Faith covers a lot of territory!

Faith is also intricately linked to prayer. One study involved coronary patients at San Francisco General Hospital. For 10 months, half of a group of 393 patients had people (unknown to them) praying for them, while members of the other half of the group did not have anyone praying for them.

The prayer groups consisted of people of various religions who were given only the most general information about their subjects and their health. The groups were asked to pray each day (no instructions on how to pray) for the patients. Each patient assigned to the prayer group had from five to seven people praying for him or her.

The results: The patients who had people praying for them were five times less likely to need antibiotics and three times less likely to have pulmonary edema than those who were not prayed for. Those who were prayed for did not need endotracheal intubation (artificial airways) and fewer prayed-for patients died.

Although the faith involved here was that of the those who prayed and not (necessarily) of those who were prayed for, this study clearly shows the power of faith and prayer.

If you have faith in a supreme being, or the power of hypnosis, or the power and benefits of meditation, the point is that you have faith in something. It may even be faith in yourself to be an active part of your healing.

A quote from Emerson reminds us that "they conquer who believe they can." We have already talked of the value of hope. Now if you want a double dose of something extra effective, try putting hope, faith, and prayer together. Hope helps start your journey or your road to recovery; faith keeps you going.

None of us knows for certain how much time we have. We may think that we don't have time for months and years of therapy sessions. We may need and want to get down to our core a little sooner. We may want to bypass the protective layers and see that Hope Diamond up close and personal.

Personal Strength

There are times when you will want an entire army helping you fight your cancer, including but not limited to your doctors, partner, support group, and medicine. There is strength in numbers! But there will also be times when you want to be "one on one" with your cancer and just knock the living daylights out of it. If you could put on a pair of boxing gloves and climb into the ring with your cancer, because you are so angry, there will only be one survivor, and that survivor won't be the cancer.

You may never understand the why of your breast cancer. You may simply need to go on with your life, and going on with your life takes personal strength.

You have had to learn to be strong for your family, friends, and co-workers. And, by now, you have learned that you have to be strong for yourself, too. All these people care for you and want to help, but the bottom line is that unless someone else has gone through what you are going through, they

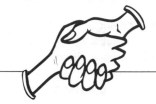

Helping Hand

Always remember—even as you pass through surgery, chemotherapy, radiation therapy, and hormone therapy—that "this too shall pass."

Tales from the Trenches

Penny not only wanted to "participate in her recovery;" she wanted to pick up the banner and lead the charge. She wanted to be the "Joan of Arc" of cancer. She was "Penny of Pittsburgh," and she did all she could, with others and by herself, to fight this disease.

217

really will never know what it is like. And, you never want them to know. The nice thing about this kind of strength is that you do not have to go to a gym and sweat or feel the burn. Women gain personal strength differently. Some read the stories of the women in the Bible. Now there are some pretty strong women! They not only bucked the "good ol' boys" system, they risked their lives in doing so.

Others gain strength by expressing their inner being in different manners. One woman rescued dogs and trained them to work in the hospices. Another became a part-time comedian (although I think most of us are that). Still another took art lessons. You begin to find that your world is a reflection of you. (It's call mirroring.) If you are angry, so is your world. If you are happy, so is your world. If you are strong, so is your world.

Claiming your personal strength, I think, will help you face the challenges that await you. Strength has a place in all things.

Take It from Us

Don't neglect everyday joy. Keep a positive attitude. Positive people have better immune systems. Smile. Find some joy in every day. Take up ballet for exercise ... the music is great, too. Plant a garden. Grow an orchid. Take walks. Have picnics.

The Least You Need to Know

➤ What works for one does not work for all. Find what works for you.

➤ Visualization, meditation, and hypnosis are just a few of the techniques available to help you tap into, and calm, your inner strength.

➤ Your attitude affects your immune system—the one system in the body that you need on your side at this time in your life!

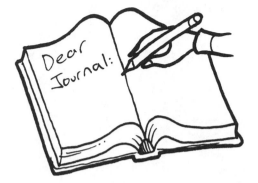

Chapter 19

Support Tools

In This Chapter

➤ Print and nonprint sources of inspiration

➤ The why and how of journaling

➤ Asking for help from family and friends

➤ Professional support for the tough times

How do you stay positive, remain in control, and continue to be there for your family? (Especially when you'd rather go have a good cry, feel out of control, and need your family to be there for you?) That's a big question with no easy answer. But survivors have shared their stories, saying, "This worked for me." So in addition to the formal and informal support discussed in the previous two chapters, you may want to check out a few other tools of the support trade.

In this chapter, we'll take a look at some books, tapes, and movies that offer support. We'll consider the purposes for and techniques of journaling as a form of support. Then, because it's often so hard for us to ask for help, we'll figure out easy ways to do so. Finally, we'll take a look at what professional support is available to you if and when the time comes.

Another Voice

Think about these words from an ancient Sanskrit proverb:

> Look to this day,
> For it is life,
> The very life of life.
> In its brief course lie all
> The realities and verities of existence,
> The bliss of growth,
> The splendor of action,
> The glory of power—
> For yesterday is but a dream,
> And tomorrow is only a vision.
> But today, well lived,
> Makes every yesterday a dream of happiness
> And every tomorrow a vision of hope.
> Look well, therefore, to this day.

What wonderful words of inspiration and encouragement! The words of an accomplished motivational writer or speaker can lift us across the abyss of gloom and doom and land us lightly in the land of waterfalls and rainbows. Whether the words are as old as papyrus or as fresh as this morning's dew, they spark inspiration.

Although there are literally thousands of books and tapes that fall into the category of "support tools," not quite so many offer the gender-specific, subject-specific support tool you're looking for in the midst of your battle with breast cancer. When we asked survivors for their favorites, they bombarded us with lists, and a few authors and titles popped up as regularly as Saturday morning after Friday night. The top 10, in alphabetical order:

➤ Ayers, Lauren K., *The Answer Is Within You* (Crossroad Publishing Company, 1994)

➤ Brack, Pat and Ben, *Moms Don't Get Sick* (Melius, 1990)

➤ Brinker, Nancy, with Catherine McEvily Harris, *The Race Is Won One Step at a Time: Every Woman's Guide to Taking Charge of Breast Cancer & My Personal Story* (The Summit Publishing Group, 1995)

Take It from Us

Don't think you have to do it all yourself. Many folks say that inspiration comes from within. Well, to an extent, that's true, but when you're diagnosed with breast cancer, you feel like somebody kicked everything out of you. So, for the duration, at least, consider other sources of support. Then you can use 100 percent of your energy for healing.

➤ Canfield, Jack, and Mark Victor Hansen, *Chicken Soup for the Soul* (Health Communications, Inc., 1993 to present) (A series of titles)

➤ Carlson, Richard, *Don't Sweat the Small Stuff Collection* (Simon & Schuster and Little, Brown, 1997 to present) (Books and tapes)

➤ Halvorson-Boyd, Glenna, and Lisa K. Hunter, *Dancing in Limbo: Making Sense of Life After Cancer* (Jossey-Bass Publishers, 1995)

➤ Rollin, Betty, *First You Cry* (HarperCollins Publishers, Inc., 1992) (Book and film)

➤ Siegel, Bernie, *The Bernie Siegel Audio Collection* including *How to Live Between Office Visits* (1993); *Peace, Love and Healing* (1989); and *Love, Medicines, and Miracles* (1986) (Also in book form)

➤ *Voices of Healing Audio Series, Conversations with Breast Cancer Survivors and Those Who Love Them* (Voice Arts Publishing Company, 1997)

➤ Yalog, Ina L., ed., *Straight from the Heart: Letters of Hope and Inspiration from Survivors of Breast Cancer* (Kensington Publishing Corp., 1996)

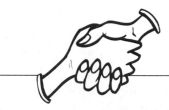

Helping Hand

Laughter is one of the best coping mechanisms. Hit the video rental store and go straight to the comedy section. Rent the silliest slapstick you can find, invite a few friends to share in the merriment, and giggle until you jiggle.

Tales from the Trenches

As you listen and/or read for inspiration or motivation, jot down those on-target phrases that you really relate to. One survivor said she used sticky notes to post reminders of inspirational ideas all through her house—on the bathroom mirror, on the cabinet doors, on the refrigerator, on the telephone, on the TV remote—anyplace she'd likely see these regular reminders that life is precious.

In addition, why not keep an ongoing list in your notebook or journal?

In addition to these favorites, find others at your library or bookstore under the headings of alternative medicine, self-improvement, inspiration (usually part of religion), or in the audio section. You'll find lots of choices.

Journal Jottings: Jabs and Gems

While we often turn to other's words for support and inspiration, our own words usually carry a superior value. Really, it's true! Before you throw up your hands and swear you cannot, will not, and do not want to write, hang with me for a few more paragraphs.

Many survivors recommend keeping a *journal*. If you decide to keep a journal, we recommend that you use a different book than the one in which you keep your medical records, names and phone numbers, and questions and answers. It's also different from a diary, which often simply records daily events. There's no prescribed format for a journal, and folks write irregularly, sometimes every day, sometimes every few days, sometimes weekly. So it has no set form, no set writing time, and—most important—no audience but you. It's just as personal as your notebook, diary, or favorite underwear.

From the Book

A **journal** is a periodical record of thoughts, emotions, and reactions to the writer's experiences. It's different from a diary because it usually doesn't record daily events in a chronology, the way a diary does.

Right Write Rite?

So why keep a journal? Consider the following reasons:

Maybe you're a really private person and can't comfortably share your thoughts and feelings with others, especially strangers in a support group. Still, you'd like an outlet for your thoughts. That idea may have shades of *The Bridges of Madison County,* but maybe in your small community there's absolutely no one you can turn to who would understand what you're going through.

Maybe you feel pressured to remain strong in the eyes of your family and friends when inside you're coming unglued. You can scream, bitch, curse, pout, and vent your anger and frustration all you want in a journal: No one else needs to hear or know.

Maybe you find introspection a great way to cope. By writing about your feelings, opinions, beliefs, hopes, fears, questions, problems, and accomplishments, you can actually promote wellness. If you get the anger out, examine your depression, and step right into the thick of your emotions, you're likely to help yourself put much of it behind you—behind the covers of your journal.

Tales from the Trenches

Nine years ago, Helen journaled her way through breast cancer. "When I wrote it [my journal], it never entered my mind I'd make it for nine years. Now I see no reason why it won't be nine more—maybe several times over. It's so positive for me when I re-read it now."

Her only previous experience with breast cancer had been with folks who, before the advent of regular mammograms, discovered the cancer too late. "My journal was comforting. It let me get rid of my anger. I said things there I couldn't say to my family. I had to be Superwoman to my family; I'm real in my journal."

Maybe you need to celebrate life, to take note of all the little things that make you smile: your granddaughter's dimples, your son's brown eyes, the first daffodil, a cardinal in the snow, a cup of green tea, your worn wedding band, your grandmother's gravy boat, those little things that define your life. Your journal lets you make as many lists as you'd like, every day, if you wish.

Maybe you need to get organized. Some of us are veteran list-makers, but a journal lets us write not only the list but remind ourselves why the to-do list amounts to anything more than a hill of beans.

Finally, maybe you just want to be able to explain more clearly to your family and friends how you feel or what you're thinking. By writing your thoughts on paper first, you can go through a sort of dress rehearsal of what you want to say, crossing out, rewriting, rewording, until you have something like what you want to say face to face. Then, when the time comes, you're more fluent.

Get Set, Go!

Maybe you can see that a journal might really offer you some much-needed support. So how do you get started?

You need nothing more than a notebook and pen or pencil. Some folks buy beautiful journals at the specialty stationery shops or bookstores, and I have to admit I love writing in those gorgeously bound books. They make me feel really special. But I also feel some sort of hidden pressure to use perfect penmanship and the same color ink on every page. Maybe that's okay, but you might enjoy writing just as much in a spiral-bound from Wal-Mart. Of course, if your fingers fly across the keyboard faster than you can push a pen, you may prefer journaling at the keyboard.

Some folks say they need the discipline of setting aside a certain afternoon or evening to do their writing. Others say, "No, write when you feel like it." See what works for you. But no doubt you'll discover many different reasons to want to write: when you have an overwhelming fear that the chemo isn't working; when you've reached a milestone, like losing your hair (or having it start to grow back); when something has upset you or sets you down, like the insensitive sister-in-law who asks if you've updated your last will and testament; or when the world overflows with such incredibly wonderful sunsets and lush wildflowers that you just have to make note.

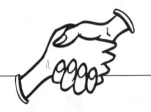

Helping Hand

If you have trouble getting your thoughts on paper, try using a tape recorder. Imagine yourself talking on the phone to yourself. If you want to transcribe the tape into a paper journal later, fine. In the meantime, your journal is auditory!

Whether or not you keep your journal under lock and key, tucked away in a drawer, or buried in a secretly coded file on your hard drive, knowing that it's personal relieves you of any pressure of writing well or even accurately. You don't care if you misspell a few words or don't apply every punctuation rule that Miss Beanbottom tried to teach you in seventh grade.

Along for the Ride

If you need help getting started, try a few of these suggestions:

➤ List words that describe the feelings you've had in the past day (week, month).

➤ Imagine where you want to be a year from now. Tell about it.

➤ Finish this sentence: "I'm most worried about …"

➤ Finish this sentence: "I'm most happy about …"

➤ Describe how you felt when you were first diagnosed and compare it with how you feel now.

➤ If there was one message you could send loud and clear to your husband/son/daughter/best friend, what would it be?

The more you get in the habit of writing, the more often you'll catch yourself thinking, "I should write that in my journal." You may find yourself toting your journal along to chemo or when you figure you'll be stuck in a waiting room somewhere.

… And You Shall Receive

Sometimes support tools come in the form of people. You'll hear folks say, "Let me know if I can do anything," and you shrug off the seeming hollowness of the offer.

Well, sisters, stop the shrugging. You'll likely need someone to run the kids here and there, baby-sit, run errands, rake leaves, cut the grass, or cook a few meals. If you're married and your wonderful guy takes on the role of Mr. Mom, you are blessed. But keep in mind that he's under nearly as much stress as you are, so don't hesitate to ask others to help with the errands.

When someone has said, "Let me know," that's your opening line. No harm in saying, "You know, I'd just love it if you'd take me shopping for a wig." Or, "I'd love someone to play cards with me next Thursday while I'm getting my chemo. Would you?" Or, "Charlie's trying to get the yard cut and trimmed, but I really need him to go with me to the oncologist. Do you know someone who could help Charlie so that he can help me?"

Tales from the Trenches

Because food is an ongoing daily topic even when you don't want it, survivors share some great ideas: One told about her sorority alum sisters who took turns bringing a family meal every evening for a week after each chemo treatment. Another had the same experience with her church group. One told about a thoughtful friend who gift-wrapped 20 area carryout menus and checked daily to see if, when, and where she could pick up and deliver. Another noted that sometimes the casseroles friends brought were too large for her and her husband, so she'd divide it and freeze half—but only on days she couldn't convince her friends to stay for the meal they'd brought.

Because we gals have mostly been caregivers, we sometimes have a hard time either accepting help or knowing what to ask for when others want to help. If you fall into any of these categories, try one of the following:

➤ If someone is willing to prepare and bring in a meal, invite her (and maybe her family) to stay and eat with you. Not only do you have a ready-to-eat meal but you'll also have stimulating, change-of-scenery conversation.

➤ When someone offers to help, ask her to pick up something from a carryout menu and join you for lunch or dinner.

➤ On good days, when you feel like getting out, accept someone's offer to help by inviting them to go with you to a museum, art gallery, restaurant, or drive along the lake, through the park, or around the neighborhood.

Take It from Us

On occasion the offer "I'll do whatever you need" turns up empty. One friend asked to take me to lunch. With a drain hanging from me and no means yet to fill out one side of my bra, I wasn't quite ready for public appearances. "Give me a little time; then we'll go," I suggested. She never called back. My fault or hers? I'll never know.

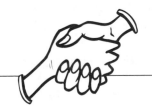

Helping Hand

One wonderfully thoughtful gal gave her friend a set of home-made "coupons" to be redeemed at will. The coupons included, among others, one for Help with Housework, Call Me Collect, I'll Take the Kids, Lunch on Me, Movie Matinee, A Walk in the Mall, Prayer Support, I'll Bring You a Home-Cooked Meal, Free Book, and Music Therapy.

➤ If someone asks "What can I do?" ask her to go with you to your next appointment and read to you while you're taking chemo. When you share books, you share a part of life and lots of treasured moments.

➤ When there's shopping to be done for birthday and holiday gifts, accept help when someone offers. Ask if they'll pick up nine gift certificates for your grandchildren's Christmas gifts. Voilà! Your shopping is done!

➤ If someone is willing to spend an afternoon, ask her to go with you to shop for something femininely pretty, like a lacy camisole or ruffled nightie.

➤ If you've chosen to wear a prosthesis, when your best friend offers help, ask her to go with you to help make the right choice.

➤ When someone says, "I'll do whatever you need," ask if she does windows; then, joking aside, ask if she'll run the vacuum or dust the living room.

➤ On really tough days, accept someone's offer of help by giving him or her your grocery list.

➤ Accept help by asking others to entertain your children for an afternoon. It's a tough time for the kids when they can't have special days because you and hubby are overwhelmed with the here and now.

➤ If someone offers, ask him or her to choose a good rental movie and join you for an evening's entertainment. Suggest you'd prefer a comedy to a tear-jerking drama.

➤ When an appropriate someone offers, ask if he or she would help your husband so that he has more time to help you. Maybe it's cutting the grass, raking leaves, trimming the hedges, weeding the garden, or getting the oil changed in the car.

It's the little things that count, so they say. Indeed, all those little things—getting the oil changed in the car, weeding the flower bed, dusting the family room—are the things that add up to a total of overwhelming. You need support to avoid (or over-come) the overwhelming. It's simple. If you accept help with the little things, you'll have time to deal with the one really big thing in your life right now. And that's all that really matters.

When the Fiddle String Breaks

Sometimes we all find ourselves stretched to the limit; but during your battle with breast cancer, your "limit" undergoes a severe test. When things get too much for you and your family, even with the fine support of others around you (or, worse yet, with-out support from others), you may need to consider professional help.

Your local hospital or clinic will have a *social worker* or can at least refer you to one. That person most likely has a Master's degree in social work and, depending on your state's laws, may have some kind of state license or certificate. He or she is prepared to help you meet a broad range of challenges, including the bottom-line stuff (like your insurance, financial concerns, and accounting matters) as well as the touchy-feely areas (like your emotional turmoil, deepest fears, and family relationships).

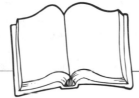

From the Book

A **social worker** usually has a Master's degree in social work and may or may not hold a state license or certificate. A **counselor,** sometimes also called a social worker, may not have a Master's degree in counseling and, depending on your state, may or may not have any state license or certificate. A **family counselor** is a counselor who specializes in working with the family unit. A **psychiatrist** is a medical doctor who can administer medications as part of your treatment. A **psychologist** has a Doctorate, but the degree may be in psychology, anthropology, education, or a host of other subjects.

You may find your medical dream team refers you to a *counselor* instead of a social worker. Although the terms "social worker" and "counselor" are sometimes used in-terchangeably, a counselor may have less training than a social worker. For example, a counselor may not have a Master's in counseling and may or may not have any training in psychology. Most states offer no specific certification or licensing for counselors, but ask about your own state's requirements. Your medical team can recommend someone it thinks is a good match for you and your immediate concerns.

Group counseling and self-help classes are other options to consider. Depending on how you feel about spilling your guts to strangers, choose the one best for you. (The primary difference between group counseling and a support group as discussed in Chapter 17, "Groupies: Yea or Nay?" is the training of the facilitator. In group counseling, the facilitator is most likely trained in group or family counseling.)

You can also find other kinds of professional support in a self-help class. These classes have a single focus, like helping you cope with breast cancer, and most run six to eight weeks, meet once a week for a couple of hours, and have a weekly "lesson," followed by discussion and questions. The American Cancer Society sponsors one such self-help series called "I Can Cope." While the classes deal with all forms of cancer, the sessions are generic enough to be meaningful to you. The speakers are as diverse as the communities that host them, so you may be hearing a doctor or a fellow survivor on the evening the class discusses coping with pain. For the time and place nearest you, call your local ACS or nationally at 1-800-ACS-2345.

Finally, when you realize that you, your husband, and/or children may be facing an extended crisis, consider family counseling. Your local county health organization and/or your medical team can recommend a licensed *family counselor* who can help you sort through the confusion and put you in touch with other avenues of professional help, from dealing with pain to dealing with dollars. Ultimately, if you're getting too close to the breaking point, get medical help. Your team can recommend a *psychiatrist* or *psychologist,* depending on your needs. The quicker you gain equilibrium on the home front, the quicker you can turn your total energies to the healing process.

In addition to counseling in all of its forms, many women have found the ultimate support tool in their religious beliefs. Regardless of your religious persuasion, you must know that others have found solace there. See Chapter 18, "Mind and Body: Spiritual Support."

Wherever you turn for support, survivors have affirmed, you'll find more than you expect. You'll get cards, notes, phone calls, and e-mails from folks you haven't heard from in years. Now they're there for you. You'll also meet a whole new group of friends, members of the sisterhood, who will also be there for you. May you find the same support at your every turn.

The Least You Need to Know

➤ Motivational and inspirational words in books and on tapes punch up a deflated attitude.

➤ A top-notch avenue for coping runs between the pages of a journal.

➤ When folks ask, "What can I do to help?" let them help you, then enjoy the satisfaction they derive from the experience.

➤ Professional help may be the best alternative when things get too tough.

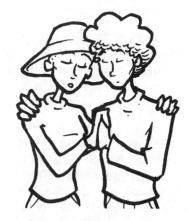

Chapter 20

Easing Others' Pain: Walking the Mile

> **In This Chapter**

➤ Watching for signs of others' distress

➤ Doing what you can when you are able

➤ Creating a "new" normal life for you and your family

➤ Asking for what you need

➤ Learning to be strong for others

When are things going to get back to normal? Eventually, your friends won't be the only ones asking that question; you'll be asking that of yourself. In fact, it's often easier for you to think of things getting back to normal than it is for your friends because they take their cues from you. Your loved ones can't wait to hear one or more of these magical lines coming from you:

➤ "Let's plan a party for someone's birthday."

➤ "Let's go on a picnic after church."

➤ "Let's go to a movie after supper."

➤ "Let's plan where we want to vacation this summer."

In this chapter, we'll talk about the steps you can take to reach that goal sooner rather than later.

Easing into Normalcy

Chances are, you're not quite ready for any of these "let's go" scenarios right now. You're probably having more good than bad days but those bad days still creep up on you and you still must struggle just to get through them. What's even more difficult for you is seeing the pain in the eyes of those who love you—the pain that comes from seeing you suffer physically and emotionally as you cope with the challenge of recovery.

Take It from Us

Don't beat yourself up when you make plans you can't manage to complete. Remember, you're likely to have a few days when you just don't feel like your old self and may have to cancel plans. Your friends and family will certainly understand, so banish the guilt and move on.

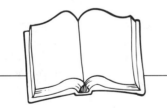

From the Book

Normal has several definitions. One definition is "conforming to a typical pattern, level, or type." Another definition is "not affected, immunized, or changed by experimentation." In one case, your life is very normal; in another, it is not.

Up until this point, you've probably been feeling so rotten that it took all your strength and your self-focus to get through an hour, let alone a day. Now that you're getting back on track, you may be able to get past that self-focus and consider the needs of those around you with some sense of balance and clarity. You might even be able to help ease the frustration and challenges your loved ones have been experiencing during, and sometimes because of, your illness.

Your ability to help others through this time will do much to deepen your relationships and it may help you to realize that you're not the only one who's suffering emotional stress. The people who love you also feel pain, and have been changed by your experience with breast cancer. Your family may have been one of the reasons you kept going when you were at your darkest moments. Now they may need your help to cope with their own emotions.

Another Mile: Finding the Strength

It's safe to say that your life will never be the same. As much as you try to restore what was "normal," it will be a new normal for you and your family and friends. The word "cancer" will sound different to your ears, and the news that someone you know has cancer will trigger strong emotions. You may feel that, from now on, people will look at you differently whenever the subject of cancer comes up. Because every breast cancer survivor has her own unique qualities, there are no simple formulas for dealing with these new feelings and perspectives. You, and your family, have walked a road of hope and hopelessness, of bravery and horror, of pity and anger. In most cases, you walked this road together. At this point, they may well be waiting for you to take the lead.

Now is the time to muster courage and focus on the new future you want to create and live. Now is the time to create your new *normal* life.

Now is the time to share with your loved ones what you've learned through this process of change and growth and healing, and for them to share with you. Now is the time for you and your family to stop distancing yourselves from each other, walking on eggs, or testing the waters. Now is the time to start new relationships if those you had have failed.

Now is the time to help yourself by helping others. It is in giving that you receive.

So, How's Your Husband?

Partners share both pain and sorrow just as they do hope and joy. In most cases, your husband (or significant other) has been your mainstay of support, and you've tried to be his.

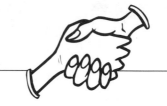

Helping Hand

Know that there *is* an end! The disruptions that you and your family have experienced won't last forever! Use the countdown system. Only three more chemo treatments. Only one more week of radiation treatments. Only one more school function that you can't attend. It is extremely important for you and your family to know there *is* an end to this.

Men, especially, are doers, not thinkers or emotional sharers. They feel best when they can *do* something concrete to fix whatever is broken. Chances are, then, your husband has felt a bit helpless during your struggle with breast cancer, because there simply is nothing he can do to fix your situation. As soon as you're able, it's important that you recognize that your husband may be feeling left out, helpless, and anxious all at the same time. In addition, he may find it difficult—if not impossible—to express his emotions to you, and therefore may seem withdrawn, even uncaring. And, as irrational as it may seem, your husband may also feel somehow responsible for your condition, that somehow, something he did or didn't do affected your health in a profound way.

If you suspect that your husband may be harboring these feelings—and even if you're not sure—you might want to sit down and try to draw out his feelings.

Indeed, men tend to put on a front for others, and whatever it is that they are feeling or going through, they pretend to the outside world that it's no big deal. I know there are probably exceptions, but most men have been just as worried and stressed as you are; they just handle it differently. Instead of talking about it, or crying, or even withdrawing, they cling to their daily routines and stay busy as a way to cope with the changes that are occurring to their wives and families.

Always keep the doors of communication open between you and others. Some men do have close male friends that they share with. Encourage your husband to spend time with his friends.

Tales from the Trenches

I thought my husband was handling my chemo well. He took off every third Friday and went to the clinic with me. He watched, but said little. The day I took my last chemo drip, he came home, sat down in the recliner, went to sleep, and I could not wake him. It was as if he were in a temporary coma. I realized he was just worn out dealing with the chemo. His breathing was steady, and he did not look as if he were suffering, so I just watched him sleep and waited for him to awake. At 2:00 A.M., 11 hours after he fell asleep, he woke up.

Takin' Care of Business

Because your husband will probably continue to work at his job as much—or even more—than he did before you became ill, it's also important for you to take an interest in his professional life. That's especially true if he is facing special challenges at work—is there an important meeting coming up or a deadline he's facing? If so, lend him some extra support—even though you may be facing some of your own challenges. If you're able, take on some extra responsibility at home to make his life at this time a little less fraught. In fact, this is the perfect time to call upon your friends, children, and support groups to pitch in.

Behind Closed Doors

Please pardon the pun, but things are probably still "touch and go" in the area of sexual intimacy. Are you responsive or taking the lead? Are you watching for signs of need or interest?

Although having cancer may have thrown some roadblocks into your relationship—temporarily—you'll now have a chance to help bring it back to a normal—sometimes even improved—state. But even now, when you're feeling stronger and ready to enjoy your intimate relationship again, you may find it difficult for both you and your husband because you're simply unsure of how to act.

Maybe you're both not particularly interested in sex at this time. Before your illness, you may have accepted that very normal situation without giving it much thought. Now, however, you're both liable to assume that temporary disinterest actually means rejection. But if your husband appears to be very interested in you sexually, you might not think it's just because he loves and desires you—which is what you would have thought before your illness. Now, you could interpret his interest as a selfish need for the physical act of sex.

Take It from Us

Be alert to changes in your husband's behavior for indications of how he is feeling. Men are more action people than word people. If your husband is at your "beck and call," it might mean he's really anxious about your condition. If he's working at his home computer or cleaning out the garage, he could be less anxious about you and your prognosis. Actually, him being busy or involved in something other than your recovery is a good sign to you that he thinks things can get back to normal.

As you can see, when it comes to sex after breast cancer, both you and your partner are likely to feel as if you're walking a very fine emotional tightrope. During this time of transition, what are your options?

First, you should do whatever you can to feel comfortable, emotionally and physically. If you've had surgery and remain uncomfortable with your body, you'll want to first discuss your feelings with your partner—and your partner should be willing to discuss his with you. To meet your physical needs, you may want to wear some type of clothing during sex to cover healing or missing tissue. You may want to try a new sexual technique(s) that is comfortable for both you and your husband. You may want to use "estrogen-free" vaginal lubricants to be more comfortable.

To say that the first attempt will be awkward is an understatement! Be patient with each other. Maybe this a situation where we need to keep "practice makes perfect" in mind? If you are having difficulty talking with your partner or accepting a "new" sexual relationship with your partner, please ask your doctor to refer you to a sex therapist for counseling.

Calling It Quits!

Usually, a couple can work through the troubles and share the burdens like a well-oiled machine; however, if a relationship was on the rocks before the cancer, it may not survive.

When you hear of a marriage that has failed in these circumstances, you may assume that it was the husband's idea to leave. This isn't always the case. It may be due to a woman's loss of self-esteem or, conversely, on a new sense of her own strength and identity. Some women try to spare their partners the struggle and potential grief that may attach to a diagnosis of cancer.

Take It from Us

If you and your husband have decided to end your marriage and you have been covered under his insurance policy, please check out your insurance possibilities. A new insurance policy will consider your breast cancer as a preexisting condition and treatment might not be covered. Don't stay together just for insurance reasons, but do consider all your options.

And How Are the Kids?

Have you been watching your children to see if they have recovered? Have your friends or the teachers at school helped keep you informed? Are you checking for signs of stress? When it comes to stress, do you know what is normal for a child or teenager and what isn't?

As facile as it may sound, it's very true that the first step in easing your children's pain is to get to know who they are and how they react to stress—and believe it or not, the first time you really get to know your children may be as you face your illness together. Of course, how you discuss your cancer and how involved they become in your illness will depend on their ages, their maturity levels, and your own needs. Knowing that they are going through much of the same as you and your husband, what are some things you can do to ease their emotional pain?

➤ Allow them to live as normal a life as possible.

➤ Remind them that you, or no one else, expect them to grieve all the time.

➤ Set a time limit, say three or four months, when you will need their help. They seem to handle things better when they are working within boundaries.

➤ If they have a school/social conflict with something that you have asked them do to, try not to force them to make a decision between you and it. This is a good time to ask friends or other family members to help.

➤ Don't rely on them too heavily for emotional support. No matter how adult they may seem from time to time, they are still children.

➤ Don't force them to talk. There will be times when they want to talk and times when they don't. In this case, let them take the lead.

Don't just talk to them; talk with them. Watch for signs of the unusual. If they are having trouble or distancing themselves from you, please seek help from members of your support group or a reliable counselor.

Tales from the Trenches

Charlotte said that watching her children's reactions was like a twinge from a broken bone. Years ago, she had broken her ankle. Even though it had healed, and she had forgotten the pain, every now and then, she'd step in a hole or on an uneven part of the sidewalk, and she'd get a twinge reminding her. Sometimes, when looking into her children's eyes, she'd get that same kind of twinge, reminding her that things just weren't the way they used to be.

Helping Others Help

Helping can be a two-way street. I guess that's why we reap what we sow, what goes around comes around, and one hand washes the other. If you're like most women, you derive a sense of pleasure and satisfaction from helping others. Now, however, you must learn to help others to help you. How many people have asked you what they can do to help you through this crisis? And how many times have you shrugged off their help, wanting to handle things yourself, not wanting to be a burden, not knowing how to accept their generous gift of friendship and time? That attitude is an admirable one in many ways, but it can hold you back from getting the help you need and it prevents the people who love you from giving of themselves, which is the way they can help to heal themselves of the emotional pain and frustration they feel about your illness.

Tales from the Trenches

Bonnie's friends wanted to help; they were just waiting for the "word." And Bonnie needed their help, but, when she got around to last-minute calling, they weren't at home or had something else that they had to do. She finally wised up and made a list of what she needed help with, talked with her friends (in advance), and got on their schedule. All it took was planning.

Going Beyond Personal Borders

In addition to personal friends and family, you can also reach out to national organizations, churches, and support groups.

The benefit of asking for help from an organization trained to give it to you is that you can avoid feeling as if you're a "burden" on those close to you.

These groups are there to give your family support as well, which may help to ease the stress that would otherwise fall on the family unit. Think of it this way:

➤ By calling a cancer-care organization or other support group, you are not pleading with someone who has no interest or feels put upon. You are dealing with people who chose to take on the responsibility of helping you and your family.

➤ These helping people not only come to your aid, but may also help your loved ones in their efforts to support you.

➤ These people can teach you how to ask for help and to accept it when it comes.

➤ When you see the joy that others derive from helping you, you may realize that your family and friends will enjoy the same sense of satisfaction—if only you'll let them help you.

Whatever you can pay someone to do, do. Whatever you can get help with, do. Whatever you can temporarily postpone, do. This is your new "to do" list, and right now, it's great!

Words and Actions ... and Hugs

So many of us have the same needs: kind words, actions that show we care and haven't given up, and the ever-popular hug that helps keep us connected with others.

My mother paid me the ultimate compliment. She told me that I made coping with cancer look easy. I guess working to keep my life running as smoothly as possible was my way of trying to ease my mother's pain. I realized early on, as many breast cancer survivors do, that the only thing worse than having breast cancer is loving someone who does. The fear, the worry, the grief is still present but it's outside and it's something we can't fight. I'm almost sure you've come to this conclusion yourself and I hope that reading this chapter has given you a way to let those who love you inside, at least a little bit.

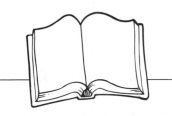

From the Book

To **celebrate** means to observe with ceremonies, to perform, to announce. With what you've been through, every day is worth celebrating!

Now, however, it's time to *celebrate*. You have a reason to celebrate when you've healed from your surgery, when you pass your two-year mark, when you pass your five-year mark, and when you complete any of your therapies.

You have a reason to celebrate getting your family back to normal or creating a new, comfortable normal for them and you. You have a reason to celebrate living through and with this disease, easing your own pain, and easing the pain of others.

The Least You Need to Know

➤ There comes a time when you need to focus less on yourself and more on those around you who've been trying to help.

➤ Although the lives of all involved will never be the same again, you can create a new "normal" life, and get on with it.

➤ When your family's lives become a little more complicated than usual, you'll need to provide them with a little special attention.

➤ If you have difficulty helping to ease others' pain, go to an organization that can help you develop a workable plan or approach.

Part 5

The Aftermath: Its Many Parts

It's probably safe to say that every woman comes out the other side of breast cancer a different person. Yes, you're physically different, but you're also emotionally different. You have a new set of priorities. The shocking new world is no longer new to you, and life takes new meaning from the change.

In this part of the book you'll learn about the physical changes, from the controversy and details about breast reconstruction, the ups and downs of prostheses, and how the new you can dress more comfortably. And you'll also learn about the new emotions, the turmoil of dealing with recurrences and, sadly, in some cases, a loss of life.

Finally, we end with a trumpet call to arms, a plea and a set of suggestions for serving as a volunteer/advocate to help stop this debilitating disease called breast cancer.

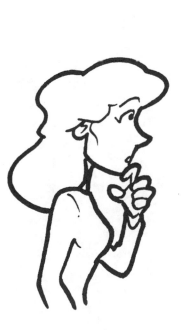
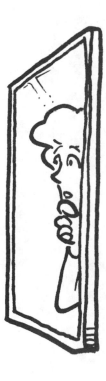

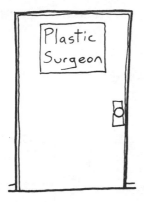

Chapter 21

Back to the Bikini: Reconstruction

In This Chapter

➤ Great debate over reconstruction

➤ Three common kinds of reconstruction

➤ Issues about nipple reconstruction

➤ Happy—and not so happy—results

You've had a mastectomy, and the decision to do so was based on medical information. Whether or not you choose breast reconstruction, however, is strictly personal. Whatever you decide is right, and it's nobody else's business. Still, knowing what others have decided and how they feel about their decisions may help you make yours. In this chapter, we'll consider the great debate over reconstruction; we'll describe the three most common kinds and how they're done; and we'll meet the survivors who sport the latest bionic look as well as those who chose otherwise or face unhappy results.

So You Want a Remake!

As a result of the Women's Health and Cancer Rights Act of 1998, insurance companies must pay for *breast reconstruction* following a mastectomy resulting from breast cancer. That law has significantly impacted the business of breast reconstruction; and, at least as a partial result, *plastic surgeons* have refined their techniques. Reconstruction is now common practice.

Chances are, if you've had a mastectomy you qualify for a remake—especially if your cancer was removed by the mastectomy. If you're reading between the lines here, you recognize that some reconstruction could conceal a recurring cancer, or at least make it more difficult to detect and/or treat. But those situations are rare; so it's not an issue unless your doc says it is.

Tales from the Trenches

When she learned she would have a mastectomy, the first thing Aurelia did was to catalog-shop for vests. "My mother had had a terrible time with her prosthesis; it was always riding up. So in the back of my mind I was considering [having] reconstruction later, after I'd healed. Then I talked to Carol Rogers, co-founder of Woman to Woman. She'd had a TRAM flap 10 years earlier, simultaneously with her mastectomy. My doctor hadn't even mentioned that I could have immediate reconstruction." Now, four years later, she's thrilled with her remake. "My ugly Caesarian scar is gone; my nipple is actually tummy skin; and my remake looks better than the real one!"

If you're considering reconstruction, you'll need to choose a plastic surgeon, and you'll want to be just as careful choosing him or her as you were choosing any other member of your medical team. If your plastic surgeon is a perfectionist, you'll have a pretty outcome with neat scars. And how do you find the perfectionist? Consider this plan:

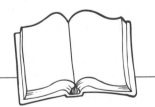

From the Book

Breast reconstruction refers to the surgical remake of the breast after a mastectomy. The medical person who does the reconstruction is called a **plastic surgeon.**

➤ Check their membership in the American Society of Plastic and Reconstruction Surgeons. Reputable docs proudly post their membership documents in plain view.

➤ Ask how many breast reconstructions he or she has done in the past year. For the same reasons you wanted a surgeon who specializes in breast surgeries, you want a plastic surgeon who specializes in breast reconstruction.

➤ Ask what type of reconstruction is right for you and why.

➤ Study the pictures. Plastic surgeons worth their scrubs have photographs of their work. You won't see faces, only chests and breasts.

It's almost like catalog shopping, deciding what looks good to you and what doesn't. Would you be satisfied if you looked like the pictures?

No matter which doctor or which means of reconstruction you choose, you'll need to come to grips with the fact that you get only two real breasts in a lifetime. No reconstruction, no matter its superior quality, is like the real thing. The general purpose of reconstruction is to make you look good in your clothes. Naked, I doubt you'll ever fool anybody.

The Great Debate: Yes

Those survivors who chose reconstruction by and large said they made the choice for vanity reasons. In their clothes, they want to look the way they've always looked. For various reasons, they didn't want to accomplish the look with a prosthesis (see Chapter 22, "Boob in a Box: Prostheses," for issues about wearing a prosthesis). Survivors who are physically active didn't want to be hampered by a prosthesis that bumps against their chest wall when they chase a tennis ball. Other physically active folks cited problems with swimming, rafting, canoeing—all of which require a water-suitable prosthesis and/or an alternate breast form for when they change into dry clothes. In fact, some physically active women who initially chose a prosthesis later chose to have reconstruction for these very reasons.

Survivors consistently mentioned two other matters. First, age may be a primary factor in some women's decision. In general, the younger the woman, the more likely she is to choose reconstruction. Second, breast size seems to be a factor. Rather flat-chested women don't seem to mind the missing breast as much as someone in a EE cup does.

Other serious considerations come into play, too. Your age, health, anatomy, and tissue available determine the type of reconstruction best for you. Whether or not you're willing to have foreign materials (like implants) placed in your body makes some decisions easier.

And another part of the great debate focuses on possible recurrences. If you have reconstruction, will it obscure early detection of a recurrence or a new cancer? Will the reconstruction in some way damage tissue, thereby actually causing a recurrence? In case of a recurrence, will treatment be more difficult? Valid questions, all. The answers are less clear. However, according to some plastic surgeons' literature, as far as anyone knows, reconstruction has no known effect on recurrence. And usually reconstruction doesn't interfere with treatment if cancer recurs.

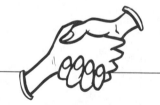

Helping Hand

Consider a breast reduction in the other breast if you're an especially large-breasted woman. In the end, your breasts may not look the way they've always looked; they may look better.

The Great Debate: No

Some survivors skipped breast reconstruction and have never looked back. In large part, their reasons for deciding against the procedure were consistent: They wanted to focus on their fight against cancer and couldn't face the additional surgery—or even the three or four additional surgeries—necessary for total reconstruction. (Depending on the type of reconstruction you choose, it can double to quadruple surgery time.) They also felt the extended recovery time for the additional surgery could impede their fight against the cancer.

Other issues: Any surgery carries possible risks and complications, like bleeding, fluid collection, scar tissue, and problems with anesthetics. More surgery adds more scars and, depending on the kind of reconstruction, the scars can be significant—all the way across your abdomen or along your back. Since scars can limit what you wear, they're an issue. (And if you smoke, nicotine slows healing, thus making worse scars.) Of further concern: You always risk infection with surgery, and if you have an infection and/or a reaction to implants, you may lose the implant or the transplanted tissue can die. Scar tissue can thicken and make the breast feel hard, even painful. Additional surgery may then be necessary to remove scar tissue and/or an implant. If you're taking chemo, all these issues of infection compound.

Tales from the Trenches

"I know I'm a woman. I don't need breasts to prove it," proclaimed a young woman whose mastectomy at age 33 made her a prime candidate for reconstruction. "If I have reconstruction, maybe they wouldn't find a recurrence in time. It's an unknown." She opted out.

Karla agrees. "Six months after my mastectomy, my surgeon suggested reconstruction. I kept putting it off; and then a year after my first surgery, I had a recurrence in the scar. Then I was glad I hadn't messed with it. It might—or might not—have made the detection harder, but [in my case] it would certainly have made the treatment harder."

The Generic Plan

Surgeons follow two approaches to reconstruction: immediate or delayed. Many plastic surgeons work directly with your surgeon and perform the breast reconstruction simultaneously with your mastectomy. You wake up with a new breast and never see yourself flat. That's immediate reconstruction.

You can also choose delayed reconstruction, which involves a separate surgery at some point after your mastectomy. You might decide to wait because you're not prepared to make a decision about reconstruction in the middle of all the turmoil of learning that you have breast cancer. It's also possible that you may have other health conditions that would complicate reconstruction, like obesity, high blood pressure, diabetes, or cigarette addiction. So, yes, you can have reconstruction later. Even years later. Radiologists will tell you, however, that radiated tissue tends not to heal well for some time after therapy ends. So if you choose not to have immediate reconstruction, and if you have radiation, you'll need to wait a couple of years to have the most satisfactory healing conditions for delayed reconstruction.

The general routine for reconstruction goes something like this: The first part is done under a general anesthetic and involves the creation of the breast mound—the most complex part. Follow-up procedures, usually months later and with a local anesthetic, include creating the nipple and areola. Both of these procedures, of course, are optional. Some folks skip both; some get the nipple and skip the areola. Do what's right for you after discussing the matter with your doc.

Before you make a final decision about either immediate or delayed reconstruction, check with your insurance company. Because of the 1998 law, insurance usually covers reconstruction after a mastectomy, but what type of reconstruction and how much coverage varies from state to state. So check ahead of time about any limitations. They may pay for one procedure but not another. And you don't need any more surprises right now. Not for a long, long time.

Take It from Us

Don't forget to massage! Estelle says the trick to eliminating problems with scarring is to massage the implant and surrounding area. "My husband helps by massaging me every evening. When we were gone to Europe for two weeks, we were so busy we skipped the massage. By the time we got home, I was in pain. It took two weeks to get things loosened up again."

It's worth mentioning, too, that many folks who have reconstruction choose to have surgery on the remaining healthy breast to get an even match—surgery to enlarge, reduce, or lift. As a result of the 1998 law, most insurance companies will pay to create the symmetry. But it goes without saying (doesn't it?) that these additional surgeries also leave more scars.

As you read about the three most common methods of breast reconstruction, know that every surgeon does personal variations. The following details, however, should give you enough information to ask the right questions.

Look Out, Dolly Parton: Implants

Of the three kinds of reconstruction, the use of implants is the most common. Implants are *silicone* bags that the doc fills with either silicone gel or *saline*. Think of them as zippered bags filled with saltwater. The implant goes under the muscle where breast used to be. You know how chicken breasts have that little slot you can stuff? Well, you have the same kind of slot in your chest muscle, and that's where the implant goes. But since that isn't where your breast used to be, the muscle and skin have to stretch to accommodate whatever size you're aiming for. (You can be a Dolly or a Twiggy.) So, in order to stretch the muscle, the plastic surgeon will likely take you through a two-step process.

Depending on the kind of implant you have, you may have an expander inserted to stretch the skin prior to the insertion of the permanent implant.

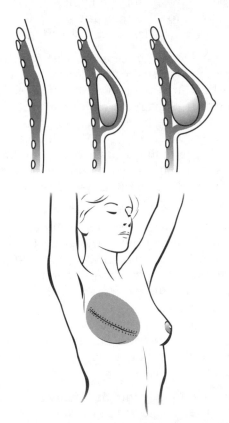

The first step is to insert something called an *expander*—an empty bag to which the doc initially adds about 200cc of saline and periodically, through a port, adds another 60 to 100cc over the next several weeks or months. Sometimes the expansion is uncomfortable, even painful, because you're getting stretched across already tender tissue. When you're stretched enough, you'll go back for a second surgery. Then the surgeon takes out the expander and puts in the implant. (Some expanders also serve as the permanent implant. Ask.) The implant itself is silicone, but what goes into the bag is silicone gel or saline, a natural saltwater solution harmless to the body. Before you make your decision about an implant, however, ask questions of your plastic surgeon:

➤ What are the risks associated with an implant?

➤ What are its limitations?

➤ How long will the implant last?

➤ What events can cause it to rupture or leak?

➤ What happens to me if it ruptures or leaks?

➤ Will a rupture or leak cause lymphedema to flare up?

➤ How will I recognize a leak?

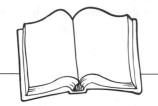

From the Book

Silicone is a synthetic material used to make implant bags and, in some cases, used in gel form to fill the bags. **Saline** is a saltwater solution. An **expander** is a temporary implant used to stretch the tissue so it will accommodate a full-size implant.

Tales from the Trenches

Survivors say if your implant changes appearance, feels different, becomes painful, numb, hot, or tingling, it may have ruptured or begun leaking. In addition, thickened scar tissue can start squeezing the implant, so the breast may feel hard. Of course, if it gets too hard, you'll need to have the implant removed and/or replaced. Some women have had their implants turn sideways or otherwise slip from position. If you notice any irregularity, see your doctor immediately.

36A or 36C? Making a Breast

For folks who don't want implants, plastic surgeons can make a breast using tissue taken from other parts of the body, a process called *autologous tissue reconstruction*. When the surgeon moves the tissue to the chest without detaching it from its original site and keeping the original blood supply, it's called a *flap*. The flap uses skin, fat, and muscle from your abdomen or back that is tunneled to your breast site and formed into a mound. Some flaps hold an implant; others don't. Another type of autologous tissue reconstruction takes tissue from your abdomen, thighs, or buttocks and transplants it to the breast. During the transplant, your plastic surgeon has to re-connect blood vessels and thus must be knowledgeable about *microvascular* surgery as well.

From the Book

Any kind of **autologous tissue reconstruction** rebuilds your breast with tissue from another part of your body. The tissue is called a **flap** if it remains attached in its original location and maintains its original blood supply. If not, and tissue is trans-planted, **microvascular** surgery connects blood vessels.

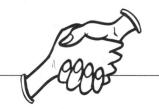

Helping Hand

Know your stuff! Here's a tough question: Why affect healthy working components of your body for a cosmetic outcome? That's what you're doing with either a TRAM or LATS flap reconstruction. Be sure you can answer the question to your own satisfaction.

Of course, with any kind of autologous tissue reconstruction, you will have scars at both sites—at the breast and wherever the tissue comes from. As a result, recovery takes longer than with an implant. On the brighter side, however, if the flap comes from your abdomen, it's like getting a tummy tuck. So let's take a look at the two most common flap constructions.

Belly Dancer: From the Front

Of the two most common flap reconstructions, the TRAM is more popular, mostly because of its more natural-looking shape and droop. TRAM stands for transverse rectus abdominis myocutaneous, referring to the source of tissue for your new breast. Basically, the surgeon takes a piece of your tummy, runs it up behind your skin, and creates a breast. The surgery takes several hours and adds significantly to your recovery time—sometimes as long as six weeks. It does carry the disadvantage of weakening your abdominal muscles, and sometimes you need a mesh-like material fastened inside to hold your innards in place. Because it's so serious, you'll want to ask some rather direct questions:

➤ How long does this surgery take?

➤ How long will it be after surgery before I can stand up straight?

➤ How long will recovery take?

➤ Should I donate my own blood beforehand?

➤ How much scarring will I have and where will it be?

➤ What risks are involved?

➤ What are the chances that the tissue may die after it's rerouted to my breast?

➤ Now that part of my abdominal muscle has been moved to my chest, what abdominal problems might I face?

➤ What will my new breast look like?

➤ How closely will it match my other breast in shape and size?

➤ How soon can I return to normal activity?

Let's face it: Some surgeons are better than others. If possible, then, you'll want to talk to folks who've been through the surgery with the same surgeon. Ask for that opportunity. Be cautious if you're denied.

Tote That Bale: From the Back

The other kind of flap reconstruction is called a LATS flap, referring to the muscle from which it comes, the latissimus dorsi, which is in your back just below your shoulder. Just like the TRAM flap, the LATS flap reconstruction moves the skin, fat, and muscle under the skin to the front of the chest wall. Depending on your size, the flap may be adequate, but usually a LATS flap reconstruction creates a nest for an implant. So if you want to avoid an implant, you're probably limited to the TRAM.

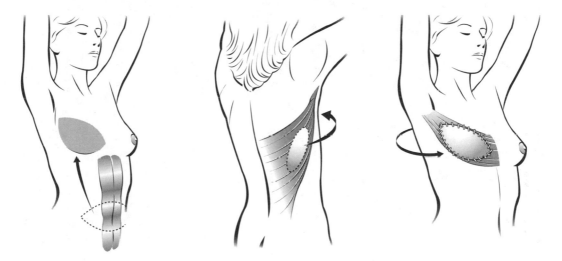

The TRAM flap reconstruction tunnels abdominal skin, fat, and muscle to the chest to form a breast mound. The LATS flap tunnels tissue from the back to form a breast mound.

In addition to the questions we list above for the TRAM flap, you'll want to ask two additional questions about the LATS flap before you make a decision:

➤ Will I require an implant with a LATS flap?

➤ Now that my back muscle has been moved to my chest, what back or shoulder problems may I face?

You may make more sense of the similarities and differences among the three kinds of reconstruction by studying the following chart.

Top Twenty Issues with the Three Common Kinds of Breast Reconstruction

Issue	Implant	TRAM Flap	LATS Flap
1. Length of surgery, simultaneously with mastectomy	three to four hours	five to six hours	four to five hours
2. Length of hospital stay	one to three days	three to five days	two to three days
3. Number of incisions	one	two	two
4. Number of drains	usually two	usually three to four	usually two to three
5. Extent of pain	some; expander in stage I sometimes quite painful	very painful; most severe in abdomen, not chest	painful
6. Extent of scarring (note that nipple replacement may add scarring to one or more parts of the body)	across, above, or below breast mound	across or around breast mound; across abdomen from hip bone to hip bone.	under breast mound; football-shaped incision, about 6" × 2" on back below shoulder
7. Recovery time	about two weeks; second surgery about one week	may take six weeks to walk fully erectly; tightness in abdomen can last a year or more	about three to four weeks
8. Initial physical limitations	can't raise arm over 90 degrees for about one week; can't lift for two weeks; can feel tight in chest area for several months	can't raise arm over 90 degrees for about one week; can't lift for two weeks; can't drive for two weeks; can't stand erectly for sometimes six weeks; difficult to sit up or get out of bed for one week; no abdominal exercises for two months	can't raise arm over 90 degrees for about one week; can't lift for two weeks; can't drive for two weeks; can feel tight in chest area for several months
9. Possible problems	may suffer from infection around implant; may have capsular contracture; may become hard; implant can leak and impact lymphedema	transplanted tissue can die; seroma (fluid pocket that forms after drain removal) may form	may suffer from infection around implant; may have capsular contracture; breast may become hard; implant can leak and impact lymphedema; transplanted tissue can die; seroma (fluid pocket that forms after drain removal) can form

Issue	Implant	TRAM Flap	LATS Flap
10. Use of foreign material	implant bag filled with saline solution	may include mesh added to the abdomen	implant bag filled with saline solution
11. Shape of reconstructed breast (without nipple)	firm mound; does not relax to side when reclining	most naturally shaped mound with natural droop; will relax to side when reclining	firm mound; does not relax to side when reclining
12. Sensation in reconstructed breast	generally numb; no sexual stimulation	generally numb; no sexual stimulation	generally numb; no sexual stimulation
13. Body size	not usually an issue	need adequate body fat and abdominal tissue	not usually an issue
14. Effects of chemotherapy and radiation therapy	radiation therapy can cause skin to tighten around implant; chemo hinders body's ability to fight any infection; thus no chemo until healed	chemo hinders body's ability to fight any infection; thus no chemo until healed	radiation therapy can cause skin to tighten around implant; chemo hinders body's ability to fight any infection; thus no chemo until healed
15. Long-term issues	implant generally lasts 10 to 15 years; periodic additional surgery required to replace implant	no implant to deteriorate	implant generally lasts 10 to 15 years; periodic additional surgery required to replace implant
16. Matching the healthy breast	may require lift, enlargement, or reduction of healthy breast	may require lift, enlargement, or reduction of healthy breast	may require lift, enlargement, or reduction of healthy breast
17. Effects of active life	protect from impact	may have weakened abdominal muscles	protect from impact
18. Weight change	implant can be reduced or expanded surgically	gain/loss usually same in TRAM tissue as in remainder of body	gain/loss usually same in LATS flap as in remainder of body; implant can also be reduced or expanded surgically
19. In case of a future mastectomy	can do another implant	almost always must do different kind of reconstruction	can do another LATS
20. Insurance coverage	usually	usually	usually

New Nipple News

No matter what kind of reconstruction you choose, you'll have to decide whether or not to have nipple reconstruction. Survivors we talked to couldn't reach a consensus about the procedure, although some said given the chance, they'd never do it again. Others, however, said it was no big deal, that it was the finishing touch to a reconstructed breast.

In some cases, the doctor creates the nipple by bunching and stitching together a little skin to resemble a nipple and later tattooing the areola for color. In other cases, the surgeon grafts a piece of skin from the groin to create the nipple and areola. (You can pluck any pubic hairs that grow in; usually they don't grow back.) We even met one lady whose surgeon removed her nipple and areola, grafted it to the inside of her leg, and when her reconstruction was done and healed, removed the graft from her leg and re-grafted it to her breast. It was, of course, a perfect match, but she admitted her leg was sore much longer than her breast. And one woman, unwilling to endure one more surgery, decided to have a butterfly tattooed in place of the nipple and areola. In short, you'll find almost every imaginable solution to the nipple and areola reconstruction. Ask enough questions to know what to expect; then make your decision.

Take It from Us

Don't rush your decision about reconstruction. One woman said she'd had to make so many decisions she couldn't even face going grocery shopping anymore. If you feel the same, perhaps that's a good reason for having delayed reconstruction. You can make decisions at your own pace.

What the Happy Customers Say

On a continuum from "It's wonderful" to "It's horrible," we asked survivors to rank their results of reconstructive surgery. The answers compiled into an astonishing pattern. Survivors ranked all three common kinds of reconstruction from one end of the continuum to the other. As nearly as we could tell, the results seemed to be connected to two primary variables: the plastic surgeon's ability and the survivor's expectations of the outcome.

Women who are pleased with their reconstruction are almost evangelistic about it. They know none of us have exactly the same set of circumstances, but they are so thrilled that they can't imagine any other alternative. They look great, feel great, and lead active, busy lives. They knew up front that their bionic boob would be different from their natural one. They knew up front that they wanted to look good in their clothes but that naked, they would fool no one. Their positive attitudes radiate confidence in their remake.

The Rest of the Story

Others, however, are less than satisfied. As one woman said, "I'm satisfied, but I'm not happy. It looks good, but it doesn't feel good." Others admitted their expectations were undoubtedly too high. Others have had failed surgeries that have left them bitter.

Probably one of the most important messages survivors passed along is that a reconstructed breast is numb. While you may regain some feeling as years go by, they're not natural feelings; and the bionic breast no longer gives you sexual stimulation. In fact, the breast will be firmer and rounder than your natural breast. It won't sag or hang to the side when you lie down, although the TRAM comes closer to the natural breast than other options. True, the scars fade over several years, but they never go away entirely.

Finally, in spite of your mastectomy and the apparent removal of all breast tissue, you will probably continue to have mammograms on both breasts. If you have an implant, with or without the LATS flap, you'll want to get your mammogram where the folks know the special techniques necessary to get a reliable reading.

Whether you choose to look like Dolly or Twiggy, the very fact that you have the option makes this battle somewhat more bearable. We have, indeed, come a long way, baby!

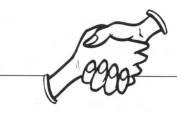

Helping Hand

Know that it is possible that a breast reconstruction can interfere with detection of a recurrence of breast cancer or of a new cancer. Interference is interpreted by the Food and Drug Administration as either a hindrance or a delay. Reconstruction makes clear mammograms more difficult.

Tales from the Trenches

"I'll never have to wear a bra again," Ruthie exclaimed. She's had two mastectomies, with a LATS flap after each. "When I'm 75 and lying on my back on the beach, people will walk by and say, 'She's too old for implants.' My breasts are perky and always will be." On the other hand, Jody now has one perky breast and one saggy one. "What do I do?" she queries. "The surgeon wants to lift the healthy breast, but I just hate the thought of anybody cutting into something healthy." It's another issue with breast reconstruction.

The Least You Need to Know

➤ Important arguments about the advantages and disadvantages of breast reconstruction need your attention.

➤ An implant is the most popular method of reconstruction.

➤ The two most common kinds of natural tissue reconstruction are the TRAM flap and the LATS flap.

➤ While some folks swear by their bionic boobs, others have not found happiness.

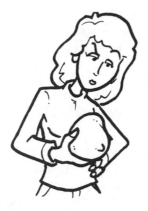

Boob in a Box: Prostheses

Bobbie is a professional model. When breast cancer took her off the runway and marched her onto the battlefield, her career went on hold—but only briefly. Mastectomy over, prosthesis in place, she was back on the runway in less than a month. Just as she had before, she modeled shimmering strapless gowns, fashionable bathing suits, and even some lingerie. For a long time, no one knew she was wearing a prosthesis, not even the other girls in the dressing room. Too good to be true? No! And the best news is that a prosthesis can work as well for you.

According to the most recent statistics, about 80 percent of the women who undergo a mastectomy choose some nonsurgical option to reconstruction. In this chapter, we'll discuss the advantages and disadvantages of prostheses, suggest the best time to be fitted, explain the various kinds of prostheses, and offer hints for looking great in the meantime. (Of course, if you weren't a model before your surgery, a prosthesis probably won't make you one afterward.)

Ups and Downs: Prosthetic Issues

If you had a lumpectomy, you have a very different need from someone who had a mastectomy. You may have remarkably good cosmetic recovery from your lumpectomy, but it's possible you may find yourself a bit lopsided. The breast is still intact,

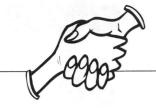

Helping Hand

Wait until after your radiation treatments to start wearing your prosthesis. Your skin will be tender, probably like a sunburn, and a prosthesis will irritate the area. Even after you've healed, you may decide not to wear your prosthesis at home or out working in the yard, but instead use either a leisure form or some other stuffing in a comfortable bra—or nothing at all—and save your prosthesis for dress-up.

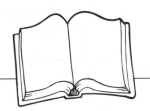

From the Book

A **breast prosthesis** is a breast form made of silicone, fiberfill, or other material. Almost all are designed to be worn inside a special bra; however, new forms are being developed that do not require a bra. A **breast enhancer** is a small form that fills out the breast shape after tissue is removed, such as during a lumpectomy.

but it just doesn't measure up to par. You'll be looking for something called a *breast enhancer,* a small form that fits under, over, or beside your breast to fill out the shape and make one breast match the other. Some of the enhancers are silicone; others are fabric. Some fit into fashion bras; others need some sort of bra pocket—perhaps one you add yourself—to hold it in place.

Even if you had reconstruction, you may find a breast enhancer beneficial. Frequently women discover that the perky new breast is no match for the saggy old one. Breast enhancers will even the score and help you avoid further cosmetic surgery to balance your appearance.

If, on the other hand, you had a mastectomy, you probably need a complete *breast prosthesis.* Everything has its ups and downs, and breast prostheses are no exception. The two biggest complaints are that they are hot and heavy. In part, the complaints are related to breast size. For instance, if you wear a size 42D bra, you will have a very different prosthetic situation than if you wear a 32A. In either case, however, choosing a breathable, lightweight prosthesis can lessen both the heat and weight. Fortunately, the industry has much more to offer than it once did, and that's terrific news for women who, for whatever reason, choose not to have reconstruction (see Chapter 21, "Back to the Bikini: Reconstruction").

Agony and Ecstasy: Being Fitted

Most professional prosthetic fitters recommend that you wait at least six to eight weeks after surgery to be fitted with a breast prosthesis or enhancer. They cite several reasons for the delay. First, you will be quite tender along and around your incision for at least six weeks, maybe longer. If a bra rubs any part of the incision, you may experience discomfort for several months. Trust me, it doesn't feel a bit good to try on prostheses when your skin is tender.

Second, you may have swelling, which dramatically affects how the prosthesis fits now—and doesn't fit later.

Third, radiation therapy can cause swelling and soreness, which in turn affects bra size. Fourth, if you were post-menopausal and taking hormone replacement therapy, you will probably notice that with the absence of the HRT, your intact breast will shrink. That, too, affects bra size and any matching prosthesis. And finally, sometimes chemo causes big changes in your weight, both up and down.

When you're healed, you've reached a stable weight, and your doctor agrees that you are ready to be fitted, he or she will write a "prescription" for a prosthesis. Most insurance companies require the doctor's order before they pay for the prosthesis—but most insurance companies, including Medicare, do pay—thanks to the Women's Health and Cancer Rights Act of 1998.

Sellers of the Goods

When the time comes for a fitting, you'll be asking, "Where do I go to find the breast form right for me?" If you live in a large community, you'll find breast prostheses in the lingerie section of large department stores, in lingerie specialty stores, in orthetic and prosthetic shops (also called O&Ps), and in a growing number of small shops generally referred to as mastectomy boutiques, of which there about 400 or so in the United States. Some communities offer shop-at-home services. Check the Yellow Pages in your phone book under headings like "Mastectomy Forms and Apparel," "Breast Prostheses," "Prosthetic Devices," "Artificial Breasts," or "Surgical Appliances."

Take It from Us

Before being fitted, ask about insurance. Some companies allow one prosthesis a year; others, one every two years. Most pay a percentage for post-surgical bras; some, a dollar limit; the number yearly varies. If you've had a weight change, most allow a prosthesis more frequently than stipulated, but your doctor must prescribe. Ask, too, for a list of in-network providers (who usually offer better benefits).

How do you choose where to shop? It's really a matter of personal comfort. If you shop at a large department store, you'll probably find a certified fitter available, although she may not be on duty during all hours the store is open. But you can walk in and browse through the lingerie like any other woman without calling attention to your personal needs. At an O&P shop, you'll be in the same waiting room as folks needing all kinds of prosthetic devices. Try not to let this make you uncomfortable. Stay focused on yourself and your recovery and you'll make it through your shopping experience just fine. If you visit a mastectomy boutique, you'll find a warmer and more comfortable environment, lots of feminine amenities, a sensitive and compassionate staff, and certified fitters. Of course, it may be more obvious to passersby why you're shopping there.

If you live in a smaller community where there are none of the outlets described above, you can turn to mail order and online companies. In Appendix D, "Sources of Prostheses and Post-Surgical Clothing," you'll find a list of several major manufacturers and their toll-free numbers. By calling them, you can learn the location of the retailer nearest you. You'll also find listed Web sites and mail order shops. Because Web sites change overnight, you'll also want to check your Internet's Yellow Pages for mastectomy forms.

Take It from Us

Wherever you purchase your breast form, make sure you get a written guarantee. Most guarantees are good for two years, but if you're especially physically active, your form may not hold up. Keep your sales receipt, guarantee, and insurance forms.

Consider calling your hotline volunteer to ask about the reputation of prosthetics dealers and/or manufacturers. And consider traveling to a location with a wide selection rather than settling for whatever you're first shown. The more brands a store carries, the better your choices.

Having a Fit over Fits

Breast prostheses are expensive. The off-the-shelf or non-custom silicone products generally range from $250 to $350 with custom-made ones running as much as $3,600 to $4,800 or more. (The custom products cost more because they're designed and made just for you. More work costs more dollars. But if your surgery left your chest less than even, a custom-made job may be just the trick. If you can afford it, why not go for the best?) No matter whether your insurance pays all or part of the cost, you want to be sure you have a prosthesis that fits properly. If it doesn't, no matter who paid, you'll be really unhappy.

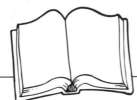

From the Book

A **fashion bra** is the kind you've always worn. If it's a great-fitting bra, you can turn it into a post-surgical bra by sewing a pocket (one you make or one you buy) into either or both sides. A **post-surgical bra** has a pocket built in each cup to hold a breast form in place; thus any post-surgical bra functions for any woman, no matter which breast has been removed—or if both breasts have been removed.

The best way to avoid disappointment is to make sure the fitter is certified and knowledgeable. Then shop around. When one fitter comes up with her best recommendation, get her name, make a note of the model, size, and style she recommends, and thank her for her help. Then go elsewhere to compare. Try several brands to find the best style. For instance, some forms have a nipple, others don't. Some are flat where they fit against your chest; others are concave. Some are tear-shaped, triangular, or asymmetrical. Some fit satisfactorily into a *fashion bra;* others require a *post-surgical bra* for a satisfactory fit. (For more about post-surgical bra options, see Chapter 24, "Fashion Fling: New Clothing Priorities.") Each style fits differently and, therefore, feels more—or less—comfortable. Until you try them on, you can't know which is best for you.

Tales from the Trenches

Jody Brennan explains, "Eight out of ten women wear an ill-fitting bra. Most of us don't think about a perfect fit; we just buy what's comfortable. If we look good in it, that's a bonus! But more is involved in a good fit, especially after surgery. Now your needs differ, and most bras aren't suited for a breast form.

"There's a saying: 'Sometimes it is harder to fit the mind than the body.' If you expect to stay in the same bra you've worn for years, you're facing disappointment. A good-fitting bra is critical to a good-fitting prosthesis, so be prepared to buy a new bra and make a change."

Remember the adage, "Expectations breed frustrations." No matter which prosthesis you choose, nothing will exactly replace the breast you lost—no matter how good it looks or feels. So be realistic about your expectations, and you'll be much happier.

When you go for your fitting, follow these hints:

➤ Make an appointment, even if you call the day you go in. Having an appointment will relieve the stress of having to wait or—worse yet—finding that the fitter isn't in that day. (Many are part-time employees.)

➤ Allow plenty of time, usually an hour to an hour and a half, maybe longer.

➤ Make sure your fitter is certified. She usually has her certificate posted somewhere. If you don't see one, ask.

➤ Judge the fitter's personality. Some fitters presume to know all and can tell you what fits you best; others want to help you find what feels best. Opt for the latter.

➤ Bring your doctor's prescription and your insurance card with you. Some stores will process your insurance paperwork for you. It will also save you sales taxes.

➤ Bring your best-fitting bra with you. Most of us have a favorite, and if it fits well, you may not need to buy post-surgical bras at $35 or more apiece. A good-fitting bra, however, is essential to a good-fitting prosthesis, so be prepared to make a change if necessary.

➤ Wear or bring with you a form-fitting sweater or shirt, one with horizontal stripes or plaids. It will help you see whether the prosthesis is a symmetrical match to your intact breast and whether it sits evenly.

Take It from Us

Be sure when you purchase a post-surgical bra or prosthesis that any bills, checks, and/or receipts are marked "surgical." Otherwise your insurance probably won't pay.

➤ Take a measuring tape to help check symmetry. Stretch the tape from one breast tip to the other and see if the tape looks straight. Measure from the notch in your collarbone at the base of your neck to each breast point and see if you measure equal distances.

➤ Discuss any special needs with your fitter, especially if you're into swimming, dancing, athletics, or any other activity that may affect a decision about a prosthesis.

➤ Ask about exchanges. Many stores will not exchange a breast form once it's been worn.

➤ Consider bringing your husband or a close friend whose opinion you trust. He or she may help you feel confident about your decision.

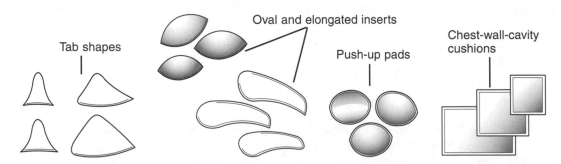

When you've had a lumpectomy, you may find beneficial a breast enhancer in one of several shapes, including (from left to right) tabs, oval and elongated inserts, push-up pads, and chest-wall-cavity cushions.

Partial Parcels

Breast enhancers come in at least a half-dozen shapes. Some fill space under the breast; some fill above the breast; some fill the side of the breast; some fill space from lymph node removal; some cup over the full breast. Most are worn inside a good-fitting bra of your choice, although some need a pocket to ensure that they stay in place. Whichever shape you need, you'll find it available in several materials and in a variety of colors to match skin tone.

The Full Load

If you've had a mastectomy, you'll find breast prostheses in a variety of shapes, styles, and colors. Let's try to make sense of the array of options.

We need to say up front that controversy rages over the importance of the weight of a prosthesis. On the one hand, many maintain that women who don't replace the weight of a breast lost to mastectomy will face possible curvature of the spine, a drooping shoulder, neck pain, backache, and/or loss of balance. On the other hand, there are those who say there is no scientific proof of those effects, and that the prosthetics companies have sold us a line by publicizing them. In fact, by supporting a three-pound breast form from the shoulder, we're asking for trouble with lymphedema (see Chapter 13, "The Big Arm: Lymphedema"). What's the difference, they ask, whether you carry a three-pound shoulder bag or a three-pound prosthesis on your shoulder? The answer, we argue, is that you carry a shoulder bag only intermittently but that the prosthesis is always with you.

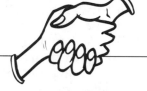

Helping Hand

It's reasonably clear that if you're a 44D, the issue of prosthetic weight is different for you than if you're a 32A. Be aware that your breast weighs anywhere from a pound to four or more pounds. When it's gone, your body may notice.

Standard Style

For years, the standard breast prosthesis has been a silicone form designed to feel and move like the real McCoy. It comes in multiple colors to match your skin tone and in three basic shapes:

➤ **Triangular**—to suit most situations in which less breast tissue has been removed.

➤ **Teardrop**—to fit women whose surgeries removed some underarm or clavicle tissue.

➤ **Asymmetrical**—to accommodate substantial underarm excisions.

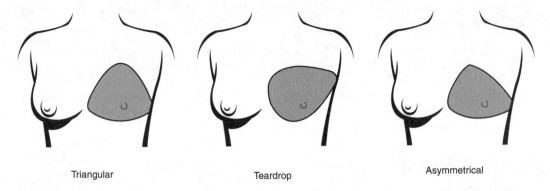

Triangular   Teardrop   Asymmetrical

The three basic shapes for breast prostheses are triangular, teardrop, and asymmetrical.

The weighty silicone forms help prevent muscular problems that some women experience in their back, shoulder, and/or neck. Soft and pliable, they move, feel, and weigh like the real thing. Most women say they feel huggable in a silicone prosthesis. Unlike liquid-filled prostheses, they won't leak if punctured and, unlike lighter or unweighted forms, they won't ride up in your bra. And cleaning is simple. Just wipe with a slightly sudsy cloth, rinse, and pat dry. Always put it back it its box when you're not wearing it.

But it does take getting used to. At first it may feel heavy—too heavy—and perhaps cause irritation if you try to wear it all day. Instead, wear it for only a few hours at a time, gradually increasing the wearing time as you gain comfort.

The biggest complaint, of course, is that silicone forms are hot. You'll now find pads on the market that you wear between the form and your chest wall; they wick away the moisture. Because you feel drier, you'll also feel cooler.

Two new kinds of silicone forms have recently hit the market. The first is a softer silicone form that provides a match for what the company so tactfully calls "more relaxed breast tissue." For those of us who sag, the new form is more like us. The second item in the news is a soft-backed form made of flowable silicone gel. Its special trick? It molds to the body for a perfect fit. Since most of us nowadays aren't perfectly flat after a mastectomy, these may fill the bill.

Lighter, Cooler Forms

More recently, the silicone form is getting competition from lightweight forms, some as much as 60 percent lighter (and lots cheaper—priced from $20 to $150). Generally, the lightweight forms are better for exercise, swimming, and hot weather. Made of polyester, fiberfill, or foam, some are weighted; others aren't. Generally, the fibers are breathable and, therefore, cooler. One lightweight form is made of a hollow silicone shell with a polyester foam insert. Those with added weight, usually in the form of a small lump embedded in the fiber, tend to better stay in place. Unweighted forms tend to ride up during physical activity. Usually, they can be washed by hand and must be left to air dry. Unless the manufacturer specifies it's okay, don't put them in the dryer or use a blow dryer.

One kind of lighter, cooler prosthesis comes permanently fitted into its own bra. While you never have to wonder if the breast form will stay in place and keep you looking symmetrical, you do have expensive bras (about $130 each) and laundry day is a hand operation.

Stick-On

Stick-ons? No, we're not talking pasties here. Some of the breast forms that are loosely called "stick on" use a Velcro-like strip that you glue to your skin with a special gel adhesive that has long been in use in the medical world. The strip in turn has a Velcro-like surface that corresponds to the gel along the edge of the breast form. It's *self-adhesive* and *self-supporting*—for short periods of time without rigorous activity. If you're out for a game of tennis, though, add the bra. Fortunately, however, a fashion bra is just dandy—no need for the industrial-strength, post-surgical jobs. The advantage is the elimination of bounce against the chest wall. And with some styles, you can go braless and still look great.

The disadvantage is that you'll have to keep buying the skin-support strips, each of which cost $3 or $4 and lasts about a week. Be aware, however, that some women have found some of these to be less than 100 percent secure, probably due in large part to the necessity of using exactly the right application process and maintaining clean surfaces—on both you and it. And if you sweat, well, it's probably slippy-slide. Braless could be serious then.

Another kind of stick-on prosthesis is self-adhesive but not self-supporting and does away with the strip glued to your skin. Rather, it has its own permanently sticky circumference that adheres to clean skin. It's too new for us to give you much insight into its success, but you won't go dancing wearing a stick-on without a bra.

Take It from Us

If you itemize expenses on your tax return, the cost of breast forms and bras with pockets may be tax-deductible. Likewise, if you have a bra altered to accommodate a breast form or your post-surgical condition, that, too, may be tax-deductible. But if you don't get receipts, you're out of luck. So get 'em!

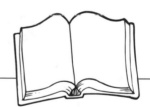

From the Book

Self-adhesive breast forms are those that stick directly to your skin, usually with some kind of glue-like substance developed to use directly on the skin. A **self-supporting** breast form is one that is adequately self-adhesive to stay in place without the support of a bra.

265

Custom-Made

Custom-made prostheses are making names for themselves. One company advertises a "third alternative" and refers to "external reconstruction." A trained consultant makes a plaster cast of your torso and intact breast. Next, artists use the cast to sculpt a mirror image for your prosthesis: the same shape, size, and color as you, including the areola and nipple.

Another alternative in the custom-made line offers an impressive product created by using a three-dimensional scanning device that measures your entire chest wall and incision site, including your intact breast, if you have one. Then, with high-tech flair, images are altered to either construct a form that matches your intact breast as it hangs naturally or altered to replicate the shape of your breast inside the cup of your bra. Matching your skin color and nipple design are added benefits. Pricey, but gorgeous.

Because custom-made products are new on the market, insurance information can be vague. Your doctor can help, especially if he or she will argue for the medical necessity of a custom-made product as a result of poor post-surgical cosmetic recovery. You'll have to ask lots of questions.

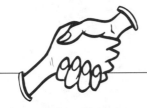

Helping Hand

If your insurance pays for your post-surgical bras and/or breast prostheses and/or enhancers now, it probably will not pay for any kind of reconstructive surgery in the future. Be sure to check out the facts before you file any claims. Ask for the facts in writing; keep them on file. Insurance companies merge and consolidate and change policies. Stay on the safe side.

Swim Prosthesis

Chlorine and salt can quickly damage many prostheses, and swimming will most certainly expose your breast form to one or the other. Always ask whether or not your prosthesis can be worn while swimming and, if so, what special care it may need. Be sure to find out if your guarantee is still good if you wear the prosthesis for a swim. On the other hand, inexpensive swim forms (usually less than $20) will give you an alternative to risking damage to an expensive one.

Before the Real Thing Comes Along

You can't crawl under the porch for six weeks or longer while you wait to be fitted with a proper prosthesis. Within a day—or even the same day—of your

Tales from the Trenches

In the first few days after my mastectomy, I found the perfect use for all those old shoulder pads stuffed in the back of my drawer. Tucked into the pocket of a baggy T-shirt, they gave just enough suggestion of a shape that I managed to feel reasonably inconspicuous.

surgery, you'll be ready to get out and around, even if it's just for a walk around the block. So what do you do to look presentable?

Many women start with a post-surgical camisole, an attractive feminine camisole with a soft cotton-lycra top portion made with pockets designed to hold soft fiber forms. A Reach to Recovery volunteer may show up in your hospital room with a temporary cloth form that you can stuff to your personal specifications by using any kind of soft fiber filling available at your local craft or fabric store (I bought a big bag for a dollar).

Other folks wear a T-shirt to which they pin a soft form and then wear another loose-fitting shirt over that. A ready-made alternative comes in soft stretchy T-shirts with a built-in bra pocketed to hold soft breast forms. Yet another option comes in the form of soft bras, typically called leisure bras, pocketed to hold soft forms that exert no pressure on your incision site. Many of these bras have front openings so that you can easily fasten and unfasten them even with the typically limited range of arm motion that post-mastectomy women experience.

Thousands of women are quite comfortable with their prostheses. Like any other change in life, it takes getting used to; but most women who choose a prosthesis over reconstruction know that it's much simpler to replace a prosthesis than to replace an implant. And they'd rather buy a different size breast form than to surgically enhance a sagging breast to make it match a perky reconstructed one. Still, it's a personal decision either way.

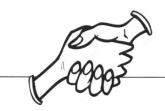

Helping Hand

During these first few weeks, you'll probably be self-conscious of your flat side (or sides). In all likelihood, however, most passersby aren't going to notice. We probably flatter ourselves that every pair of eyes we pass checks out our features. Of course, I'm assuming you'll not be wearing a form-fitting knit sweater. Save that for later.

The Least You Need to Know

➤ Breast enhancers and breast prostheses meet the needs after either lumpectomy or mastectomy surgeries.

➤ Prostheses come in a wide variety of shapes, forms, and colors.

➤ Shop for the right fit in both prosthesis and bra.

➤ Even before you're ready for a standard prosthesis, you can still look terrific.

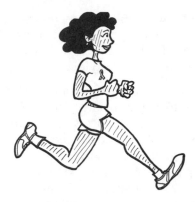

Chapter 23

Life Goes On: Physical and Emotional Changes

> **In This Chapter**
>
> ➤ Getting it "back" together
>
> ➤ Improving your visuals
>
> ➤ Winning your own mind games
>
> ➤ Living in the now

After having faced the surgeries and treatment for breast cancer, many survivors go on to make major changes in their lives, changes to enrich life that now weighs more precious. Some make dramatic changes in their physical lives, altering their diets and exercise routines to improve their general health and vitality. Some make dramatic changes in their emotional lives, pinpointing and then striving for what brings them daily joy and peace. In this chapter, we'll outline some physical and emotional alternatives that may help you create a healthier, more satisfying life for yourself and your family.

From the Mirror: The Outward Signs

The mirror reflects a great deal about any physical changes you may want to make, from a change in diet to a change in hair and skin care. Let's look at all three.

An Apple a Day

The first step in taking care of the physical you is a good, sound, nutritional diet. Your body talks to you about those excess calories you gobbled down or the lack of citrus in your tummy. And the mirror reflects the message. But no subject is more fraught with contradictions and imperatives than diet. A trip to the health section of any book-store will tell you that there are nearly as many different theories about proper nutrition as there are consumers. It goes far beyond the scope of this text to provide you with all the options open to you as you begin to create a healthy lifestyle.

However, learning about *nutrition* is important for everyone. Poor dietary habits, such as eating too much fat and not enough fiber, are related to serious health problems, including heart disease and certain cancers. Although the exact connection between diet and cancers is still unclear, there are certain guidelines that you can follow. Maintain a healthy weight for your body frame, eat a balanced diet by increasing your low-fat fibers and decreasing your fat intake, take daily vitamins, reduce alcohol consumption, drink eight glasses of water daily, and use sugar in moderation.

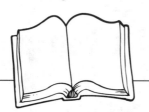

From the Book

Nutrition involves the inter-related steps by which a living organism assimilates food and uses it for growth and for tissue repair and replacement.

Today, most experts agree that a healthy diet is one that focuses on fresh fruits and vegetables, fish and lean meats, low fat, and high fiber. Needless to say, what you need to maintain your health and proper weight is highly personal, and we suggest you discuss your eating plan with your doctor or a qualified nutritionist if you have any questions or concerns.

Tales from the Trenches

Karen remarked, "Breast cancer made me do an about-face. It was the first time that I realized I wouldn't be around forever. I wanted the days I had left to be fun. I wanted to be active and able to live life on my own if I needed to. Just as soon as I felt good and had my doctor's blessing, I saw a nutritionist to change my diet, began an exercise program, and enjoyed each day. I now feel healthier than I ever had before. I have been blessed."

Silken Tresses

If your treatment included chemo, you probably lost your hair. If so, you're likely in the market for a wig.

Call your local hair salons to see if they sell wigs or can refer you to a salon that does. Check the Yellow Pages under "Wigs" or "Hairpieces" for businesses that specialize. You can also check the Internet for wigs. On the other hand, if you can't afford a wig (and some are considerably less expensive than others), contact a local cancer organization. Many survivors, after completing treatment and regaining a full head of hair, donate their wigs to such organizations.

You'll find two basic kinds of wigs on the market: those with synthetic hair and those with real hair. Obviously those made of real hair are more pricey, but you can find some truly lovely synthetic pieces that will make you feel just as pretty. And speaking of pretty, depending on your preference, you can choose a wig that looks like your own hair (and maintain your privacy) or decide instead on a different color and style (and be a new you).

For comfort's sake, you'll probably not wear your wig every waking hour, choosing hats or scarves instead (see Chapter 24, "Fashion Fling: New Clothing Priorities," for more ideas). And unlike folks with permanent hair loss, you'll not wear your wig for more than a half-dozen months or so. Still, over that short time, you'll need to take care of your wig in order to keep it looking great, and that care depends on whether it is synthetic or real hair. Pay special attention to the cleaning directions (which will come with the wig or which the stylist and/or salesperson can detail for you) and follow those directions to the letter. Then, once your own hair has grown back in, consider donating your wig to a cancer organization to help someone in a similar situation.

Instead of wigs, some survivors claim greater comfort with a *cranial prosthesis*. Designed for folks who have little or no hair, the prosthesis sports a truly soft skullcap, so soft you can wear it for 18 hours without being too uncomfortable. You'll need to find a stylist who specializes in them in order to get a good fit and a good match with your own hair.

Regardless of your "temporary" hair decision, I doubt if any of you who have had "no hair" days will ever again complain about a "bad hair" day. It's another of those priority changes!

But now that your own hair is coming back (and it may have come back in a different color or texture), you'll want to take special care of it. Sleep on silk pillowcases; they don't tug as cotton does. Buy the best salon products (they have passed FDA approval as opposed to over-the-counter products) to protect your hair. Wear hats to protect the texture and color from sun damage. To increase the circulation at the roots, learn to do scalp massages with the pads of your fingers, not your nails. Products that contain peppermint and eucalyptus help promote healing and also increase circulation, so you may want to look for hair products containing these ingredients.

Finally, a word to the wise: See a professional for hair styling and treatment as often as you can afford to. Ask your stylist to check your scalp for anything unusual for you such as a scalp rash, more than normal breakage, or no signs of new hair growth.

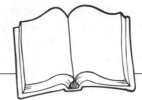

From the Book

A **cranial prosthesis** is a hair-piece basically designed for people who have little or no hair. The skullcap is softer, more elastic, and less scratchy than a wig because, in most cases, a wig is made assuming that the wearer has hair to help pad the scalp. The cranial prosthesis should be ordered while you still have your hair because it is ordered by length and color. Once it arrives, a stylist who specializes in cranial prostheses cuts and styles it to match what you currently have. In most cases, people will never guess you are not sporting your own hair.

Fish Scales and Hide: Skin Tone

If you've undergone radiation, it's probably taken a toll on your skin, and you'll probably want to get it back into shape as quickly as possible. Consider the following:

➤ Get a massage. Massages relax the muscles and joints and help increase the blood circulation in the massaged area.

Take It from Us

Watch your paperwork! Handling paper can abuse the nails and cuticles. Paper is made of wood, so it's abrasive. If you do handle paper a great deal, keep the nails and cuticles creamed. Using a letter opener will also save your hands and nails.

➤ Protect damaged skin by wearing soft, loose clothing, by bathing with cornstarch, and by patting (not rubbing) when you wash and dry it.

➤ Avoid irritants such as perfumes, coarse or raspy household products or materials, and direct sunlight.

➤ Use exfoliating creams to remove dead skin cells (which helps eliminate dry scratchy skin) and then replenish the skin with oily creams that penetrate the skin.

➤ Wear gloves when using abrasive cleaners.

➤ Avoid nail products that have a high concentration of acetone. They dry the skin around the nail bed.

➤ Drink eight glasses of water every day to replenish lost moisture.

Exercise: Keep on Keepin' On

After your surgery, your doctor should talk with you about exercise. You'll want to focus on regaining your normal range of motion in the arm affected by surgery. These exercises usually consist of simple activities like squeezing a rubber ball or walking the wall with your fingers, and some can be done in bed while you are beginning recovery. (For more details, see Chapter 9, "Between Surgery and the Rest.")

In addition to these crucial, but highly specific exercises, you may also decide to improve your overall level of fitness by exercising your whole body. If you enjoy team sports, tennis or volleyball may be the way to go (once you get your strength back). If you're a more solitary exerciser, you might decide to walk or jog alone. *Aquatic therapy* is another option, and you may even be able to find special water aerobics classes for breast cancer survivors through your local YWCA or cancer organization. Working out in the water puts less stress on the joints and, for the survivor, strengthens the shoulders and increases range of motion.

From the Book

Aquatic therapy is a rehabilitation (to restore to use) therapy done in a heated pool. Water helps keep you buoyant and eliminates impact on the joints.

Of course, before you start your exercise program, check with your doctor. Then, choose an exercise that fits your lifestyle and that you enjoy. Exercise helps release endorphins into your body, and endorphins are the chemicals in your brain that act as painkillers. Need we say more?

Healing Body and Soul

You came into this world as a package deal with both body and soul. However, there are times when you forsake one or the other; and when you are under stress (such as when you are diagnosed with breast cancer), it's really easy to forsake one or the other.

What's happening to you now, as you're dealing with breast cancer, can truly affect your body and soul. You have simultaneous physical and emotional reactions to the situation. You need to know what will help you cope and then what will help you move on.

Sleepy Time Gal

Before breast cancer, you may not have taken "getting a good night's sleep" quite so seriously. Now that taking care of yourself is a high priority, you'll want to find a way to get a good night's sleep on a regular basis. Sleep is not only an escape from illness, sadness, and depression, but it is also a time of healing. When the body is at rest, it can focus more energy on healing itself.

Since some folks find themselves unable to sleep, especially during certain parts of their treatment, consider this: Even if you're not asleep, your body can rest. It's a one-two process. First, lie where you're most comfortable (and that may not be in bed if you've just had surgery or if you're experiencing certain side effects). Second, relax and quit worrying about not falling asleep (an act that in itself will likely prevent your falling asleep). You can't be fretting about yourself or someone or something else. Let your mind rest as well by focusing on the positive and the pleasant. (For more, see Chapter 18, "Mind and Body: Spiritual Support.")

Of course, you'll feel better if you can actually sleep, and sleep soundly. To help you get that good night's sleep, develop some bedtime rituals to get you in the mood: a cup of cocoa, a few pages of a novel, meditation, or even soothing music. And remember that taking afternoon naps can hamper a good night's sleep. So try to be like the bunny, and just keep going as long as you can. When you finally are tired and do lie down, sleep will usually come. The tossin' and turnin' will be saved as a golden oldie.

Tales from the Trenches

Kathleen believed that hot flashes helped in the rehabilitation of her right arm because she spent most of the night throwing the covers off and then pulling them back on. She suggests that you not only layer your clothing but also layer your bedding. Use a top and bottom sheet and several all-cotton blankets under a spread. Cotton is more easily and more quickly washed, and depending on how hot or cold you are, you can cover with one or several layers.

Hot Woman—or Hot and Sweaty?

With or without breast cancer, at some point hot flashes are certainly part of your life. They are uncomfortable. They are embarrassing. They are distracting. And they simply are! What can you do? Your doctor can prescribe medications, or you can consider soy products and herbs, although neither of these are proven remedies. When those options don't work, try an attack plan:

➤ Wear cotton clothing from the skin out; it helps absorb perspiration and makes you feel cooler.

➤ Wear layered clothing.

➤ At bedtime, skip the long bathrobe; instead wear a bed jacket over sleeveless or short-sleeved pajamas.

➤ Keep your house and office cool. When you feel as if your inner temperature is 110°, an outside temperature of 65° is a big help.

Eventually, you may be back to your old "hot mama" self, but for a while, unfortunately, you'll be just hot and sweaty.

Sex and Intimacy

Sex and intimacy are certainly flip sides of the same coin, but they're not the same. Intimacy is a private association of our deepest nature.

Doctors and psychologists verify that certain things in your life will affect your sex drive. Those of you with a load of stress in your lives will be thinking, "No kidding!" But stress is only one factor that can affect your sex drive. Other psychological factors include depression, anxiety, fear, fatigue, some medications, and, yes, physical or medical problems. And just for the record, dealing with breast cancer may quite likely, at least at one point or another, involve all of the above.

It's normal for your sexual desire to diminish from time to time. In most cases, it does pick right back up. But in light of your treatment, you may no longer be typical of "most cases." Right now you may have more need for intimacy—hugging, cuddling, kissing, holding hands—than for sex. Your breast cancer and/or disfigurement may have shaken your self-esteem, and even thinking about a sexual relationship may put you in a state of panic. You know that "time heals all wounds." Time will usually heal the emotional wounds and scars of breast cancer just as it does the physical scars from the surgery.

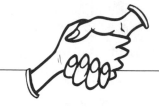

Helping Hand

Learn to make accommodations. At one point in your life, having sex might have involved sexy underwear, enticing music and lighting, and suggestive videos. But it doesn't always have to be that way. Being in a hot tub together, making out at a drive-in, or just snuggling in bed watching a movie can certainly be sexy, too.

Take It from Us

Recognize all the things that make you sexy. Your laughter, smile, caring nature, and even intellect are part of your sexiness. It's a package deal. Just losing part of your breast, and an inch or so of tissue—or even all of your breast—doesn't take away everything else that makes you sexy.

Find new products that will help you feel sexy. Lacy nightgowns with built-in bras may make you feel more comfortable than gowns with spaghetti straps, or no gown at all. (See Chapter 24, "Fashion Fling: New Clothing Priorities" for more details.)

Concentrate on other good qualities such as your laughter, eyes, legs, and so on. Make the most of them.

While you are enjoying intimacy with your partner, think about and discuss those sexual issues. Are you worried that your partner may be unfaithful? Discuss it. Are you afraid of being rejected? Discuss it. Just worrying about something won't make it go away; in fact, worrying can make things worse, even blow things way out of proportion. If you and your partner are uncomfortable discussing these issues, you may want to sign up for a few sessions with a sex therapist. Your doctor can recommend one.

If you are single and your friends are interested in "fixing you up," don't allow them to force you into something you are not ready for. Timing is so important; so be patient with yourself and ask others, partner or friends, to be patient with you, too.

Attitude Adjustment

Having breast cancer has become an ever-present part of your life, but still it isn't your whole life. For most of you, it's a significantly unpleasant detour from what you had planned or expected. And as with any detour, you have to look at your map and find a new way. Finding a new way to approach how you live your life—or whatever is left of it—changes your priorities.

What's the bottom line to your life? When you sort through all of life's events, what really matters? Your changing priorities may make you uncomfortable for a while. Seeing a new side to things usually does, and your battle with breast cancer may have brought you face to face with some tough new questions:

➤ What legacy am I leaving?

➤ What future am I planning?

➤ Can I deal with the changes I'm envisioning?

➤ What's truly important to me?

➤ What can I do to make my life better?

➤ How can I work the "new me" into the old routine?

You may have heard, "Change is inevitable; growth is optional." You've changed; now you'll most likely choose the option to grow. Although time does seem to heal all wounds, the wounds often leave scars that make you different.

Stan, my husband, is a perfectionist. He likes everything perfect; and, in this world, perfection is hard to find. One Saturday morning we got our bank statement in the mail. It was off by several hundred dollars. He was furious. He walked into my home office, threw the bank statement on my desk, and said, "Suzanne, I can't believe you are not upset about this. This is a problem." I said, "No, breast cancer is a problem. This is an inconvenience."

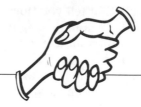

Helping Hand

Set your priorities. In the past, you probably focused first on doing the "should's" and "must's" for everyone else—your children, husband, parents, friends—or maybe even for your job. In doing so, sometimes you probably forgot the "should's" and "must's" for yourself. Now, as you battle breast cancer, you'll find it necessary to change those priorities, for only by taking care of yourself can you ever hope to return to taking care of the others near and dear to you.

A problem presents you with uncertainty and is usually difficult to handle—like breast cancer. An inconvenience is more of a temporary lag in your comfort level. Frequently, an inconvenience is a mountain-out-of-a-molehill situation. In fact, when you filter life's experiences through your new set of priorities, you'll find that most of what others call "problems" are nothing more than daily irritations or inconveniences. After you've been through the battle with breast cancer, Chicken Little moments take on the air of the ridiculous. It's part of your change in priorities.

Never a Wasted Day

Just as some folks have confused problems with inconveniences, I also think they sometimes lose delight in their lives. What, lately, has given you great joy?

I know most of you would feel great joy if you won the lottery, but, as I understand it, the odds of that are very slim. However, the odds of feeling great joy listening to songbirds, eating rich, creamy pudding, and spending time with friends are much more in your favor. You can feel great joy in the simple things of life: the things you've so often taken for granted. What did you do today that was delightful?

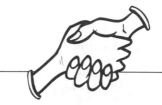

Helping Hand

Spend your time wisely. With each situation, event, and person, you could be making a memory right now.

But days are made of minutes, and minutes are made of seconds. And while 60 seconds doesn't seem like a lot, when you've been diagnosed with breast cancer, 60 seconds becomes 60 *precious* seconds that you don't want to waste.

You've seen the trivia books that tell you how many hours of your life you waste standing in line, being on hold, and driving from one place to another. Yet time is your ultimate commodity. And your changing priorities help you focus on spending your time more wisely. That includes taking as much time for yourself as you can, doing what you love to do. And since today is the first day of the rest of your life, you may enjoy the suggestions from survivors who found ways to make the most of their days—every day:

➤ Make visual changes—ones you can see—to remind you of the new you or a new hobby that you want to do.

➤ Stop watching depressing, violent, and negative TV shows.

➤ Don't offer to do something unless you really want to do it.

➤ Find time for solitude to keep in touch with yourself and what you are doing.

➤ Take five-minute breaks every two or three hours to rest and refocus.

➤ Think things through and decide with care how you want to spend your time.

➤ Develop a plan for your life.

➤ Enjoy doing things, not just finishing things.

➤ Look back on each day and rejoice in what you did that made you really happy.

There's an end to all things, even to your breast cancer treatments. And once they're finished, it's time to go on to the new you. You'll make the physical and emotional changes more easily by following the suggestions of wonderful, warm women in the sisterhood. According to them, as you've heard throughout this chapter, you'll help yourself most by a simple positive plan: Heal, cope, rejoice, and pass along to others what you have learned. We hope we've done our part to help.

The Least You Need to Know

➤ Once you've gone through breast cancer, you'll likely examine both your physical and emotional lives in anticipation of changing priorities.

➤ Focus first on meeting your physical needs, for then you can move on with your life.

➤ Be patient with yourself; for even though you'll make changes in your life, you can't change everything overnight.

➤ Spend each minute wisely, enjoy the time, and be happy about making memories for yourself and others.

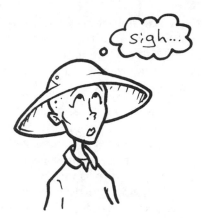

Chapter 24

Fashion Fling: New Clothing Priorities

> **In This Chapter**
>
> ➤ Possible changes in clothing needs
>
> ➤ Different bras—fashion or surgical
>
> ➤ Suggestions for fashionable comfort
>
> ➤ Meeting swimwear needs

Whether you've been most comfy in jeans and baggy sweatshirts or tailored business suits and panty hose, chances are, after your surgery and follow-up treatments, you'll continue wearing what you've always worn. Some exceptions, however, may pop up; so before you make new purchases, you may want to learn from other survivors what's worked best for them.

In this chapter, we'll talk about some temporary changes you may need to make in your daily wardrobe. Then we'll talk about the most important change you'll likely face: your all-time favorite bra may be a real letdown (in more ways than one). Next, we'll tell you why, even if you've had a mastectomy without reconstruction, there's no reason to stay away from the beach or the pool. Finally, you'll find out why you'll want to pay more attention to that little fabric-content label when you buy new clothes.

Now and Later

Let's start with now.

Whether you've had a lumpectomy or mastectomy, surgical incisions make for pain, sometimes for a month or more. And unfortunately, sometimes the incision falls right where your bra fits—and rubs. In addition, if you've had radiation, it may have left you with the equivalent of a nasty sunburn. In spite of the lotions and other special skin care we've told you about, you may find you're *waaaaay* too tender for that tight elastic of even your favorite bra. So, dear friends, you may want to follow the crowd. Lots of us reverted to the braless years of the 1960s and found relief.

To compensate for our modesty, however, (after all, the 1960s are long past and most of us are probably now more reserved and decidedly more droopy), many of us turned to a popular and even fashionable style: layers. Even in the heat of summer, we went to layers, like a light cotton vest over a T-shirt, or a rather snug sleeveless shirt under a loose-fitting short-sleeved one. Why two T-shirts? Well, you see, if you've had a mastectomy without reconstruction, the double duty lets you pin to the bottom layer a soft temporary prosthesis (or one or more of those shoulder pads you've had stashed in the back of a drawer). The loose top layer provides full deception, and you're home-free! Nothing rubs, and nothing shows.

Take It from Us

After a bilateral mastectomy and reconstruction, one survivor reports, "My new perky 36B breasts are so firm, I can go braless in slinky, sexy dresses without anyone knowing."

Of course, after a mastectomy without reconstruction, if you have any shirts with breast pockets, you'll come to have a greater appreciation of the name! You can stuff a temporary prosthesis (or those shoulder pads again) into the pockets and go merrily on your way.

It's my personal philosophy that you can never have too much denim. Fortunately, those long, shapeless denim jumpers have remained reasonably fashionable for quite some time now (probably because most of us don't want to let go of them). They offer another means to layer. Layers cover up lots of imperfections (and the braless condition), especially if the outer garment is pretty much shapeless itself!

Tales from the Trenches

One survivor wrote, "At first the scar was so sensitive I couldn't stand to have anything touch it. When I had to go out, I wore a little scrap of a no-bra bra and a polyester puff, and as soon as I was back in the car, I snatched the puff out. I was so miserable that I began to think I'd never wear clothes again. Then suddenly, the burning sensation went away."

Most of us have uneven breasts to begin with, but now maybe they're worse—whether it's the temporary result of surgical bandaging or the long-term result of a fairly drastic lumpectomy or a mastectomy. In any case, the unevenness will be more noticeable if you're wearing plaids, stripes, or symmetrical patterns. Instead, choose solids, diagonal stripes, or multiple colors in an overall pattern. Think about it: Hunters and soldiers understand the real definition of camouflage. Learn from them, but transcribe the idea from drab to delightful!

And don't forget scarves! Whole books describe the things you can do to accessorize with scarves, and we survivors learn quickly that covering up is one of them! So dig out those forgotten scarves, especially the really large ones, and go for gorgeous. Everyone will be so busy noticing how feminine you look in the swath of silk over your shoulders and covering your chest that the rest will go unnoticed!

Later, after your incision has healed and the radiation burns have subsided, you'll probably wear what you always wore, at least as far as outer garments go. After all, once you've had reconstruction and/or after you get your prosthesis, you'll have your figure back. (See Chapters 21, "Back to the Bikini: Reconstruction," and 22, "Boob in a Box: Prostheses," for more details.) In years past, when radical mastectomies were the standard, surgery dramatically changed a woman's clothing needs. Fortunately, radical mastectomies are now rare; and you can still go for the slinky evening gowns, the fetching bathing suits, or the sexy sheer blouses.

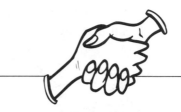

Helping Hand

If you've had reconstruction and/or reduction to achieve more even breasts, you may find yourself shopping for a different dress size. One woman reports laughing aloud in the dressing room the first time she tried on a dress and found—surprise!—that her usual size no longer fit. As a result of reconstruction and reduction, she had dropped two dress sizes—not to mention her more manageable chest size.

Not-So-Mad Hatter

If you've had chemo, chances are you lost your hair—or at least a lot of it. While we discuss wigs elsewhere (see Chapter 23, "Life Goes On: Physical and Emotional Changes"), we would be negligent not to mention hats as part of your fashion statement. Some survivors told us they wore hats just to cover their hair loss, that it was only a cosmetic convenience that was cheaper than a wig or cranial prosthesis. Others, especially those who live in cold climates or dealt with the effects of chemo during the cold winter months, said hats helped keep their heads warm—whether they found themselves inside, outside, or even asleep.

Hats of all kinds are readily available from discount stores, department stores, and the most fashionable boutiques. For instance, you may want to consider some of the following fashion hats:

➤ Wide-brimmed straw, felt, or other fabric hats that double to keep the sun off your face and neck (an important feature if you're undergoing radiation therapy). Try them on before you buy. Hatmakers assume you have hair, so some may prove uncomfortably scratchy on your tender scalp.

➤ Billed baseball-type hats that provide some shade for your face and eyes. They don't cover up much on the back of the head, and some may have scratchy seams. Those with a wacky or amusing logo or phrase, however, add a touch of humor that many survivors enjoy. Some new ones add ponytails that give an illusion of hair.

➤ *Cloche* or *scrunch* for a casual look. Some fabrics, however, can add an elegant touch for church or other dressy occasions.

➤ *Tam* or *boater* for a more tailored look. Suit your personality with the style best for you.

Some hats, however, are either more effective or designed especially to disguise hair loss (see the accompanying illustrations).

➤ Turbans come in many fabrics, like fleece, velvet, denim, cotton twill, and even lace. Some are pleated for fuller crowns and a more tailored look. They come both lined and unlined, the lining adding warmth and body to the shape. Some fit snugly as the result of a fitted band. Some sport attached hairpieces, like bangs.

➤ Kerchiefs provide a causal look and come with or without added hairpieces.

➤ Kerchief caps, which cover the back of the head and tie over the top of the head, offer a firm fit and an alternative look.

➤ Sleep caps, some of which are made of soft mesh, add warmth at night. They also help camouflage your baldness from your bed partner.

➤ A variety of hats and caps come with hair added, including bangs, falls, and ponytails.

Any of these hats, of course, can be accessorized with silk flowers, ribbons, scarves, braided scarves or fabrics, or fabric rosettes. You can find these accessories

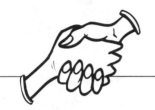

Helping Hand

Your uneven—or missing—breast may not be as obvious to others as you assume. After her mastectomy, Paula admits, "I did feel conspicuous at first, and it was a real comedown to discover that nobody noticed."

From the Book

A **cloche** is a close-fitting bell-shaped hat while a **scrunch** sports a fuller crown that, as the name suggests, has a crumpled look. A **tam** is made with a wide, round flat top, while a **boater** is a stiff hat with a flat crown and brim.

in many department stores and specialty boutiques where other post-surgical items are found. The American Cancer Society's TLC (Tender Loving Care) Catalog specializes in these items. (Also see Appendix D, "Sources of Prostheses and Post-Surgical Clothing.")

Even with all the options available in shops and catalogs, you may have difficulty finding a hat with just the right fit. And that's a big issue. After all, if that hat doesn't fit snugly, windy days can literally blow your cover. Solution? Try tucking folded paper towels inside the rim until you get the right fit.

Mentionable Unmentionables: Bras and Lingerie

For those of you who have had surgery and reconstruction, the contents of your undies drawer won't change much, except for the short haul immediately after surgery when sports bras usually feel better than other more stylish bras. Of course, if you're undergoing radiation, the operative word is "old." If not old, then at least cheap. Unless you're mapped for radiation with tattoos, your clothing may get stained. On the other hand, for those of us who have had a lumpectomy or, especially, a mastectomy, the undies may shift toward the utilitarian (especially if you now have one breast size 36B and the other 36DD). You may still find yourself checking the windows at Victoria's Secret, but you'll likely be shopping elsewhere.

A Real Lift

According to the professional fitters we talked with, most folks wear bras that neither fit properly nor provide adequate support. We'd rather not believe that—we'd rather rely on the fashion magazines and enjoy the frilly little things prominently displayed in the shop windows. Still, the facts remain.

Helping Hand

If you're handy with crafts, chances are you'll be clever enough to improvise and make your own accessories for that wonderful well-put-together look. But if you have the know-how but not the gumption, turn to your crafty friends who have asked, "What can I do to help?"

Now that you've had surgery—with or without reconstruction—your bra needs are probably somewhat different. If you've had a lumpectomy, depending on how much tissue was removed, you may have uneven breasts. You're looking for a bra that will somehow support both sides comfortably. If you've had a mastectomy but not reconstruction, you're looking for something that works with your prosthesis. If you've had reconstruction, you may now have one perky breast and one saggy breast. So you, too, are looking for a bra that will somehow support both sides comfortably.

For many folks, the first bra after surgery is the trusty, ever-reliable sports bra, especially one that fastens in the front. Snaps, however, can be scratchy, irritating on sensitive skin. Solution? Try a big cotton pad (the ones like you put on your kids' badly skinned knees) under the snaps.

Take It from Us

Remember (especially if you've had node dissection), you won't be allowed to move your arms higher than a 90-degree angle from your body for a week or so after surgery. After that, you'll need some time to stretch the tissue enough so that you can reach over your head. So if you go for the sports bra, skip the pullovers. It should fasten in the front.

From the Book

Fashion bras are those you've always purchased in all their many styles, shapes, fabrics, and colors. On the other hand, a post-surgical bra is made with a pocket behind each cup to hold a breast form. Post-surgical bras come in many styles, shapes, fabrics, and colors.

Later, you may choose to switch to a regular *fashion bra*. Some survivors mentioned popular name brands that offer comfort and good support. Those who skipped the reconstruction after a mastectomy added a sequel to the fashion bra statement: They converted the fashion bra into a mastectomy bra by sewing in their own pockets to hold the prosthesis. Some gals used a soft cotton knit to create the pockets; others spent $3 or $4 for ready-made pockets, nicely edged with a light elastic edge to help maintain shape. You'll find the ready-made pockets at the same shops that sell surgical bras and other mastectomy products. The pockets work just fine for the smaller, lightweight prostheses (or even for old panty hose wadded up to the right size).

For those of you who chose reconstruction, you may find fashion bras that have more rounded bra cups fit better than the more pointed styles. Because a reconstructed breast may have a somewhat flatter, smoother curve, a more pointed cup may leave some wrinkling. So you'll probably want to pass on the Madonna look.

Whatever fashion bra you choose, you'll likely want to avoid the underwires. While there is some controversy about underwires causing breast damage, two real problems occur after surgery. First, many folks are convinced that underwires can cause further problems if you've had lymph node removal. Second, if you've had an implant, underwires tend to rub the implant. Rubbing over the long haul equals damage. A damaged implant means more surgery. In my book, that makes the decision fairly easy. Why take the risk?

For other folks, especially those with fuller breasts, *post-surgical bras* may be the better alternative. They contain pockets in both sides (whether you need them or not) and hold anything from the lightest to the heaviest prosthesis with the assurance it won't be going anywhere until you take off your bra. Unlike the post-surgical bras from days of yore, today you'll find them in every style from the most utilitarian to quite lacy and feminine. In other words, you can still feel gorgeous in sheer blouses. In fact, many look no different on the outside from regular fashion bras.

Before you shop, consider some of the following features available in good post-surgical bras:

➤ Variety of fabrics, including cotton and polyester tricot, for the most comfortable yet attractive garment possible

➤ Variety of colors to match skin tone, including white, black, and various shades of beige and ivory (unfortunately, you'll probably not find one in red or green, or in any of the lovely pastels you'll see in a full line of fashion bras—but you can toss a white one in with a load of colored clothes and get any variety of pastels)

➤ Variety of styles, including some with camisole inserts that let you continue to wear low necklines

➤ Variety of forms, including long-line, some with wide bands, some with wide or even super-wide straps, some with leotard backs; some even strapless

➤ Back or front closures—or both, with adjustment in the back and easy on/off in the front

➤ Strap adjustments in the back, so that metal slides are well away from the delicate prosthesis

Tales from the Trenches

Some of us admit and the rest of us keep secret the bra fetishes the fashion designers have imposed upon us. You know the symptoms: As you pass through the lingerie department, you can't help fingering those lacy little things in seductive colors, wondering how badly the lace would scratch. If you've had surgery, though, you're probably living in a sports bra for that good all-over support. Perhaps you, like so many of us, wish someone out there would do a sports bra that's just a bit more exciting and colorful!

Before you make any major purchases, however, keep in mind that your bra size will probably change over the next several months or even over the next several years. First, you'll have some post-surgical swelling for at least four to six weeks, maybe longer. Until the swelling goes away, if you're like most of us, no bra feels good or fits well. Certain post-surgical treatments may also cause swelling. You may also experience some short-term weight loss or weight gain with chemo, so that affects bra fit, too. If you were post-menopausal and have been on hormone replacement therapy, you're no longer on it. As a result, you will probably experience some shrinkage in both breasts. And finally, depending on what long-term therapy you have, your breast tissue may continue to shrink. I know that's not wonderful news, but since surgical bras are a bit pricey ($30 and up—mostly up), be careful about any major initial investments. Better to wash out a few unmentionables every couple of nights than to have hundreds of dollars worth of uncomfortable, unusable stuff accumulated in the back of your drawer.

Nobody's Secret

When you're still too tender to deal with a bra, you'll find that pretty camisoles (some with built-in pockets for a featherweight prosthesis) may be the ticket to happiness. They make you feel and look pretty. Some women reported, in fact, that while they were eager to resume sexual relations with their mates, they felt too self-conscious bare-chested. The lacy camisole turned the trick (well, you know what we mean).

And speaking of camisoles, those really pretty ones in fashion colors that are designed to show under suit jackets or V-necked tops also work well for concealing some loss of tissue. Depending on how much tissue you've lost and from where it was removed, camisoles may offer a really feminine solution to some of your clothing needs. Check out the options in the lingerie department.

Helping Hand

Treat yourself to something special. Some survivors told us that on the days they felt really ugly, they got a true boost by shopping for pretty lingerie.

Other survivors reported that nighties with lots of ruffles at the top helped camouflage an uneven or missing breast and made them feel more comfortable and more desirable. (Two-piece nighties may be more comfortable—you can figure out why for yourself.) Most gals said they didn't want to wear a prosthesis to bed, even the softest, lightest prosthesis imaginable. So, unless you habitually wore a bra at night, you most likely won't want to wear one now in order to hold a breast form in place. So consider the ruffles (and check out Appendix D).

Knits and Knots and Dresses

Depending on what kind of surgery you've had, you may find yourself making some minor changes in your closet as well. There's probably no reason why you can't continue to wear those V-necked and scoop-necked dresses and tops, but you may need to make some alterations. And at least for a while, you might want to skip slinky and think one size larger.

You may also consider two-sided clothing tape. Designed originally to keep scarves in place, it works quite well to keep low-cut shells in place. One side of the tape sticks to the skin and the other to the fabric, which makes for a simple solution for avoiding that all-too-revealing view we offer others when low-cut clothing drops away from the body when we lean forward or bend over.

Tales from the Trenches

If you have a favorite V-neck dress that, when you lean forward, falls away from your body, you'll likely be showing more than you want. Louise, who has always favored V-neck styles, says you can compensate several ways. First, you can simply pin the low-necked shirt or dress to your bra so it won't fall away. You can add darts to a deep V-neck to make it fit more closely. Or you can have the garment tailored by raising the shoulder line and thus shortening the V-neck. Otherwise, you can accessorize with camisoles or fill in with a wonderful scarf.

Sleeveless garments, however, can suddenly become a big problem, especially if the armhole is large and if you've had lots of tissue removed from under your arm. You may have no alternative other than to wear a jacket over the sleeveless blouse or to wear a short-sleeved shirt under the sleeveless shirt.

If, in spite or your careful behavior, you find yourself suffering from lymphedema, you may find the need to alter your favorite garments. For instance, you may need to enlarge armholes and sleeves.

In short, if you've had lymph node removal, you'll need to make sure you're wearing nothing tight anywhere along your arm. That means when you wear cuffs that fit loose at the wrist, you must never shove them up your arm—an unconscious habit that many of us have. (See more details in Chapter 13, "The Big Arm: Lymph-edema.") So, yes, you can continue to wear your favorite turtlenecks. Just keep the loose cuffs at your wrists.

Dive In

Just because you had a mastectomy and chose not to have reconstruction doesn't mean you have to skip the beach parties or the lazy afternoons by the pool (or wear tent-like cover-ups while you're there). You'll find a number of satisfactory alternatives from which to choose.

First, swimwear often includes its own bra. That means you'll likely be able to pin a prosthesis to it. Just be sure that salt or chlorine won't harm the prosthesis you use. Of course, be certain not to puncture one that maintains its shape with some kind of fluid. And surely some of you will make your own swimwear prosthesis using polyfill, old panty hose, or other soft but springy fabrics. Then if the salt or chlorine damages it, you'll feel free to pitch it and get another.

Take It from Us

Don't use mail order unless the suit can be returned. You simply can't tell how it will fit under the arm or through the bra until you try it on. And remember that no matter which swimwear best serves your needs, you'll need a dry prosthesis for the trip home. Most prostheses that are best suited for swimming absorb some amount of water.

If you choose swimwear that includes its own bra, you can also add a pocket to one or both sides. The pocket will hold your prosthesis more easily than if you try to pin it in place. (Some tend to float up and that could be a bit embarrassing. Pockets solve that problem.)

If you don't find suitable swimwear with its own bra, hit the boutiques or specialty shops for post-mastectomy swimsuits. You'll also find them available through mail order, some more reasonably priced than others. Unlike other swimwear, these suits follow the design of post-surgical bras. Many, in fact, are made by the same companies that market the bras. Like bras, the suits are designed with a pocket on each side (even if you don't need both) into which a prosthesis fits snugly.

You'll also want to consider various necklines for your new swimwear. You may like a soft scoop, or one that fits fairly high in front. Fortunately, many fashionable suits will surely offer an alternative just right for. It's likely that your underarm scar may be the hardest to cover.

Fabrics of Your Life

There's nothing more miserable than that creeping sensation that tells you your body's heating up. Hot flash on its way. Glasses fogging up. You know that soon you'll be perspiring, and everyone else in the room is comfortably bundled up in Polartec jackets over bulky sweaters over long-sleeved shirts. As you perspire, your clothes get damp (or even plain wet), and then, a half-hour later, you're chilled. That's downright unhealthy. The answer: layers. Lots of layers (so you can rip them off one at a time until you're down to whatever). The real trick, however, is to layer with natural fibers. They breathe. They keep your body more evenly comfortable.

In short, if you have a closet full of polyester, polyester blends, rayon, nylon, acetate, or other synthetic fabrics and blends, you'll probably start changing your shopping habits. Synthetics are hot. Plain and simple. Most survivors told us that they turned entirely to *natural fabrics,* especially to cotton—summer and winter. Even cotton turtlenecks in winter.

Next to cottons, folks counted linen and wool among their favorites, admitting, of course, that linen has its perpetual wrinkled look (well, at least it does within three minutes of putting it on). Still it's a natural, breathing fabric, and some linen blends wrinkle less than pure linen.

So what about silk? It's a natural fabric. Just don't forget that you'll find insulated underwear made of silk—because it's so warm, and water or moisture leaves stains on silk. No-brainer, isn't it?

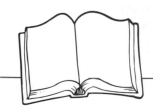

But it's not just in your closet where you'll soon decide to keep all natural fabrics. You'll probably soon choose all cotton undies and nighties as well.

From the Book

Natural fabrics include cotton, wool, linen, and silk, or any combination of these—such as a cotton-wool blend or a cotton-linen blend.

Fortunately, enough folks began requesting all-natural fabrics years ago that designers and manufacturers took note. As a result, all manner of natural-fabric clothing is readily available; gorgeous, fashionable things designed to wear from the skin out. You'll love 'em!

The Least You Need to Know

➤ After surgery, you'll make some short-term clothing adjustments for the sake of comfort and modesty.

➤ Later, you may reconsider the kind of bra and other lingerie that will work best for you.

➤ Surgery, with or without reconstruction, shouldn't keep you away from the pool or beach.

➤ Later, you'll probably wear what you've always worn with some adaptations toward natural fabrics.

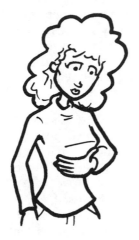

Chapter 25

Recurrence: Safe to Go Back in the Water?

In This Chapter

➤ Living with the fear

➤ What signs you should look for

➤ What to do if it happens to you

➤ Knowing it's not a death sentence

➤ Finding a new support group that can help

If there is one word that will strike terror into a cancer survivor's heart, it is *recurrence*. What's going through your mind at this point? No, this can't be happening—again. I had the surgeries! I went through all the therapies! I lost my hair and my breast! I've prayed and meditated! I'm eating healthy and exercising! What have I done wrong? Nothing. Stuff happens. And this stuff could happen to you.

Even though the news of recurrence is devastating to the survivor, it emphatically does not mean a death sentence. You just have to regroup and develop a new plan of attack. After all, the cancer cells are attacking you. You have every right to attack back! This is war! In this chapter, we'll discuss some of the strategies you can develop that will move you forward through this difficult time.

Types of Recurrence

Is there any way to know whether you'll be likely to face a recurrence? Not for certain. Of course, nothing is for certain when we talk about breast cancer. Some conditions, however, suggest a strong possibility of recurrence. If, for instance, you had a fairly aggressive type of cancer like inflammatory breast cancer or if your tumor was quite large with lots of positive lymph nodes, you have a higher probability of recurrence than someone who had a noninvasive condition does. On the other hand, there is no evidence to suggest that just because you had a more serious kind of cancer that you will, indeed, eventually have a recurrence. Just as we don't know what causes breast cancer or who will get it, we really don't know who will have a recurrence.

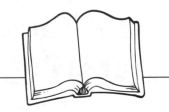

From the Book

Local recurrence is when your breast cancer comes back near or at the site of your lumpectomy or mastectomy. **Distant recurrence** is when the cancer has spread to another part of your body such as the bones, brain, lungs, or liver. A distant recurrence is cancer that has metastasized.

Likewise, we can't say when this recurrence will happen, if indeed it does. Some recurrences have shown up within months of the original surgery; others took years, maybe 20 or more. In some cases, however, the recurrence may be some leftover cells that the surgery and/or treatment simply missed, especially when the recurrence comes so quickly on the heels of the surgery/treatment. At the other extreme, of course, a recurrence that shows up 20 years later may be a new cancer, not a recurrence of the old one. While the fine-line differences may make a big difference to your doctor, the bottom line for you is the same. It's back. Again.

Doctors loosely categorize recurrences as either *local* or *distant*. As the name implies, a local recurrence is a cancer that appears at or near the site of the original tumor. A distant recurrence, on the other hand, involves a metastasized cancer that occurs in another organ of the body, such as the bone, brain, lungs, or liver.

If you had a lumpectomy as opposed to a mastectomy, local recurrence is more common and will usually occur within two years, often as a new pea-size lump or a change in the coloration (reddening) of the skin. You or your doctor may find the lump during a BSE or mammogram. Because it is "local" and has not spread into the lymphatic system, chances of recovery and containment are good.

Treatment for a recurrence may or may not vary from your initial treatment. Depending on the location and size of the recurrence, you may have another lumpectomy with or without adjuvant treatment. More than likely, however, if you've already had a lumpectomy, a recurrence will suggest the necessity for a mastectomy with or without adjuvant treatment. However, in most all cases, you cannot have radiation in the same spot as you did in the past. In addition, your treatment will depend, just as it did with your first cancer, on the stage of your cancer when it is discovered.

As strange as it may sound, even if you had a mastectomy you can still have a local recurrence, most frequently located in the scar. Because you have insufficient breast tissue for a mammogram, your only means of detection is a BSE or clinical exam. Again, a lump or redness will be a telltale sign. Treatment will likely involve surgery to remove the lump and may or may not involve adjuvant treatment.

Another kind of recurrence is less local. Although it's rare, a recurrence can occur not in the area of the breast but in the area of the lymph nodes. Again, usual treatment is a combination of surgery and adjuvant treatment.

A final kind of recurrence isn't actually a recurrence at all, but a new cancer. In this case, new cancer will appear not in the scar or its immediately surrounding area, but in another part of the breast. It's really a bit of a word game we're playing here, so whether it's technically a new cancer or not, you have cancer again. Nevertheless, the designation "new cancer" may cause your doctor to look at the condition differently and recommend a different treatment.

With any local recurrence, the first line of defense is frequently to test for any other cancer in the body, particularly in the bones, lungs, or liver. More on tests for these later.

That takes us to the other kind of recurrence: distant recurrence. This kind of recurrence tends to be a more serious challenge because it is cancer that has metastasized and spread into other body parts. A distant recurrence of breast cancer occurs most commonly in the bones, lungs, and liver and less commonly in the brain and spinal cord. Because the cancer has spread into other parts of your body, treatments vary with the type of cancer and in its intensity depending on the stage of the cancer.

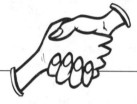

Helping Hand

Don't panic. The signs of metastasized cancer are also signs of normal, even everyday, ailments. Just because you have a headache does not mean that you have brain cancer. Just because your ankle pops when you walk does not mean you have bone cancer. Do pay attention to changes that are constant or intense, and see your doctor to either ease your mind or to catch a distant recurrence early on.

There are some common signs to look for that could indicate a metastasized cancer. However, do keep in mind that all of these symptoms could also indicate perfectly benign conditions; you have absolutely no reason to panic. Simply check it out with the doc and receive a complete, thorough examination. In the meantime, here are a few general observations about breast cancer metastases:

➤ **In about 25 percent of the cases of metastasized breast cancer, the recurrence shows up first as bone cancer.** And regardless of where the metastasis shows up first, those who die of breast cancer almost always eventually get it in their bones. Bone cancer usually causes pain similar to that experienced with arthritis. The difference between this type of pain and arthritis is that the pain from bone cancer is steady and does not go away with most over-the-counter medicines or while you are sleeping. The pain is a result of the cancer cells eating up space in the bones and applying pressure to and on them. Bones become more brittle and fracture easily. If your cancer has metastasized to your bones, a bone scan (not to be confused with a bone density test) will be the first means of detection. X-rays, CAT scans, and MRIs can also aid in detection. Radiation to the localized bone area is usually the first line of treatment. If the cancer is too widespread through your bones for radiation, chances are the doc will recommend another round of chemo.

➤ **In about 20 percent of the cases of metastasized breast cancer, the recurrence shows up first in the lungs.** Eventually, however, in about 65 percent of those who die of breast cancer, the disease ultimately spreads to the lungs. Lung cancer usually causes shortness of breath due to the damage the cancer does to lung tissues. A chronic cough may also be symptomatic. Because breast cancer that spreads to the lungs doesn't usually cause pain, the shortness of breath is the only clear-cut symptom. And because it comes on gradually, it's often difficult to diagnose. Detection is via a combination of x-ray and either needle or surgical biopsy, and the treatment is frequently chemotherapy.

➤ **About 25 percent of metastases show up first as liver cancer.** Weight loss, fever, anorexia, and gastrointestinal trouble are the initial signs of liver cancer. It's usually diagnosed through a blood test, but some medical teams will use a liver scan, CAT scan, or ultrasound. Like other metastasized cancers, liver cancer is usually treated with chemotherapy, although if the metastasis is limited to only a few spots on the liver, surgery may also be in order.

➤ **Less frequently, the metastasis may spread to the brain or spinal column.** Headaches seem to be a normal part of life for most of us, but a headache that doesn't go away could be a sign that the cancer has spread to the brain. Other noted symptoms of brain cancer are changes in behavior, such as being unbalanced when you walk. This kind of cancer is diagnosed by means of a CAT scan or MRI, and the treatment is usually radiation.

With recurrence you will probably experience the same emotions that overwhelmed you when you first found out you had cancer; but this time, fear is likely to be pervasive. You'll ask yourself questions, among them the following:

➤ Was everything I went through in vain?

➤ Is my body no longer strong enough to fight the cancer?

➤ Am I going to suffer as much through the second and third treatments as I did the first?

➤ Am I facing death—again?

➤ Am I going to die in horrible pain?

➤ Can my family and friends deal with this again?

➤ Can I deal with this again?

When these questions plant themselves firmly in your mind, ask yourself one more question: "What are my options?" To answer that question, you'll not only have to delve inside your own heart and soul to find new ways to cope with the new challenges ahead, but you'll also have to have a good long involved discussion with your doctor. He or she will help you sort out the medical options and imperatives for you—and all the same rules apply as did the first time. Bring a friend or a tape recorder with you so you don't forget the facts; ask plenty of questions and don't give up until you have the answers; and take some time to let the news sink in before you make any decisions.

Every Ache and Pain

You are upstairs collecting the laundry. With a huge bundle of clothes in your arms, you head downstairs to the laundry room. About halfway down the stairs, you feel a tremendous pain shoot through your ankle. You throw the clothes down the stairs, grab the railing, and collapse on a step in a sweat. "Oh, no." You panic. "It's gone to my bones." Or you roll over in bed and feel a twinge in your rib cage. You sit up with a start and think that your ribs are cracking. Or you're walking the dog, and your knees begin to ache. As you limp back home, all you can do is think that all you went through was for nothing.

If you've had similar experiences, you're not alone in your reactions. Although no hard-and-fast statistics exist, I think it's fair to say that fears like these overwhelm every cancer survivor at least occasionally. Indeed, reacting this way to what others would pass off as simple aches and pains is perfectly normal when you've faced the challenge of cancer in the past.

Knowing that recurrence can be a part of breast cancer, survivors become more sensitive to any minor discomfort and more anxious with any minor illness. Especially if you know your cancer had spread beyond the breast, you probably worry

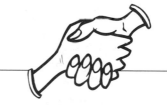

Helping Hand

Help others cope, too. Even though we survivors know that recurrence happens, it is still something no survivor, family, or friend wants to think about. Don't take their avoidance as a slap in your face. Know that their fear of "this could happen to me" is something that must be conquered over time.

Take It from Us

Don't ignore a symptom. Know your body. Notice anything that is new or different. Get it checked out. Don't stop. Be vigilant. Don't settle for answers that you don't understand or that don't make sense to you.

even more because you're aware that there is no "cure-all" for metastasized cancer. Once the cancer has spread to other parts of the body, it is more difficult—and sometimes even impossible—to stop. Even if your cancer was noninvasive, the idea of recurrence produces anxiety because you've been through so many initial treatments and you know, both mentally and physically, what you'll have to go through again. While my grandmother used to tell me that the "devil you know is better than the devil you don't know," I'm sure all of us would prefer not to spend time with any devil, especially this one. Chances are, your panic over every ache and pain will decrease with time. After two, then five, then 10 years, you may just be able to chalk them up to aging or stress or one of the other reasons you've had a twinge in the past.

Tales from the Trenches

Joan had a mastectomy about 12 years ago. Two years after her mastectomy, the cancer had metastasized and was in her bones. Later, after one hip surgery, she sat down on the bed and felt and heard the bones crack. Another hip surgery followed. Her advice: "When you have something in your body that is not normal for you—don't ignore it or be put off. Have it checked out thoroughly, to your satisfaction." No one knows your body better than you do. Listen to your body, not just for the sound of cracking bones.

Medical Check-Ups: Better Safe Than Sorry

No one likes to visit the doctor, and—needless to say—breast cancer survivors are no exception. But no matter how much you dislike your check-ups (and you may have one or two each year) keep every single appointment. If you're okay time after time, the anxiety you feel when that smell of "hospital" hits your nose will start to dissipate and you'll gain more confidence with every "all's well" determination.

And if you're not fine, if the doctor does find something amiss, you'll at least have caught it at the earliest stage possible, which almost always means a better prognosis. (For more about follow-up, see Chapter 14, "Again and Again: The Follow-Up.")

Coping with Recurrence

Before you can begin to make the medical decisions that evolve from a diagnosis of recurrence, you have to at least start to get past the whirlwind of emotions that will undoubtedly assault you. Again, it's likely that you'll pass through the same stages of emotions you did when you were first diagnosed: shock, denial, anger, grief, fear—you name it.

Perhaps the most common statement you'll make to yourself and hear from your loved ones will be "Not again." You've recovered; your hair has grown back; the routine of life is getting back to normal; you can count on a future. Then, recurrence.

Your first reaction may be to withdraw. Just as before, you're feeling a wide range of emotions and not just on your own behalf, but for your family and friends as well. You know that they had suffered with you before and you hate so much to put them through the struggle again. For that reason, it may at first be difficult to spend time with them. You may also find it tough to be around other survivors. Those who've never had a recurrence find it too easy to see themselves in your position—and resent you for bringing them face to face with that potential. At the same time, you may find yourself resentful (or at least envious) of survivors who haven't had a recurrence and continue to have that apparently bright future.

It's important, however, not to withdraw for too long. Yes, take some time to regroup and prepare yourself (as best you can) for the physical and emotional challenges you know lie ahead. But then, as soon as you're able, reach out for the help that you'll need and that you deserve.

Normally, the depression with recurrence is shorter than with your initial diagnosis. Although you have tried not to think about recurrence, the possibility is in the back of your mind. The shock is not quite as great. Your diagnosis does not mean a death sentence, and you're more knowledgeable on the subject and thus have a better idea of what to expect.

Doctors indicate that if depression lasts longer than a week, you will need outside emotional help to get you through a recurrence. A recurrence support group is a great source of help. David Spiegel's research on recurrence done at Stanford University indicates that those who participate in support groups not only had a better quality of life but actually lived longer than those who did not.

Helping Hand

In a national research trial reported in the *ACS News Today*, October 15, 1999, radiation treatment after noninvasive breast cancer tumors were removed reduced the chance of breast cancer recurring from 31 to 13 percent. If radiation therapy is not part of your treatment, you may want to talk to your doctor about it.

The Medical Outlook

You may find your recurrence or your doctor may find it during a regular visit or test. You may not be aware that anything is wrong and may even be symptom-free for quite a while, but this does not mean that you should postpone treatment. A quick reaction, after a reasonable time to let the news sink in and make considered decisions, is of major importance.

As discussed, treatment of recurrence will depend on the type and stage of your cancer, your general health, and other factors unique to you. You may require another surgery, chemotherapy, hormone therapy, or radiation. If the cancer has spread so far that no treatment is available, your doctor will help you find ways to live your life as free of pain as possible.

Fact or Fiction

With every article, news program, and scientific update, we hear new information about cancer, what causes it, who gets it, and so on. Needless to say, especially when it comes to a recurrence when emotions are likely to be running high, it's important to sort out the information you receive and only heed that which comes from the most reputable and trustworthy of sources. In addition, you must then take whatever trustworthy information you've derived and bring it to your doctor so that the two of you can evaluate the information in light of your very specific, personal condition and characteristics.

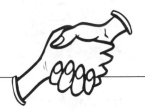

Helping Hand

Keep current. When you hear of some new treatment or recovery process, check it out through reliable cancer research sources and your doctor. This is not a time when you should have only one source or one point of view. While different opinions make horse races, our race for our cure has a better chance of winning when the odds are in our favor.

While many of the following statements probably popped into your mind with your initial diagnosis, they are persistent when you hear you have a recurrence.

Here are some basic myths you can discount right away:

➤ "It was my fault. I didn't concentrate on the treatment; I've been a bad person; I didn't get my mammogram on time."

➤ "I shouldn't have had all those massages; the increased circulation probably caused my recurrence."

➤ "I should have taken hormones; they keep breast cancer at bay."

➤ "I should have relaxed more; stress probably triggered the cancer again."

➤ "I didn't give up caffeine and smoking when I was first diagnosed and now their use has caused my breast cancer recurrence."

➤ "I should have moved away from the Sunbelt because living there has caused my recurrence."

➤ "My job caused a recurrence because I'm constantly exposed to small, daily doses of radiation."

➤ "I shouldn't have had children after my first round of treatments because then my breast cancer would not have recurred."

➤ "Having all of those regular mammograms caused my recurrence."

➤ "I should have had a mastectomy or breast reduction surgery to avoid a recurrence because my breasts are too large."

➤ "I should have never taken artificial hormones because they were responsible for my breast cancer."

➤ "If I had stuck to my macrobiotic diet, I would not have had a recurrence."

The Waiting Game

As time goes by, most cancer survivors can manage to get through most days without consciously thinking about their cancer, but the truth is, the thought of recurrence is never far from our minds.

A myth that many survivors have about breast cancer is that all you have to do is live five years without a recurrence (or only with a local recurrence) and you have your "get out of jail free card." However, recent research suggests that—at least in the case of breast cancer—there is no definitive end to the disease or to the possibility of recurrence. Dr. William Rate, radiation oncologist at Clarian Health Center in Indianapolis, states, "Breast cancer is not like lung or colon cancer where two- or five-year disease-free intervals, respectively, are considered synonymous with a cure. The rule of thumb in breast cancer studies is that longer follow-up intervals are necessary to determine true recurrence rates, and eight years is probably a minimum."

However, the truth is that many doctors are beginning to use the word "chronic" to describe breast cancer. Women who have had breast cancer in one

Take It from Us

Face this fact now: You'll never be prepared for a recurrence. If it happens to you, take some time to regroup, to gather your physical, emotional, and intellectual resources, and then get out and fight with all you've got.

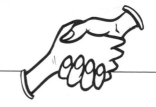

Helping Hand

Learn to let go. Joan, a survivor of breast cancer and recurrence, urges everyone to focus on what they can deal with and let go of emotions that are no longer of any use. "Anger is good if you can use it to make constructive changes. If you can't, let the anger go."

breast, for instance, are more likely to develop breast cancer in the other breast as they age. And what that means to you is that you must remain vigilant by following your doctor's orders about appointments and self-care, performing self-exams once a month, and staying as healthy as possible by eating well, exercising regularly, and reducing stress as much as possible.

Now, that's not to say that a two-year or five-year mark isn't worth celebrating. In fact, every day that you stay healthy and cancer-free is a reason to celebrate.

The emotions ride just as high with recurrence as they did with the initial diagnosis. But, there will come a time for most of us when we let go of the emotions, and our logic or intellect takes over, and we move with precision and speed to take care of ourselves—one more time.

Recurrence makes us think about two disagreeable by-products: death and pain. Pain is usually manageable. And, death? It's something that we all must face, as difficult as that may be. In the next chapter, we'll look at this tough but inevitable issue.

The Least You Need to Know

➤ Recurrence of breast cancer does happen to some survivors.

➤ There are two types—local and distant. Local is usually better when it comes to treatment and prognosis.

➤ Know that there are many facts associated with recurrence and even more fiction. Know the difference.

➤ Every day you live without a recurrence is a day worth celebrating.

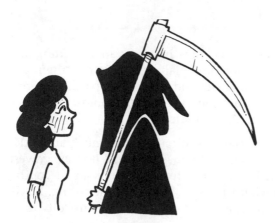

Chapter 26

Facing Death: Day to Day

In This Chapter

➤ Dealing with the fact that it happens to us all

➤ Getting your life in order once you know

➤ Deciding how you want to be remembered

➤ Making your plan for the time you have

➤ Never giving up hope

Most of us have surely experienced losing someone dear—a grandparent, parent, or truly special friend. The grief, of course, is mostly selfish; for in simple terms, we miss the departed. Certainly, as time goes on, we learn, however painfully, to adjust; but the fact remains that death makes us grieve.

When a debilitating illness such as advanced metastasized breast cancer puts death at your own door, however, your grief over loved ones lost is doubtless overshadowed by your own condition. In times like these, I remember my grandmother's sage advice. She told me, "Ain't none of us gonna get out of this life alive." So in this chapter, we'll look at death as a new presence.

The Great Equalizer

There is a good reason why so many fear death. We know nothing about it. Other than those who come back from near-death experiences talking about the "white light" and being "out of body," we have no reference about this inevitable life event. [And, it is a life event. From the moment we are born, we are dying.] There is no escape from death no matter your age, gender, race, religion, or financial status. In death, we are all the same.

The Unknown

You have gauges for other life experiences. You know how to plan a wedding because you have seen so many, or you can hire a wedding planner who knows the ropes. You know about college, pregnancy, rules of the road, and Super Bowl parties. There are guidelines, instructions, and personnel to help you get through almost any life event—but not death. There is no "real life" experience here.

To further hinder your knowledge, we as a society also don't talk much about death. It is like the old adage of "speak of the devil, and he will appear." It is the gravest of all the unmentionables. People engaged in casual conversation talk about youth, beauty, fitness, children, money, and what their spouses have done wrong. But they don't talk about death, and what you cannot talk about, you have difficulty dealing with.

Finally, because you don't know much about it, and don't talk about it, you also have no way to empathize with someone who knows they're dying. You don't know how they feel; you haven't been there. No two people live the same way; consequently, no two people will die the same way.

I'm What?

You really aren't shocked by death, but you're certainly shocked if someone leads you to believe you're dying. Indeed, we all face death in one way or another every day—on the news, through family and friends, or through the grapevine at work. But mostly you don't know when YOUR last day will be; the date's not marked in a date book or planner. If you're a cancer patient, however, you sometimes have a better idea than others do. Unfortunately, each year, nearly 250,000 people are told they have a terminal illness. And sadly, about 43,000 women die from breast cancer every year.

In some ways, knowledge is power. If you know your condition is terminal, you have a chance to plan and to use the time left as wisely (or unwisely!) as possible. And we'll talk about that part later. At the same time, however, any illusion of control you may have had over your life is now completely destroyed. You may have thought you were in control of the hours and minutes or your days with meetings, appointments, and duties. When you are diagnosed with a terminal illness, however, you sense that the control—all of it—is gone. The good news, however, is that that, too, is an illusion. You can control how you face death.

It Isn't Fair!

When your prognosis is poor, you're likely to say, or at least think, "It's not fair." And, needless to say, that's a perfectly natural reaction. But keep in mind that life isn't fair—period. A drunk driver kills a young woman and leaves her three children motherless. Is that fair? If you rob somebody in the daylight, the penalty is different than if you rob somebody in the dark. Is that fair?

Pretty soon, you'll probably get past the fact that death isn't fair; fairness really isn't even the real issue. The fact that death "is" is the issue. Perhaps that's why death is called the great equalizer and the way of all flesh. What may not be fair is that some know when the last days are, and some do not. We *recognize* death; we do not want to *realize* death.

Death's Emotional Roller Coaster

Let's see, where do we begin. As discussed in previous chapters, shock is a good place to start. Then there is anger, anxiety, depression, embarrassment, envy, fear, frustration, loneliness, numbness, panic, pity, relief, and regret. Whether you have six weeks, six months, or two years to live, you'll have the time to go through almost every one of these emotions and maybe some we've left out.

You're angry! Why me? You're anxious. How long? You're depressed. I'm going to die. You're embarrassed. Others know, and they don't know what to say to me. You're envious. People I know are going to live. You're fearful. What will it be like? You're frustrated. There is so little I can do. You're lonely. I'm in this by myself. You're numb. I am waiting. You're panicked. What will happen to my family? You feel pity. I won't be here for the holidays. You feel relief. There is an end. And, you feel regret. What could I have done differently?

From the Book

Recognize means to be aware of something. **Realize** means to make something real.

Tales from the Trenches

Abby was so tired. She had decided to keep working as long as she could, and the past four weeks had zapped her of all her strength. After an especially long, frustrating day, she was so near exhaustion that she called her best friend from the car to talk with her to avoid falling asleep. She said to her friend, "Until today, I never really understood how people could be tired of living. Now I do."

Is there a cure-all for the emotions on this roller coaster? And would you really want to stop from feeling them and simply become numb? Probably not, but there is one thing that does seem to help. If you keep going and moving and doing, the roller coaster may go just a bit more slowly or at least its highs and lows won't be as startling. When you are active, you'll feel as if you have a bit of control at least over your day-to-day activities. When you're doing for others, you'll have less time to spend thinking of yourself. When you're involved, you'll still feel that you're alive and adding value to your friends, family, and the world.

Good Grief!

Grief, that intense mental anguish, seems to be a normal part of death. When someone dies unexpectedly, grief belongs to those left behind. When you're given a time frame for your own death, naturally you grieve for yourself.

As Reverend Joy Bilger Gehring states, "More often, we can deal with death on an intellectual level, especially if we have little or no faith. It is on the spiritual or emotional level that we agonize. This is where faith comes into play."

So many wonderfully helpful books have been written by those who study death and those who face death. These books can be a great help to you as you search to recognize your feelings as you go through this process. They also provide you with the comfort of knowing that you're not alone; that your experience, though unique, has universal elements. Patterns emerge in this grief process. Dr. Elisabeth Kübler-Ross and numerous other authors describe five phases of grief associated with death and dying.

Take It from Us

Do your paperwork. Folks are now fortunate to be able to have their "right to die" made known. By making a living will, you can, if you wish, have someone pull the plug if you're suffering from a terminal illness such as advanced metastasized breast cancer. By making this decision yourself, you not only eliminate others' suffering, but you also eliminate their potential guilt feelings or their inability to make this very difficult decision.

Phase 1 is denial, shock, and isolation. Not only does the dying person experience these reactions, but so do those around them. Sometimes the shell of denial grows thick and hard to crack. Then support from others becomes more difficult. But most folks move from phase 1 to phase 2 fairly quickly.

Phase 2 is anger. WHY? Why am I dying and others are living? Why do others get so stressed out over such simple things? Don't they know where the true value of life is? Is a traffic jam or a paper cut truly that big of a deal? Many times, the more you love life, the angrier you become. The positive side of these reactions is that they typically prompt you into action. And of course, you feel more in control when you're active.

Tales from the Trenches

Mattie was so angry, and her anger was consuming her. Little things that others complained about seemed so trivial, and she knew she needed to vent if she were going to cope and move on. She developed a plan. Every day, when she came home, she set the timer on the stove for 20 minutes. For that 20 minutes she screamed, cried, and railed. When the timer buzzed, she stopped and went on with the rest of her life.

Phase 3 is the bargaining stage. Remember doing this as a kid? "I promise I'll study for the next test if I can just pass this one," or "If John asks me to the prom, I'll do volunteer work at the hospital for the rest of my life." Now, our bargains have just grown a little more serious. "Okay, I know I'm going to die, just don't let it be before the holidays, or if I pray two hours everyday, I'll live longer." Needless to say, however, the powers that be don't cut deals.

Tales from the Trenches

Cathy was struggling with depression and felt she was just drifting through her days. One afternoon, she stopped at a card store, and there she saw something that changed her attitude. It was a plaque that read "The most wasted day of all is one in which you have not laughed." She bought two of them: one for her office and one for her home. From that moment on, she dealt with her illness more successfully and tried to laugh each and every day.

Phase 4 is depression. I think this is the hardest phase to deal with. You have gone inside yourself. Others see that you're suffering; they try to help, but they don't know what to do. As a result, perhaps even unintentionally, they may avoid you, and that in turn may feed your depression. Unfortunately, there's no set time frame for depression. It could last for a day, month, or years. And, finally, no one knows what will bring you out of it. It could be something as simple as thinking, "Well, I've been depressed and nothing has changed. I guess it's time to stop." Or, it could be something as severe as the loss of a friend or family member.

Phase 5 is acceptance. When I think of acceptance, I remember the Serenity prayer, which speaks of having courage to change what you can, to accept what you cannot change, and having the wisdom to know the difference. When you finally arrive at the point of mental, emotional, and spiritual acceptance that you are dying, you can finally enjoy the precious time left and stop wasting it on what you cannot change.

Grief is part of your life, but it must have an end.

When you first begin to grieve, others are supportive, but the longer you grieve, the more people shy away. What you can't change, you must endure. Grief should never be chronic. It stops you from acting, from being, and considering that you may not have much time left, you must live and act upon what you do have.

Tying Up the Loose Ends

Of course, you'll work your way through the stages of grief at your own pace, caught up in some stages longer than others and perhaps shifting from one stage to the other and back again. In the process, however, you'll probably start tying up some of those loose ends in your life—the letters you always intended to write, the photo album you always planned to complete, or the apology niggling in the back of your mind that you know you need to make. Surely lots of folks go to their deaths never having had an opportunity to mend fences, rebuild bridges, or simply say they were sorry about something.

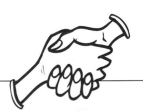

Helping Hand

Remember that this is an emotional roller coaster ride you're on, so be careful with liquor or drugs. It's possible to have a momentary slip in coping, and this time may not be the time to slip in the "great plan" of your life.

One advantage to knowing that your demise is near is that you can create closure. You have the incentive to say what you want to people today because you know tomorrow may never come. Apologizing, rekindling lost relationships, and expressing emotions may become the agenda for each day. As a result, you may be one of the fortunate few who can plan to leave this world with no unfinished business, a checkmark by each item on your "to do" list.

Finally, you can help yourself get those loose ends tied up by taking care of yourself. When you're facing death, it's easy, at times, just to let things go, things

306

like your appearance, diet, exercise, and sleep. Believe it or not, these things help you face each day with more energy, a better attitude, and an increased ability to cope. The bottom line, of course, is that you may know the end is near, but of course you don't know the exact hour or day. Every day can be precious to you. Prepare for it with your best foot forward.

Life, at best, is fragile, and seldom do we feel as if we're finished living. Show the world that! Show yourself that! Show the powers that be that! And that means taking the time to take care of yourself, even if you know your time has been shortened by your illness.

Take It from Us

Create closure if you feel some type of positive or negative emotion toward someone and you know your end is near, and you may not want to carry it with you to the afterlife and beyond. You also for some reason, may not be able to express either of these emotions, perhaps because the object of your emotion may be ill him- or herself. One suggestion for people dealing with anger is to write a letter or make a video, set it on fire, tear it apart, put it in a balloon, and let it go.

Support: The Tie That Binds

You don't come into this world alone; maybe you shouldn't try to leave it that way either. Support groups for the dying are amazingly valuable in many ways, for among members of a support group is true empathy. Here is honesty. Here is coping. A shared experience of a very select group. And, while you may be losing physical strength, with the support of your fellows, you'll probably simultaneously be gaining emotional and spiritual strength, enough to face the end with grace and candor.

So what does a support group do for you? Some support groups teach visualization, pain control, self-hypnosis, meditation, and relaxation. And, if you have ever needed these, *now is the time!* But whether the group "teaches" or talks, you'll reap the benefits. The mere act of talking about facing death is helpful. You may want to talk with your family or friends, but where you have found acceptance and passed through most of your grief process, theirs is just beginning. They may not be able to hear what you want to say. People in your support group will be able to listen with a smile and a sympathetic heart. And they may be able to share suggestions about how they've talked with their own friends and family, perhaps suggestions that will work for you.

Some Final Choices

In the same way you've made all the other choices about your treatment, so, too, you can make choices about ending your treatment. You have options. Let's look at three very important ones: living wills, hospice care, and euthanasia.

Living Wills

Earlier in the chapter we alluded to a living will. To create your living will, meet with an attorney (because it is a legal document) and make your wishes known. Basically, you can make the decision about what types of medical treatment you do or do not want. The living will can, for instance, call for the words "Do Not Resuscitate" to be put on your chart. Or it can be much more specific and list directions such as "No Artificial Nutrition." You should give copies of your living will to your doctor, local hospital, and agent (a family member or friend who is to make your wishes known or possibly assist in making the decisions if you are not able). Please discuss your decisions with your doctor and agent so that they are aware of what is to be and not to be done.

Hospice Care

Maybe at this point you've become keenly aware that your days are limited. And maybe you've come to grips with the fact that, in spite of your best efforts, you're going to need help in managing the pain. As bleak as it sounds, even at this point you have some measure of control. There are things you can do regarding the quality of your remaining days, and one of those is checking out hospice services.

While hope and healing are still taken into consideration, a hospice focuses more on care—not cure—and specifically on managing types of physical and emotional pain. Not only do you receive care, but the family and friends also receive care.

Doctors, nurses, counselors, and volunteers who work at a hospice are concerned with and provide support for everything from pain medication for the patient to grief support groups for survivors. At a hospice, you'll benefit from "unit" treatment that makes every effort to meet your needs as well as those of your family and friends.

For more information on a hospice in your area and their particular requirements and treatments, please talk with your doctor or access some of the hospice Web sites. Just as the medical protocols differ, so do the protocols of each hospice. It is a good time to check out what is right for you and your family.

Euthanasia: Cheating the Grim Reaper

Euthanasia, or the act of shortening the time of suffering before an inevitable death is not viewed the same by all. Some see it as a way to end a pain so intense that you cannot cope any longer. Some look on it as a way to be in control of something that seems uncontrollable. Some look at it as an end to sorrow because death is compared to sleep, and in that sleep, you find peace and comfort. It is a final choice, the last knot.

What Legacy Do You Leave?

An old song tells us that "everyone wants to go to heaven, but nobody wants to die." I guess that's a given. Knowing your timing, however, allows you to leave a legacy to your family, friends, or the world. You decide.

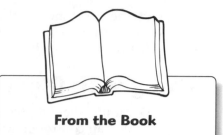

From the Book

Euthanasia is Greek for "good death" and refers to a painless, merciful death.

Bequeathing Your Body

There are many altruistic reasons for bequeathing or donating your body or specific organs to science. For some, it is to leave a legacy for other breast cancer patients. If the medical professionals have a better understanding of what happens in an unhealthy body, then just maybe a cure for whatever ails us can become a reality sooner.

Empathy, knowing how someone else feels, can be another reason why people may consider donating their body and/or organs to science. Even a cancer patient's body leaves some healthy parts—such as corneas.

Most people simply want to do good. Donating your body and/or organs for either a transplant or research is certainly a way of doing good by helping educate future medical professionals or saving another person's life. We may never know what "potential" good or benefits we can be to others.

There is also a practical side to bequeathing or donating your body: the high cost of funeral expenses. Once the body has been examined or organs have been harvested, it can be returned to the family as ashes to be saved or scattered at a spot of their choice.

Many people ask "Why?" donate their body and/or organs. Maybe we should ask "Why not?" As human beings we are compassionate and caring. Not only is bequeathing/donating a great way to leave a legacy, but it is also a great way to show that we have a concern for helping others as others have helped us.

There's No Place Like Home

Home memorial services are gaining in popularity. It used to be where funerals were conducted. We seem to come back full circle in so many things. If you really want a home memorial service, you'll want to talk with your family, requesting that the service to be held in that manner. Or maybe you'd simply prefer that after a service at a funeral home or religious facility, the mourners gather at a family home. Not only does the home memorial service work well for those who want a more personal funeral, but it also serves well for those who are not actively involved in a church or other house of worship at the time of their death.

Dying with Dignity

To each life, there should be quality and quantity. We can't do much about the quantity. We can control, however, to a much greater extent, how we live and how we die. The goal may be best summed up in the phrase "death with dignity," but then how do you define dignity in those terms? In short, the definition is a personal one. You'll decide what "dignity" means to you at this time. You'll decide how to live and act during your last days, and in the midst of all that, if you can, you should help those who love you help you muster the strength and courage to face the end. You have the privilege, too, of deciding what last memories you want to leave with others, even at your funeral. You can choose whom you want to speak, what you want to wear, what flowers you would like to have, and what music you would like played. One woman said she kept a box under her bed labeled "Funeral," and every time she heard a perfect piece of music or read a wonderful piece of poetry, she put it in the box. "There's enough there for a four-hour service," she joked.

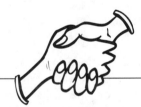

Helping Hand

You may want to create a "to do" list of what needs to be done before your death. The list may include updating a will, writing special letters, checking on bank deposits and safety deposit boxes, having co-signature cards made for accounts, and giving special things to special people. There are material possessions we cherish in this life, such as a family heirloom, an antique, a pet, a car, or a set of dishes, and it is so heartening to see the people we want to have them have them.

Faith: An Everlasting and Final Frontier

Many people, especially members of the clergy of various religions, have spoken of what a privilege it is to be with a person at the time of death. They describe a sense of sacredness that comes at the moment when a spirit passes from its earthly body.

The Greeks believed that the purpose of death was to help us reconnect with the gods. It was to get us away from the secular life and into a life divine. Faith in dying helps us stop being a solitary person and helps us become a part of the whole.

We often think about the essence of our being as who we are or how many days we have. Isn't the real essence of our being whose lives we touch and in what way?

The Least You Need to Know

➤ Grief is a natural part of the dying process. Usually it is others grieving for us; in this case, you may well be grieving for yourself.

➤ Like others, you will most likely go through the five stages of grief, from denial to acceptance.

➤ You have a wonderful opportunity that others will never have, and that is to leave this world with closure.

➤ You have choices, even now, including how and where you want to die and organizing your own memorial service.

➤ Death is a natural part of living.

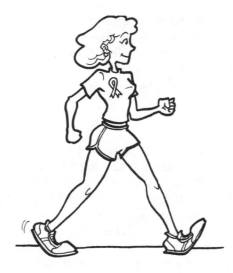

Chapter 27

Volunteers and Advocates: Working for the Cause

In This Chapter

➤ The when and how of volunteering

➤ Understanding the need and spreading the word

➤ Ways folks have raised funds

➤ How to impact legislation

➤ Showing support for advocacy

Every three minutes, someone in the United States is diagnosed with breast cancer. That's 500 a day, 185,000 a year. Until now, those statistics were just that—another set of statistics. But once you've been touched by breast cancer, either as a result of your own diagnosis or that of someone near and dear, you take a different attitude toward the statistics as well as the disease.

If you're like most women, you now are on a new mission: to bring attention and support to the fight for better treatments and, ultimately, a cure. Advocacy includes raising public awareness of breast cancer; educating women about the disease and how to care for themselves; working with policy makers to allocate state and federal monies for detection, treatment, and research; and raising funds to support groups funding research and other advocacy programs. And it all begins with volunteers— volunteers like you who add authenticity to the campaign.

In this chapter, we'll talk about some of the ways that you can repay the debt you may now feel as a result of the benefits you've received from current research. We'll suggest ways you can serve as a volunteer and as an advocate individually or in a group, how you can be a part of fund-raising, and how you can affect the Washington scene even if you live on the other side of the continent.

Repaying the Debt

You've fought the battle with breast cancer and won, and you're well on your way to recovery. You're grateful every day of your life that today's prognosis for breast cancer survivors is significantly better than it was 20 years ago. You're grateful that the treatment for breast cancer is less brutal but more effective than it was 20 years ago. You're grateful that research is regularly turning up more and more promising tidbits that suggest not only better and earlier diagnoses, but better and more successful treatment. You're grateful for all the research and the pioneering women who participated in thousands of clinical trials to make possible the treatment you had.

But you're probably also more than a little bit angry. Why does breast cancer still rob the lives of thousands of women every year? Then you look at your daughters and granddaughters. And you look at your aunts and nieces and dear friends. And you consider the 185,000 other women who will be diagnosed with breast cancer this year. Short of venting with a primal scream, you're probably ready to direct your anger toward something worthwhile. What can you do?

Tales from the Trenches

Six years ago, after having had one malignant lump and one pre-cancerous lump removed, Sylvia found it necessary to have a pre-cancerous duct removed. Yesterday, she had to have another pre-cancerous duct removed. "What a difference," she exclaimed when I talked to her this morning. "Six years ago, there was a major incision and the surgeon hoped he'd found the right duct based on the mammogram film. Yesterday, it was laser surgery guided by ultrasound. I've had a little extra-strength Tylenol, but I can hardly tell anything's been done to me." She, too, is grateful for the dramatic advances that have made treatments so much less brutal.

Wanted: Help for Free

Only if you've battled breast cancer yourself can you truly relate to a woman newly diagnosed with the disease. As a result, you're a number-one candidate for volunteering your time (and money, if you wish) to support these women. You can start working as a volunteer on a simple individual basis, working hotlines, visiting post-surgical folks in the hospital or at home, providing patient transportation to breast cancer treatment centers. You can work with the ACS Reach to Recovery to help those who will follow the same path as you and walk in the same shoes. You can send cards and notes, make phone calls, and lead discussion groups.

Volunteering is a very satisfying way to reach out to others; but before you begin extending your hand to help, make sure that now is the right time for you. Some folks start offering support to others while they're still undergoing treatment; others wait until treatment is over and they feel stronger, both physically and emotionally; others need several years to gain the perspective that gives them shoulders broad enough for others to lean on. Only you can know when the time is right.

Take It from Us

Don't let someone talk you into doing something that you don't want to do. In the long run, it will be easier to say "No" up front than to do something half-heartedly and resent the time it takes.

One on One

When you've decided the time is right, how do you make contact with newly diagnosed women? Contact your local chapter of the American Cancer Society (ACS) or breast center or cancer treatment clinic—perhaps where you yourself had treatment—and offer your services. Let them know what you're willing to do: talk by phone or in person, visit in the hospital or at home, provide transportation, or whatever. They, in turn, through mutual consent, will connect you and a newly diagnosed woman. In some large communities, the connectors hook up folks of similar age with similar diagnoses. In smaller communities that lack the luxury of choice, you may connect with anyone diagnosed, regardless of age or stage.

Next, consider some of the "do's" and "don'ts" guidelines for volunteering your time and effort to help a newly diagnosed woman:

> ➤ **Do set boundaries.** Don't volunteer for more than you can handle well or agree to do something you're not quite up to doing.

> ➤ **Don't play doctor; don't give medical advice.** You're chatting with a newly diagnosed woman to give emotional support and to show personal empathy and

understanding. You can offer suggestions about Web sites or books (like this one) for getting the right information or suggest a list of questions for her doctor.

➤ **Do stay informed about medical treatments** so that you can understand questions and concerns. Like you, this woman has heard the medical talk. Now maybe she wants layman's talk.

➤ **Don't start a "Can-you-top-this?" conversation.** You're not there to volunteer information about how your surgery went or how sick you were during chemo; you're there to remind this woman that treatment is only temporary and that she can survive—just as you have!

➤ **Do listen to her fears**—that she'll lose her hair during chemo, that she'll be dreadfully sick, that her children will suffer from neglect, that her husband might desert her, that she might lose her job. Suggest community resources for ongoing support, such as family and social services organizations.

➤ **Don't pretend to know what you don't.** Be honest and then suggest sources—like hotlines or resource centers—that can help.

➤ **Do send cards and notes.** You'll probably remember that when you were diagnosed and going through treatment you felt completely vulnerable. A card or note shows that someone cares. It's good medicine!

➤ **Don't offer platitudes, empty words, and clichés.** Don't tell someone you understand when you may not. And don't offer to do things you don't want to do if asked.

➤ **Do be sincere, genuine, and compassionate.** Be kind but truthful.

➤ **Don't forget to call before you visit someone at home.** Remember when you were ill that someone dropping by unannounced may have caught you at your worst. The visit caused more frustration than comfort.

➤ **Do offer whatever support you can**, such as bringing in homemade or carry-out meals, caring for children, doing the dishes or laundry, sharing a rented video or favorite (upbeat) book or magazine, taking her for a drive, joining in a board or card game, or engaging in plain ol' girl talk. (For more along these lines, see Chapter 19, "Support Tools.")

Using this list as a springboard, you'll think of another dozen ways to help a newly diagnosed woman.

One in a Group

Every organization functions with the help of its precious volunteers. The same is true of those organizations devoted to supporting breast cancer survivors. Barbara Russell, Executive Director of the ACS Indianapolis Metropolitan District, lists attributes, one or more of which organizations seek in volunteers. They may be people who display leadership, know businesses and the community, and/or have some type of technical expertise. They may like to plan and be involved in activities. Chances are, they can provide some type of service to cancer patients and/or family members. Certainly they enjoy working with others. And maybe they can also help raise funds and come up with new ideas.

Don't walk into volunteering for organizations, however, with blinders on. Know your strengths and understand what might be expected of you. Will you need any training? If so, how much, when, and where? Must you volunteer a certain number of hours each week or month? Will you need to drive any distance? If so, is mileage part of your contribution? What tasks will you be responsible for? To whom do you report? Is that person also your mentor? Is there a handbook or set of guidelines for your volunteer role?

So whether you're going to stuff envelopes, serve as master of ceremonies for a style show, or do data entry, your volunteer efforts will be most appreciated. And you're on your way to repaying your debt.

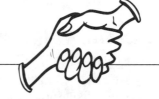

Helping Hand

News media love hot stories, so if you're on the trail of something exciting and timely, call your television stations and/or newspapers. They'll respect your privacy and you'll further the cause.

The Next Steps

As you grow politically more savvy on the subject of breast cancer, you may move on from local volunteerism to advocacy, participating in regional, state, or even national efforts. Consider these steps:

➤ If you're good at helping others learn, consider educating others about the importance of breast self-exams, annual mammograms, and annual clinical exams. You're advocating breast cancer awareness and education.

➤ Consider conducting workshops or serving as a peer leader at workshops that help others deal with breast cancer diagnosis. You're advocating breast cancer education.

➤ Take your workshop to churches, synagogues, businesses, and community organizations to teach the rest of the world about breast cancer and about how vital and vibrant we survivors are. You're advocating breast cancer awareness and education.

➤ Work with your local media to emphasize the importance of early detection; seek out already available funds for mammograms for women who otherwise can't afford them; then take your message and your money to the communities at greatest risk. You're advocating breast cancer education with funding to support your plan. Now you're really getting into it!

➤ When the available funding runs out, start raising funds to cover the remaining costs. Now you're ready for group advocacy, where you'll have strength in numbers.

From a little volunteering at the local hotline to national fund-raising, your advocacy can make a difference in the lives of thousands.

Talk the Talk; Walk the Walk

So let's get into the thick of this business of advocacy. Where can you begin on the advocacy scene? Start at home with folks you know. For example, Reba is a teacher whose colleagues for the most part had been negligent about their annual mammograms. After her mastectomy, any time she could, she showed off her bionic boob by giving a true-false test. Slipping off her jacket, she'd ask, "Which one's real?" Then, with only ladies present, she'd disrobe. "Now you know. And it could happen to you. Get your mammogram. Now." Brazen? Well, yes. But her colleagues finally came to grips with the fact that we can talk about breast cancer and we darn well better do something about early detection. "Within a year, every single woman at our school had had her mammogram," Reba reported. She was working as a breast-cancer awareness and education advocate in the place she knew best—at home.

You may also find yourself comfortable starting at home in the political arena. Write or call to make sure your locally elected state and federal representatives endorse breast cancer as a significant funding issue. At the moment, government spends embarrassingly few dollars compared to the 185,000 women who get breast cancer every year. Add to that sad statement the fact that since the 1970s, the number of diagnosed cases of breast cancer has risen dramatically. The last decade has seen the most dramatic increase. It is, indeed, a sad state of affairs.

But let's make it worse. In spite of the hundreds of thousands of women affected every year, breast cancer has no known cause and no known cure. Sure, early detection is important for recovery, but early detection isn't prevention. Furthermore, depending on whose statistics you tout, somewhere around 43,000 women die every year of breast cancer.

So what evidence can we cite that shows your efforts are not in vain, that, in fact, advocacy works? Since breast cancer advocates organized in 1991, federal funding for research has risen from $90 million to over $650 million in 1999—a total of over $1 billion. It would never have happened without advocates, folks like you making phone calls and writing letters to their legislators. As a direct result of the National

Take It from Us

The label "high risk" that some folks like to use to suggest that breast cancer is somehow all in the family explains only about 10 percent of the cases. The other 90 percent remain unexplained. Only if we can get adequate breast-cancer research funding will we ever know the answer.

Breast Cancer Coalition's 2.6 million-signatures campaign, President Clinton met NBCC's demand and committed to a National Action Plan on Breast Cancer, which insists that government, science, private industry, and consumers work together toward common goals. In addition, NBCC launched a number of educational programs to train advocates and raise political and voter awareness. So, yes, advocacy can make a difference. *A big difference.*

What are the ultimate goals of most advocates? Consider this far-reaching question: Does every woman have access to regular clinical exams and mammograms and, if diagnosed with breast cancer, can every woman get the treatment she needs and get the same quality of treatment available to anyone else? The answer to virtually every part of that question is "No." The miserably immoral fact is that while mammograms are available to almost everyone who makes an effort to find resources, if she's diagnosed with breast cancer, she may be left dangling on her own (perhaps nonexistent) resources. Advocates want to change that picture and all it implies—awareness, education, political change, and funding.

Not Just You Against the World

With hundreds of thousands of women united as they now are, the advocates are beginning to make a big difference. Consider some of these groups (listed in alphabetical order) to which you might add your support:

The American Cancer Society Breast Cancer Advocacy functions as a special section on advocacy issues. You're probably already quite familiar with the organization, but check out the special part of this huge organization that focuses on advocacy. Their Stride for Life walks/runs in cities throughout the country raise money for cancer research. Details at www.cancer.org/bcn/advocacy.html.

The Breast Cancer Fund was formed in 1992 to "innovate and accelerate the response to the breast cancer crisis." Its objectives are four: "to replace mammography with more accurate screening technology that does not expose a woman's breasts to radiation, even in low doses, over decades of her life; to shift from a reliance upon toxic chemotherapies to the use of less- or nontoxic treatments that enhance the body's disease-fighting capacity; to uncover the environmental links to breast cancer and eliminate preventable causes of the disease; and to achieve universal access to the best available detection, treatment, and prevention

Helping Hand

Advocacy comes in a wide array of forms. Climb Against the Odds pitted 11 women against the 20,230–foot summit of Mt. McKinley, the highest mountain in North America. Although bad weather halted their final ascent, the inspirational part of this story is that four of the climbers were breast cancer survivors. The story of their climb aired on public television and videos are available through The Breast Cancer Fund, the recipient of the proceeds.

strategies." To raise funds, TBCF focuses on physically challenging events to empha-size recovery and engages in high-visibility events to increase awareness. Check it out at www.breastcancerfund.org.

The National Alliance of Breast Cancer Organizations includes an advocacy com-ponent. As the name suggests, it's a group of groups, and under the same umbrella, it can weather the vast Washington storms. You can learn more about its advocacy at www.nabco.org.

The National Breast Cancer Coalition strives to increase funding for high-quality peer-reviewed breast cancer research. Its aim is "to increase access for all women to high quality care and breast cancer clinical trials, and to increase the influence of women living with breast cancer in the decision making that impacts all issues sur-rounding breast cancer." That's you, folks. Check out its Web site at www.natlbcc.org.

Sisters Network is a national organization supporting African-American breast cancer survivors and is "committed to increasing local and national attention to the devas-tating impact that breast cancer has in the African-American community." You can find more at www.sistersnetworkinc.org.

Take It from Us

When you're ready to check out more advocacy groups and their respective issues, go to the De-partment of Defense Web site for a list of advocacy groups: www.bcdg.org/. Click on "Orga-nizations and Services" and browse through a list of about 50 groups with links to dozens more. Look for the highlighted words "Outreach," "Raise Funds," and "Lobby."

The Susan G. Komen Breast Cancer Foundation, widely recognized for the Race for the Cure held in cities across the United States and now internation-ally, was founded by Susan Komen's sister Nancy Brinker. The fund-raisers support breast cancer aware-ness and breast cancer research, with 75 percent of funds remaining in their respective communities for local programs and 25 percent for national projects. Learn more at www.komen.org.

Y-Me provides peer counseling, information, educa-tional programs, and support meetings for breast cancer patients, their families, and friends. It's educa-tional advocacy on a grand scale. See more at www.y-me.org.

This very short list suggests that some groups are pri-marily advocacy groups but that many, many groups have advocacy components. We can't list all of the groups here (but you'll find much longer lists in Ap-pendix E, "Informational Web Sites," and Appendix C, "Support Groups"); however, these should help get you started along the path toward whatever contribu-tions you hope to make.

Funds for Research

When we began asking folks how they raised money for breast cancer awareness, education, research, or whatever, we were left in awe. If their extraordinarily creative ideas and multimillion dollar results don't inspire you, you're far too cynical for your own good. Listen to some of these amazing stories:

Community Functions

In Cripple Creek, Colorado, a co-worker at Bronco Billy's Sports Bar and Casino undergoing treatment for breast cancer came to work one day devastated that she'd be losing her hair to chemo. One of her fellow workers said, "You know, I ought to shave my head so she won't be alone." And a patron piped up, "I'll give you 50 bucks if you do." And the idea grew. Within a few weeks, Bald for the Cure was organized and 32 men, women, and kids—all with sponsor's pledges in hand—shaved their heads. They raised $10,000 to fight breast cancer.

A North Jersey group does an annual Pink Tie Ball (yes, the guys hang up their black ties for pink—at 45 bucks each). The affiliate was founded on a promise "to make a difference" to a 10-year-old girl who had lost her mother to breast cancer. It takes from 50 to 60 volunteers (about half of whom are survivors) a full year to plan the extravaganza, paying attention to details as if they were planning a wedding. The first year, the event raised $350,000, the second year over $700,000, and the third year well over $1 million. Not bad for an evening gala!

The American Tae Kwon Do Association sponsors Board Breaks for the Cure Day. In honor of Mother's Day, Charles Schwab and Company created the idea for Commissions for the Cure. Danskin sponsors the Women's Swim, Bike, and Run Triathlon Series with proceeds going to battle breast cancer. Goldsmith Seeds has Plant for the Cure. Hallmark Cards for the Cure allows store owners to make a million dollars' difference in the fight against breast cancer. The Home Sewing Association, with 2,000 fabric and craft retailers and 400 manufacturers, suppliers, and merchants, sponsors Sew for the Cure with a $1 million goal. Wyndham Hotels and Resorts sponsors Dream for the Cure. Lots of companies donate a portion of their sales to the battle—sales of shoes, sunglasses, bras, jewelry, sweatshirts, and on and on.

And there's Bike against the Odds, a six-day bicycle ride through southwestern Montana. Pike Hike took 1,000 folks 12 miles up Mt. Tamalpais north of San Francisco. Other Pike Hikes took hundreds up Crested Butte in Colorado and Mt. Washington in New Hampshire. And there are too many other special events to count—golf, bowling, tennis, softball, biking, snowshoeing—all to raise funds to fight breast cancer. And this is just the short list.

Inspiring? You bet! So your imagination is the only limit to fund-raising ideas.

Political Campaigns

Fund-raising is a major form of advocacy, but your impact in the political arena is every bit as important. You'll find yourself watching more and more carefully any legislation that affects breast cancer diagnosis, treatment, or research. You'll start watching your elected officials' voting records. You'll start listening more carefully to campaign speeches, listening for something about breast cancer. You'll probably start making calls to campaign headquarters, asking questions about a candidate's stand on the issue.

When the candidate is an incumbent, you'd like to know his or her voting record on issues affecting the fight against breast cancer. Sometimes voting records are a bit tough to decipher, and, when asked, many elected officials have a tendency to blur their public responses. So if or when you suspect your federal legislators may be bending the truth about their voting records in terms of funding the fight against breast cancer, here's a lie detector test: Check out the National Breast Cancer Coalition (NBCC), which posts the voting records of every congressperson and senator on issues related to breast cancer. Call toll free 1-800-622-2838 or access it at its Web site www.natlbcc.org.

Finally, call the White House Comment Line at 202-456-1111 and explain your concern about breast cancer research funding. The more often you call, the better. If the White House hears the same message week in and week out, it may soon start to register! (And there's a real person at the other end of the line.)

Tales from the Trenches

According to a recent news release from NBCC, its 60,000 members know that breast cancer is a political issue and will use the ballot box accordingly says Fran Visco, president, National Breast Cancer Coalition. For a copy of NBCC's Voter Guide, call the hotline at 1-800-622-2828 or access it through NBCC's Web site www.natlbcc.org.

Take It from Us

The total federal budget for all cancer research—not just breast cancer—is less than the cost of one stealth bomber. Two questions: How many stealth bombers do we need? Is it more important to build another bomber or to improve healthcare? Let your elected officials know how you feel.

Here's How

Before you can convey a message, you have to understand it fully and know which details—the facts and figures—will be most likely to get attention. Then narrow your scope. You can't just write an elected official and say, "You need to do something about breast cancer." Instead, zero in on an issue that needs changing, perhaps money to research the potential environmental causes of breast cancer. Get the facts and figures. Find out who has authority—state, local, or federal. Then decide just what change you want to make and how it can be done. Put the specifics into a letter or a visit.

Keep the Letters Coming

If you're ready to write your legislators and tell them what you think, here's how:

➤ Before you write, do your homework. Know the facts. Get the statistics. Understand the background.

➤ Make your letter short and to the point. Keep it to one page, either typewritten or neatly handwritten.

➤ Be polite but firm, citing solid information to support your position.

➤ If your letter concerns a piece of legislation, name the bill and give its number. Be specific about your concerns and explain in plain words how the bill will affect you and others facing breast cancer.

➤ Don't be afraid to tell your own story. It adds real punch to your message.

➤ It's okay to remind your reader that his mother, sister, lover, wife, daughter, aunt, niece, colleague, or friend is at risk for breast cancer, and that the older they are, the greater the risk. (And if you're writing to a woman, well, she shouldn't have to be convinced. But she'll probably need to be.)

➤ If you think a bill is wrong, say so; but explain why by naming the likely bad effects. Explain clearly how you want the bill changed.

➤ Don't ask for support. That's too vague. Ask instead for a "Yes" or "No" vote.

➤ Ask for the legislator's point of view. You can't demand a "Yes" or "No" vote, but your pointed question about why he or she can't vote as you suggest may cause someone to rethink an issue.

➤ Always include your name and address—and make it legible.

Good letter writing can have significant impact on policy. (And if the matter is urgent, you can fax or e-mail a letter quicker than you can mail it through the USPS.) Make yourself heard!

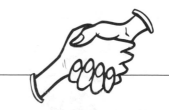

Helping Hand

If you belong to a national group, you can add power to your letter by saying that 30,000 other breast cancer survivors share your idea, or that your idea is endorsed by 20,000 members of such-and-such professional group.

Knock on Doors

Education and discussion can be much more productive than confrontation. Your elected officials need solid facts to get any legislation through, so you can help supply them with the facts to fund the fight against breast cancer. If you can visit personally with your legislator, you can look him or her right in the eye and explain what it means to be a breast cancer survivor. Then you can arm him or her with the rest of the facts. (Note that the implication is that you yourself know the facts and have adequate communication skills to convey not only the facts but their importance.)

From the Book

A **telephone bank** is a group of volunteers who, especially near election time, take phone calls from constituents, compile the information, and pass it along to the candidate for whom they are volunteering.

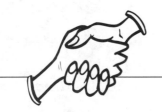

Helping Hand

A dollar from the purchase of every copy of this book will be contributed to breast cancer research. So by making this purchase, you've already taken the first step in advocacy!

If for some reason you feel a little too intimidated to meet personally with your legislator, try volunteering at his or her *telephone bank* during the next political campaign. It's a good way to get an inside track to the way things work in politics.

So how do you arrange a visit with your legislator? You'll call for an appointment (all legislators are listed in your local phone book) or find out when he or she will be in your area and make a local appointment. Don't be upset if you see only an aide. That person may actually be better informed about specific issues, but above all, an aide does the briefing for the guy or gal who actually casts the vote. Thus, aides can be truly great allies. Cultivate their trust and support.

A thank-you note after your visit is not just a matter of courtesy. It also grants you the opportunity to repeat key details and stress the importance of breast cancer research. Further, it gives you the chance to ask for a response, some kind of follow-up from your visit.

Whether or not you visit your legislator personally, keep in touch. Call regularly and keep track of your calls with dates and times. Ask questions. Then keep a record. What were his or her responses? Promises? Suggestions? Queries?

What do you ask? Consider the following:

➤ What legislation has been introduced to deal with the ongoing breast cancer epidemic?

➤ What have you done in terms of breast cancer legislation since the last time we talked?

➤ Have you learned anything new since we last talked on (whatever) date?

Faces in the Crowd

Attending a huge event supporting the fight against breast cancer can be an emotionally charged experience for survivors, their families, and friends. Over 400 survivors, each carrying one pink balloon for every year she had survived and each outfitted in a pink shirt, filed through the throng of 10,200 participants to mass in front of the stage. The scene was last year's Race for the Cure in my hometown. I'm not ashamed to say that tears flowed. Most were joyous tears, celebrating friends and family who were survivors. But some were tears of pain, with runners and walkers wearing signs commemorating the loss of loved ones. And some were no doubt tears of frustration, accompanying that lurking question of why 400 women in a community of only 150,000 should be facing breast cancer.

The 5K race was a serious race for some, and those folks crossed the finish line before the last of the remaining 10,200 walked across the starting line. But for those of us walking, it was not a race against the same clock that timed the winner in just over 15 minutes. We walked in a race against the clock that measures out our lives. The fact that we raised almost a half million dollars that day may help give us, or at least those who follow us, a little more time on the clock.

The Least You Need to Know

➤ Volunteering lets you repay your debt to those who came before you by helping those who come after you.

➤ Breast cancer advocacy includes supporting breast cancer awareness, education, policy making, and funding.

➤ You can choose from among individual and/or community advocacy opportunities.

➤ Being a part of a larger advocacy organization lets you add strength in numbers.

➤ Concise but well-substantiated letters and personal visits to elected officials can have an impact on policy.

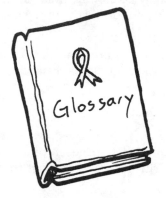

Glossary

acupressure A kind of massage in which a practitioner applies pressure to specific body pressure points.

acupuncture A treatment that involves inserting thin needles into specific places to relieve pain and treat illnesses. Some survivors have found it useful in relieving the side effects of chemo.

acute A term referring to something that is short-term and occurs during the time of treatment.

adjuvant therapy A systemic therapy used when your doctor suspects cancer cells may have escaped into other parts of the body, even if no detectable cancer remains after surgery.

advocate One who speaks or writes in support of a cause, such as breast cancer awareness, education, political policy, and research.

alpha-cradle A positioning device used to keep you in the correct position at all times while undergoing radiation therapy, providing accuracy for your treatment because the location and depth of your cancer site is different than almost everyone else's.

aspirate To insert a needle and withdraw any fluid and/or cells, especially from a cyst.

atypical hyperplasia An excessive formation of tissue unlike that in the surrounding area.

axillary A term that refers to the area under the arm, the area where the lymph nodes lie that are most closely associated with the spread of breast cancer.

baseline mammogram The first mammogram used as a frame of reference for later mammograms in order to detect any changes.

benign Not cancerous.

bilateral mastectomy   Removal of both breasts; may be modified radical, simple, or any other form of mastectomy, and may use the same or different surgeries on each breast.

bioflavonoid   A substance, found in some plants such as broccoli, cabbage, and cauliflower, useful in the maintenance of the walls of small blood vessels and in lessening the intensity of hot flashes.

biopsy   The removal of tissue to be examined for malignancy.

block   The template made for the accurate measurements of your treatment area. The block is inserted into the x-ray machine (linear accelerator) each time you receive treatment so that only the affected area is treated with radiation and not the vital organs.

blood marker study   A blood test that measures the tumor count in your blood; a high count indicates a possible recurrence of cancer.

bone density test   A test that measures how strong (dense) your bones are and recognizes—by comparison with future tests—bone density loss, a treatable condition if caught early.

boundary   A term that not only indicates a border but also a limit.

BRCA1 and BRCA2   Genes that normally make proteins that keep cells from growing abnormally. But if they mutate, that protection is gone.

breast enhancer   A small form that fills out the breast shape after tissue is removed, such as during a lumpectomy.

breast prosthesis   A breast form made of silicone, fiberfill, or other materials. Almost all are designed to be worn inside a special bra; however, new forms are being developed that do not require a bra.

BSE   Breast self-exam.

chemotherapy   A cytotoxic (cell-killing) drug used to treat a disease. For those who are diagnosed with breast cancer, chemotherapy is a drug(s) used to treat breast cancer.

clear margins (also called **negative margins**)   A term that refers to benign tissue surrounding a malignant or pre-cancerous mass, showing that the malignancy has not spread.

clinical trial   A research study conducted with patients to evaluate a new method of preventing, detecting, diagnosing, or treating a disease.

closed discussion group   A group accessed at a sponsoring organization's Web site; requires a password for participation and thus protects privacy.

complementary treatment   Therapies that help manage stress and discomfort, ease side effects, or provide a nutritional boost.

complex decongestive therapy (CDT) A combination treatment consisting of manual lymphatic drainage and the use of compression garments, along with exercises and nutritional guidelines.

contralateral mastectomy Removal of a healthy breast for symmetry; considered cosmetic surgery.

core needle biopsy A biopsy taken with a large needle to remove a core of tissue for examination.

counselor A person who may not have a Master's degree in counseling and, depending on your state, may or may not have a state license or certificate, who is prepared to help you one-on-one with coping skills.

cyst A fluid-filled lump, usually not cancerous.

DEXA (Dual Energy x-ray Absorptionometry) scan A test designed to measure the calcium level in the bones.

diagnostic mammogram A follow-up (second) mammogram taken if a lump or visible abnormality is found.

digital mammography machine A machine that projects the breast image on a screen and allows for manipulation of the image to give the best view of the breast tissue.

distant recurrence When the cancer has spread to another part of your body such as the bones, brain, lungs, or liver. A distant recurrence is cancer that has metastasized.

drain A bulb-shaped apparatus attached to a tube through which fluids drain from the surgery area. The tube is inserted through a tiny incision and attached in place by a single stitch.

ductal carcinoma in situ (also called **intraductal carcinoma**) Usually considered a pre-cancerous condition and is confined to the milk ducts.

estrogen A female sex hormone produced mainly by the ovaries. It can also be produced by fat, the adrenal glands, and the placenta.

euthanasia The Greek word for "good death"; refers to a painless, merciful death.

excisional biopsy The removal of a suspicious lump along with a rim of tissue for pathological examination.

facilitator A person who guides a support group without interfering. The facilitator may be a medical person and/or a breast cancer survivor.

faith A confident belief that does not rest on logical or material proof.

fashion bra The kind you've always worn. If it's a great-fitting bra, you can turn it into a post-surgical bra by sewing a pocket (one you make or one you buy) into either or both sides.

fibrocystic breast (sometimes called **fibrocystic disease**). A benign condition, not a disease at all, that occurs when fibrous breast tissue becomes dense; it often combines with the formation of small cysts.

first-degree relative Someone only one step away on the genealogy chart, such as your mother, your daughter, or your sister.

genetic mutation A change in gene structure that is abnormal. Some mutations contribute to various diseases, including breast cancer.

goal A purpose toward which an endeavor is directed; an end; an objective.

hormone receptor Tissue that is sensitive to hormones and can thus be treated with hormonal therapy.

hormone replacement therapy The oral administration of the hormone estrogen which, if used, usually begins with the onset of menopause.

hyperthermia A treatment, sometimes used in conjunction with radiation therapy, where super-heated rods are implanted into a recurring tumor.

hypnosis An artificially induced state of deep relaxation in which a person is responsive to suggestions.

immunity An inherited, acquired, or induced condition to a specific disease-causing agent such as bacteria.

incisional biopsy (sometimes called a **wide excision** or **wedge excision**) The removal of a wedge of tissue from a very large lump for pathological examination.

in situ The malignancy or pre-cancerous condition is confined to the site, i.e., within the ducts or lobules. The opposite of in situ is infiltrating or invasive.

intravenous A term meaning "in a vein." In the case of chemotherapy, intravenous means an injection in a vein—usually in the hand or arm—directly from a syringe or from a bag containing a mixture of drugs.

intravenous line (IV) A tube inserted into a vein into your arm or hand.

invasive cancers Cancers that have grown outside the ducts or lobules.

journal A periodic record of thoughts, emotions, and reactions to the writer's experiences; does not usually record a chronology of daily events as does a diary.

listserve A list made up of a group of folks who share a common interest and communicate by e-mail; every listserve subscriber receives all other subscribers' queries and posts, usually free.

lobular carcinoma in situ A pre-cancerous condition confined to the milk lobules.

local recurrence When your breast cancer comes back near or at the site of your lumpectomy or mastectomy.

local therapy Treatment of the tumor with surgery and/or radiation.

lumpectomy The removal of a lump of malignant or pre-cancerous tissue along with a margin of tissue.

lymph nodes Glands found throughout the body that help fight bacteria and serve as a filter of lymph fluid. Cancer frequently spreads through the lymphatic system and shows up in lymph nodes. With breast cancer, many of these nodes are located in the armpit.

lymphatic system A system made up of lymph fluid that flows throughout the body and passes through lymph nodes to be purified, fighting infection and providing immunity to disease.

lymphectomy A surgery in which lymph nodes are removed.

malignant Cancer cells are present.

mammogram A low-radiation x-ray that takes pictures of the breast from the top and side.

mastectomy The removal of a breast.

medical oncologist A cancer doctor who specializes in the administration of chemotherapeutic drugs.

menopause A time when the body stops producing hormones (between ages 40 and 50), and begins what is commonly known as "the Change." Once you have stopped having periods for a year, you have reached menopause.

metastasis A term referring to the spread of cancer, as from the breast to some other organ or body part.

metastasized A term that refers to a cancer that has spread, by way of the lymphatic system or bloodstream, to areas of the body other than the cancer site.

micro-calcification Tiny calcium deposits. Scattered deposits are likely benign. A tight cluster of calcium deposits is usually associated with malignancy.

modified radical mastectomy Removal of the breast and nodes but not the chest muscle; usually now replaces the radical mastectomy.

negative lymph nodes Lymph nodes that test benign; i.e., they show no sign of cancer.

negative margin Tissue that does not contain malignant or pre-cancerous tissue.

noninvasive carcinoma A term used to refer to either ductal carcinoma in situ or lobular carcinoma in situ.

nutrition The interrelated steps by which a living organism (a person) assimilates food and uses it for growth and for replacement of tissue.

331

osteoporosis   The deterioration of bone density leading to brittleness and an increased risk for broken bones.

palpable   Able to be felt.

pathologist   A medical doctor who specializes in analyzing tissue to determine the presence of disease.

phantom feelings   Real sensations that seem to come from a body part that has been removed, a result of remaining nerve endings sending messages to the brain.

plastic surgeon   A doctor who performs reconstructive surgery to rebuild a breast that has been surgically removed.

port (properly a **portacath**)   A small plastic tube or metal container placed under the skin and attached to a catheter inside the body. Fluids enter and exit the body through the port by the use of a special needle.

positive lymph nodes   Lymph nodes in which cancer is detected.

positive margin   Tissue containing malignant or pre-cancerous tissue.

post-surgical bra   A bra that has a pocket built into each cup to hold a breast form in place; thus any post-surgical bra functions for any woman, no matter which breast has been removed—or if both breasts have been removed.

pre-menopausal   The age before the "change of life." Usually, before the ages of 40 to 50.

primary lymphedema   Lymphedema that results from unknown causes and can be present from birth.

progesterone   A hormone produced by the ovaries and partly responsible for the menstrual cycle.

prognosis   The prediction for the course of the disease and your chances of recovery.

prophylactic mastectomies   Mastectomies performed on high-risk women who can best be protected by removal of an apparently healthy breast to prevent a likely occurrence of breast cancer.

quadrantectomy   The removal of a portion of the breast, although the term may or may not refer to the removal of a full quarter of the breast.

radiation oncologist   A cancer doctor who specializes in the administration of radiation therapy.

radiation therapy   The use of high-energy penetrating rays of subatomic particles to treat disease.

radical mastectomy   Removal of the breast along with both chest muscles and all axillary lymph nodes; now considered an outdated treatment.

radio frequency   A wave of energy that, when stopped or absorbed in the body, gives up in the form of heat.

radiological technologist   A person who has been trained on and specializes in the use of x-ray equipment.

radiologist   A doctor trained to read the x-ray (picture) and decide which shadows and dots are suspicious and which are not.

range of motion test   A test that records the amount of arm movement that is normal for you; then, after surgery, your medical team will know when you've fully regained use of your arm.

reasonable accommodation   A change in job duties to help you during your cancer.

recurrence   To happen, come up, or show up again. As a survivor, recurrence means that our breast cancer has returned after we have been given the "all clear" sign.

relaxation techniques   Therapies that rely on deep, even breathing and exercises to relieve stress.

risk factor   Something that increases your chances of getting a disease.

screening mammogram   An annual routine mammogram for women over 40 (although some experts still say over 50) to detect any changes in the breast by comparing the screening mammogram to the baseline mammogram.

second opinion   An opinion that comes from a second doctor or surgeon who re-examines you, your mammogram, and your biopsy, and gives a diagnosis and suggested treatment regimen. You can then compare this new opinion with that recommended by the first doctor or surgeon.

secondary lymphedema   Lymphedema that is acquired as the result of surgery, radiation, infection, or trauma.

segmental mastectomy   The removal of a portion, or segment, of the breast.

Selective Estrogen Receptor Modulators (SERMs)   Hormones used to work against breast cancer by helping to systematically kill and/or arrest the growth of cancer cells.

self-adhesive breast   A breast form that sticks directly to your skin, usually with some kind of glue-like substance developed to use directly on the skin.

self-supporting breast   A breast form that is adequately self-adhesive to stay in place without the support of a bra.

sentinel node biopsy   A biopsy that identifies and tests the single lymph node that receives the first drainage from a tumor.

simple (or total) mastectomy   Similar to the modified radical mastectomy, but without the removal of axillary lymph nodes.

333

social worker   A person, usually having a Master's degree in social work and may or may not hold a state license or certificate, who is prepared to help you one-on-one with coping skills.

stage (of cancer)   An indication of how far cancer has progressed.

Stage 0   Pre-cancerous (in situ) conditions.

Stage I   Small, localized cancers, usually curable.

Stage II   Small tumor with positive lymph nodes, or a larger tumor with or without positive lymph nodes.

Stage III   Large tumors with positive lymph nodes.

Stage IV   Tumor with obvious metastasis.

stem cell rescue (also called **bone marrow transplant**)   A procedure used to treat advanced stages of breast cancer with such high doses of chemotherapy that, without the rescue, would be fatal. Bone marrow is removed prior to treatment and regenerated through stem cell support or transplant.

stereotactic guided biopsy   A biopsy taken by using x-rays from two directions to guide the needle.

subcutaneous mastectomy   Removal of most breast tissue; keeps nipple and outer skin; fills space with an implant; controversial because of amount of breast tissue remaining, thus increasing the chance of recurrence.

surgical biopsy   The removal of a small lump of tissue for pathological examination.

systemic therapy   Treatment that goes through your bloodstream (or system), such as chemotherapy and/or hormonal therapy.

telephone bank   A group of volunteers who, especially near election time, take phone calls from constituents, compile information, and pass it along to the candidate for whom they are volunteering.

ultrasound   A completely painless exam that sends sound waves through body tissue. The waves go through fluid but bounce off solid lumps.

ultrasound guided biopsy   A biopsy taken using sound waves to guide the needle.

white blood cell count   A test that indicates how many white blood cells you have and how quickly your body is returning to a normal level. During chemo, the count drops dramatically; afterward, it should return to normal levels.

white blood cells   Cells your body produces and uses to fight most infections.

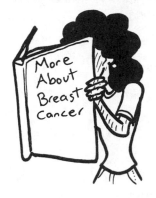

Further Readings

During our research, we found many books on topics related to breast cancer. While each book offers good information, we do not endorse every piece of advice that is offered. This list is certainly not comprehensive, but neither is it overwhelming. Each book contains its own list of "further readings" which can direct you to additional information in a specific area.

Action Guide for Healthy Eating. National Institutes for Health, 1995.

Americans with Disabilities Act: Information for People Facing Cancer. American Cancer Society, 1999.

Anderson, Patricia J. *Breast Cancer: A Patient Guide.* Creative Health Services, 1999.

Babcock, Elise NeeDell. *When Life Becomes Precious: A Guide for Loved Ones and Friends of Cancer Patients.* Bantam Books, 1997.

Benjamin, Harold H., Ph.D. *The Wellness Community Guide to Fighting for Recovery from Cancer.* Putnam Books, 1995.

Berger, Karen, and John Bostwich III, M.D. *A Woman's Decision: Breast Care, Treatment and Reconstruction.* Quality Medical Publishing, 1994.

Brack, Pat. *Moms Don't Get Sick.* Melius Publishing, Inc., 1990.

Breast Cancer Facts and Figures 1999–2000. American Cancer Society, 1999.

Breast Cancer Resource List. National Alliance of Breast Cancer Organization, 1997/98 Edition.

Brinker, Nancy, with Catherine McEvily Harris. *The Race Is Run One Step at a Time.* Summit Publishing Group., 1995.

Burt, Jeannie, Gwen White, and Judith R. Casley-Smith. *Lymphedema: A Breast Cancer Patient's Guide to Prevention and Healing.* Hunter House, 2000.

Capossela, Cappy and Sheila Warnock. *Share the Care: How to Organize a Group to Care for Someone Who Is Seriously Ill.* Fireside, 1995.

Cassileth, Barrie R. *The Alternative Medicine Handbook: The Complete Reference Guide to Alternative and Complementary Therapies.* W.W. Norton & Company, 1998.

Crenshaw, David A. *Bereavement: Counseling the Grieving Throughout the Life Cycle.* Continuum Publishing Company, 1990.

Dossey, Larry, M.D. *Healing Words: The Power of Prayer and the Practice of Medicine.* Harper Paperbacks, 1993.

Exercises After Breast Surgery. American Cancer Society, 1990.

Facing Forward, A Guide for Cancer Survivors. National Cancer Institute, August, 1999.

Gaynor, Mitchell L., M.D. *Healing Essence.* Kodansha International, 1995.

Greenberg, Mimi, Ph.D. *Invisible Scars: A Guide to Coping with the Emotional Impact of Breast Cancer.* Walter & Co., 1988.

Harpham, Wendy Schlessel. *Diagnosis Cancer; Your Guide Through the First Few Months.* W.W. Norton & Company, 1997.

Lang, Susan S., and Richard B. Patt, M.D. *You Don't Have to Suffer: A Complete Guide to Relieving Cancer Pain for Patients and Their Families.* Oxford University Press, 1995.

LaTour, Kathy. *The Breast Cancer Companion.* William Morrow and Company, Inc., 1993.

Lerner, Michael. *Choices in Healing.* The MIT Press, 1994.

Lightner, Candy. *Giving Sorrow Words: How to Cope with Grief and Get on with Your Life.* Warner Books, 1991.

Love, Susan M., M.D. *Dr. Susan Love's Breast Book.* Perseus Books, 1995.

Mayer, Musa. *Advanced Breast Cancer: A Guide to Living with Metastatic Disease.* O'Reilly & Associates, 1998.

Peale, Norman Vincent. *The Power of Positive Thinking.* Prentice Hall Press, 1987.

Porter, Margit E. *Hope Is Contagious: The Breast Cancer Treatment Survival Handbook.* Fireside, 1997.

Radiation Therapy and You: A Guide to Self-Help During Cancer Treatment. National Institutes of Health, 1999.

Rinzler, Carol Ann. *Estrogen and Breast Cancer.* Macmillan, 1993.

Schover, Leslie. *Sexuality and Fertility After Cancer.* John Wiley & Sons, 1997.

Siegel, Bernie S., M.D. *How to Live Between Office Visits.* HarperPerennial Library, 1994.

Strauss, Linda Leopold. *What About Me? A Booklet for Teenage Children of Cancer Patients.* Cancer Family Care, 1986.

Stumm, Diana, PT. *Recovering from Breast Surgery: Exercises to Strengthen Your Body and Relieve Pain.* Hunter House, 1995.

Taking Time: Support for People with Cancer and the People Who Care About Them. National Cancer Institute, September, 1997.

Understanding Breast Cancer Treatment: A Guide for Patients. National Institutes of Health, 1998.

Vogel, Carole. *Will I Get Breast Cancer? Questions & Answers for Teenage Girls.* Silver Burdett Press, 1995.

Weiss, Marisa C., M.D., and Ellen Weiss. *Living Beyond Breast Cancer: A Survivor's Guide for When Treatment Ends and the Rest of Your Life Begins.* Times Books, 1997.

When Cancer Recurs: Meeting the Challenge. National Institutes of Health, 1997.

When Someone You Work with Has Cancer. American Cancer Society, 1998.

Working It Out: Your Employment Rights as a Cancer Survivor. National Coalition for Cancer Survivorship, 1999.

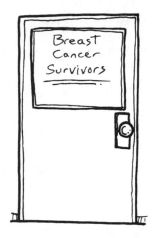

Support Groups

Check with your doctor, nurse, clinic, and/or hospital for local independent support groups. Support groups with national affiliations can be contacted through one of the following phone numbers or Web sites.

AMC Cancer Research Center
1-800-525-3777

Call for the Center's Cancer Information and Counseling Line offering easy-to-understand answers to questions about cancer; also equipped for deaf and hearing-impaired callers.

American Cancer Society
1-800-ACS-2345
Web site: www.cancer.org/bcn/index.html

Call for local groups that they or others sponsor; provides transportation to treatments as well as wigs, scarves, and temporary prostheses; specialists answer in English or Spanish, 24 hours every day.

Breast Cancer ACTION Nova Scotia
P.O. Box 34091
Scotia Square RPO
Halifax, NS B3J3S1, Canada
Web site: bca.ns.ca

This organization provides an online discussion forum and general information.

Breast Cancer Decision Guide for Military and Civilian Families
Web site: www.bcdg.org/about_the_decision_guide.html

This site is sponsored by the Department of Defense with funds appropriated for breast cancer research. Click on "interactive consultations" for guidelines specific to you; "general information" for topics to browse.

CAIRE (Center for American Indian Research and Education)
1918 University Ave., Suite 3-A
Berkeley, CA 94704
510-843-8661

The organization serves American Indian women who have—or have concerns about—breast cancer.

Canadian Breast Cancer Network
Web site: www.cbcn.ca

This is a survivor-directed nation network of organizations and individuals in both English and French.

Cancer Care, Inc.
1-800-813-HOPE
Fax: 212-719-0263
E-mail: info@cancercare.org
Web site: www:cancercareinc.org (click on "Getting Help from Cancer Care")

Cancer Care offers information and telephone and online support groups facilitated by oncology social workers; also support groups for partners, relatives, and caregivers.

Celebrating Life
Web site: www.celebratinglife.org

This site offers information about breast cancer for African-American women and women of color.

CHESS (Comprehensive Health Enhancement Support System)
1-800-361-5481 or 1-888-553-5036
Web site: www.chsra.wisc.edu/bc

Call to find the provider nearest you to grant you a password and pass code to the Web site. This Web site includes a protected online discussion group and "Ask the Experts" for personal questions.

Electronic Bulletin Boards
Here's where to go online to share information and support with other breast cancer survivors:

➤ **America Online** (1-800-827-6364); go to keyword GLENNA

➤ **Compuserve** (1-800-848-8199); go to the Cancer Forum in the Health Professional section, or GO CANCER

➤ **Prodigy** (1-800-776-3449); go to the Medical Support Board under the Cancer topic

Komen (Susan B.) Breast Cancer Foundation
1-800-IM-AWARE, Monday through Friday, 9:00 to 4:30 (Central time)
Web site: www.komen.org

Listserves
These online services are available free of charge by e-mail; for breast cancer patients, their family and friends, and health professionals; to subscribe, send an e-mail to LISTSERV@morgan.usc.mun.ca and write only the words SUBSCRIBE BREAST-CANCER in the message. Another resource is cure.medinfo.org/lists/cancer/bc-about.html.

Look Good ... Feel Better
1101 17th Street, NW, Suite 300
Washington, DC 20036
1-800-395-LOOK
Fax: 202-331-7593
Web site: www.lookgoodfeelbetter.org

This organization helps patients deal with issues of their appearance while experiencing treatment side effects.

Lymphedema
This online support group is for lymphedema sufferers; subscribe at listserv@acor.org and leave message reading only: subscribe LYMPHEDEMA YourFirstName YourLastName.

Medinfo.Org
Web site: www.medinfo.org

This site includes about 90 links, including sites for breast cancer supporters and husbands, for clinical trials, and Canadian lists; can search archives of online support group.

Mental Health Net Self-Help Index
Web site: www.cmhc.com/selfhelp.htm

This is a comprehensive listing of mental health support resources on the Web; indexed alphabetically.

National Alliance of Breast Cancer Organizations
Web site: www.nabco.org/support/

This online list includes about 350 support groups by city and state; includes Canada; with phone numbers.

National Cancer Institute's Cancer Information Service
1-800-4-CANCER
Web site: www.nci.nih.gov

Offered in English or Spanish; Monday through Friday, 9:00 to 4:30 (local time); provides a list of certified mammography providers in your area; ask these providers for support group suggestions.

341

Native American Community Board
PO Box 572
Lake Andes, SD 57356
605-487-7072

The board serves geographical area Native American women who have—or have concerns about—breast cancer.

Prodigy's Medical Support Board Under Cancer
1-800-776-3449

Sponsors an online bulletin board where cancer survivors regularly provide support and information to each other.

Self-Help for Women with Breast or Ovarian Cancer (SHARE)
1501 Broadway, Suite 1720
New York, NY 10036
Hotline: 212-382-2111 (answered by survivors)
Spanish: 212-719-4445
Business office: 212-719-0364
Web site: www.sharecancersupport.org

Peer-led support groups with hotlines where survivors answer phones.

Sisters Network, Inc.
713-781-0255
E-mail: natsis4@aol.com
Web site: www.sistersnetworkinc.org

Call for the local chapter nearest you supporting African-American women and women of color.

Y-Me National Breast Cancer Organization
212 W. Van Buren Street, 5th Floor
Chicago, IL 60607-3908
Hotline: 1-800-221-2141 (answered by survivors)
Spanish: 1-800-986-9505
Web site: www.y-me.org

Go to the Web site and click on "Support Group Meetings" for group names, addresses, phone numbers, and meeting dates and times by city and state.

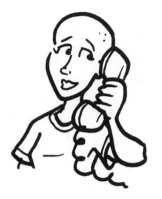

Sources of Prostheses and Post-Surgical Clothing

The following alphabetical list of manufacturers, distributors, and a few select retailers of post-surgical products is not an all-inclusive list but does suggest the many options available to you.

Check your local Yellow Pages or the Internet for additional sources of post-surgical items.

Airway
BRANDS: Airway and Truform-OTC
Division of Surgical Appliance Industries
3960 Rosslyn Drive
Cincinnati, OH 45209
Phone: 1-800-888-0458 or 513-271-4594
Fax: 1-800-309-9055 or 513-271-4747
Web site: www.surgicalappliance.com

Products: textile pads of lightweight foam, compression arm sleeves, turbans, surgical bras, lightweight and full prostheses in many shapes. Ask for distributors near you.

Almost You
91 Market Street, Suite 23
Wappingers Falls, NY 12590
Phone: 1-800-626-6007
Fax: 914-297-1634

Products: bras, swim forms, leisure forms, and multiple silicone prostheses.

American Cancer Society
2525 Ridgepoint Dr., Suite 100
Austin, TX 78754
Phone: 1-800-ACS-2345
Fax: 512-927-5791
Web site: www.cancer.org

Offers breast forms. Can provide names of prosthetics distributors in your area.

Amoena
(*see* Coloplast)

B&B Company, Inc.
BRAND: Bosom Buddy
PO Box 5731
2417 Bank Drive, Suite 201
Boise, ID 83705
Phone: 208-343-9696 or 1-800-262-2789
Fax: 208-343-9266
Web site: www.bosombuddy.com

Products: breathable all-fabric breast forms, suitable for swimming.

Camp Healthcare
BRAND: Naturalwear
PO Box 89
Jackson, MI 49204
Phone: 517-787-1600 or 1-800-492-1088
Fax: 517-789-3299 or 1-800-245-3765
Web site: www.camphealthcare.com

Products: weighted, unweighted, textured-surface, polyurethane-covered silicone, and foam/fluffy filled breast forms, as well as pocketed bras. Will send brochure and list of dealers in your area.

Capital Marketing Technologies, Inc.
BRAND: Nearly Me
3630 South I-35
Waco, TX 76706
Phone: 1-800-887-3370
Fax: 254-662-1760
Web site: www.cm-tech.com

Products: breast prostheses, enhancers, scar-reduction products.

Careguide
255 Revere Drive
Northbrook, IL 60062
Phone: 847-205-1260, 1-877-CAREKIT (questions), or 1-888-333-5520 (orders)

Fax: 847-205-1270
Web site: www.carekit.com

Products: post–breast surgery kits for single and multiple drains (endorsed by The American Breast Cancer Foundation, Susan B. Komen Foundation, and Y-Me), bras, prostheses, and swimwear.

Classique Mystique Monique, Inc.
12277 SW 55th Street, Suite 905
Cooper City, FL 33330
Phone: 954-252-3334, 1-800-327-1332, or 811-453-1351
Fax: 954-252-3336 or 1-800-736-3474

Products: bras, silicone prostheses, lumpectomy forms, swim forms, leisure forms, swimwear, and breast enhancers. Will direct you to nearest store.

Close to You
11661 Preston Road, Suite 154
Dallas, TX 75230
Phone: 214-692-8893
Fax: 214-692-8945

Products: Close to You prostheses (solidified silicone, to be worn with regular bra) and other brand prosthetics, bras, leisure forms, LymphaPress pumps, compression sleeves, including nighttime sleeves.

Coloplast Corporation
BRANDS: Ameona and Discrene
1955 W. Oak Circle
Marietta, GA 30062-2249
Phone: 770-281-8400, 1-800-926-6362, or 770-281-8501
Web site: www.us.amoena.com

Products: breast forms, bras, swimwear, and skin care. Ask for certified fitter nearest you.

ContourMed, Inc.
2821 Kavanaugh Blvd., Suite 2
Little Rock, AR 72205
Phone: 501-907-0530 or 1-888-301-0520
Fax: 501-907-0533
E-mail: info@contourmed.com
Web site: www.contourmed.com

Product: lightweight custom-made breast forms that offer a made-for-you solution constructed from three-dimensional scans; also noncustom line. Call for literature or the name of a retailer near you.

Designs for Comfort, Inc.
PO Box 671044
Marietta, GA 30066
Phone: 1-800-433-9226

Products: head coverings and hair pieces. Call for nearest retailer or ask for catalog for mail order.

Discrene
(*see* Coloplast)

Freeman
900 W. Chicago Road
Sturgis, MI 49091
Phone: 616-651-2371 or 1-800-253-2091
Fax: 616-651-8248
Web site: www.freemanmfg.com

Products: temporary weighted breast forms and silicone forms, bras, and compression sleeves. Ask for nearest retailer.

Gentle Touch Medical Products, Inc.
1160 Pine Drive
Ortonville, MI 48462
Phone: 1-800-989-5726
Fax: 248-627-7006
E-mail: info@gentlet.com
Web site: www.gentlet.com

Products: mastectomy and lumpectomy camisoles with polyfill breast form attached and front Velcro opening.

Health-Related Products
BRAND: External Breast Reconstruction
1704 Mathis Road
Greenwood, SC 29649
Phone: 1-800-845-4566

Product: builds prostheses to match your intact breast shape, size, weight, and skin color.

HPH Corporation
BRAND: HPH
4714 Del Prado Blvd.
Cape Coral, FL 33904
Phone: 1-800-654-9884

Product: silicone breast forms. Mail order only. Call for a catalog.

JC Penney Catalog
1-800-932-4115

Products: carries Jodee products, including bras, breast forms, swimwear. Call for special catalog.

Jodee Bra, Inc.
3100 N. 29th Avenue
Hollywood, FL 33020
Phone: 1-800-865-6333 (office) or 1-800-821-2767 (mail order)
Fax: 954-926-1926

Products: breast forms, bras, and swimwear. Call for nearest dealer or for JC Penney catalog.

Ladies First, Inc.
BRAND: Softee Comfort Form
PO Box 4400; 286 Salem Height Ave. SE
Salem, OR 97302
Phone: 503-363-3940, 1-800-497-8285, or 1-800-300-3940
Fax: 503-363-1985
E-mail: ladies1@wvi.com
Web site: www.wvi.com/~ladies1/

Products: post-mastectomy camisoles, support camisoles, silicone breast prostheses, and mastectomy slips. Sells mail order; call for catalog.

Land's End
1 Land's End Lane
Dodgeville, WI 53595
Phone: 1-800-356-4444
Fax: 1-800-332-0103
Web site: www.landsend.com

Products: mastectomy swimwear. Mail order only; call for catalog.

Magic and Vanity
E-mail: info@magicvanity.com
Web site: www.magicvanity.com

Products: online catalog featuring hats, swimwear, casual wear, bras, and breast forms.

Nearly Me
(*see* Capital Marketing Technologies, Inc.)

Sea-Shore
PO Box 704
Ardsley, NY 10402
Phone: 914-693-5389

Products: lightweight silicone-coated fabric prostheses and swimwear. Ask for nearest dealer.

347

Simone Company, The Leading Ladies Company
BRAND: Leading Ladies
24050 Commerce Park
Beachwood, OH 44122
Phone: 1-800-321-4804 or (in Ohio) 1-800-832-3112
Fax: 216-464-9365

Products: bras; lightweight, foam-filled weighted and unweighted prostheses. Ask for retailer nearest you.

Softee Comfort Forms
(*see* Ladies First)

Susan's Special Needs
2751 E. Jefferson, Suite 104
Detroit, MI 48206
Phone: 313-259-7832 or 1-800-497-7055
Fax: 313-259-3282
Web site: www.cancerdirectory.com

Products: wigs, hats, turbans, and mastectomy exercise wear, including sports bras, zippered sports bras, and leotards. Call for list of distributors near you.

TLC, Tender Loving Care
American Cancer Society
1599 Clifton Road, NE
Atlanta, GA 30326
Ordering address: 340 Poplar Street
Hanover, PA 17333-0080
Phone: 1-800-850-9445
Web site: www.cancer.org

Products: call for catalog featuring hats, kerchiefs, wigs, swimsuits, surgical bras, pocketed T-shirts, radiation camisoles, featherweight breast forms, silicone breast prostheses, latex breast prostheses (weighted and unweighted, suitable for swimming), and enhancers.

Underneath It All
444 East 75th Street
New York, NY 10021
Phone: 212-717-1976
Fax: 212-717-1968

Products: post-mastectomy fashions. Accommodates phone orders.

UnderThings
8055 West Avenue, Suite 106
San Antonio, TX 78213
Phone: 210-344-8983
Fax: 210-344-8986
E-mail: cowles@texas.net

Products: breast forms, post-mastectomy bras, swimwear, turbans, hats, lymphedema pumps, and compression garments.

Y-Me
1-800-221-2141

Call for names of distributors of various post-mastectomy product retailers in your area.

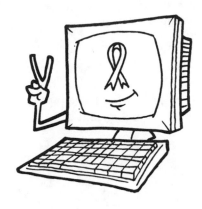

Informational Web Sites

It goes almost without saying that Web sites come and go overnight. Thus, while the following sites are up and running as we write, they may evaporate before you find them. We've chosen these sites because of their sponsorship, their content, and/or their ease in navigation. Still, depending on which search engines you use, you may find other equally valuable Web sites. Just make sure that any Web site you rely on for vital information is sponsored by a reputable facility or organization.

Acor.org
Association of Cancer Online Resources

amazon.com
Online bookstore, good listing by categories

avoncrusade.com
Avon's Breast Cancer Awareness Crusade

azstarnet.com
Mothers Supporting Daughters with Breast Cancer: networking group providing opportunities to express emotional anxiety and effects breast cancer has on a mother and her daughter

bca.army.mil
Breast Cancer Awareness and Solutions Network: group dedicated to improving awareness about breast cancer issues

bmt-talk-request@ai.mit.edu
Bone Marrow Discussion Mailing List

breastcancer.net
Breast Cancer Newsletter

bco.org
Breast Cancer Online: free independent educational service and information resource for professionals working in the field of breast cancer

bestiary.com/ibc
Inflammatory Breast Cancer Help Page: patient-generated Web site

canceranswers.org
Breast Cancer Answer Project

cancerbacup.org.uk
CancerBACUP: foremost provider in the United Kingdom aiming to help people live with breast cancer by providing information, emotional support, and counseling for patients, families, and healthcare professionals

cancerfatigue.org
CancerFatigue

cancerguide.org
CancerGuide: Steve Dunn's Cancer Information Page: patient-generated Web site helping individuals find the answers to their questions about cancer

cancerhelp.com
EduCare Inc.: dedicated to empowering women and their families with educational material about breast health

cancernet.nci.nih.gov
National Cancer Institute's CancerNet Information Service

cancertrials.nci.nih.gov
National Cancer Institute's cancerTrials Information Resource

cansearch.org
National Coalition for Cancer Survivorship: a group to empower cancer survivors

cancersurvivors.org
Information for cancer survivors

cdc.gov/nccdphp/dcpc/nbccedp/new.htm
Center for Disease Control National Breast and Cervical Cancer Early Detection Program: provides recommended screening to low-income women

centerwatch.com
CenterWatch Clinical Trials Listing Service: international listing of clinical research trials

chsvc.com
Breast Cancer Web: linking breast cancer information on the Internet

commtechlab.msu.edu/sites/bcl/index.html
Breast Cancer Lighthouse: where newly diagnosed women can explore medical information and personal stories of survivors: a virtual support group

discoveryhealth.com
DiscoveryHealth: multi-pronged path to a more vigorous life

dol.gov/dol/pwba
Online information on pensions, welfare, benefits, and administration

ecog.dfci.harvard.edu
Eastern Cooperative Oncology Group: cooperative studies of leading medical institutions

fda.gov/womens/
Office of Women's Health

feminist.org/other/bc/bchome.html
Breast Cancer Information Center: information site posted by the Feminist Majority Foundation

healthanswers.com
Health Answers: sources and information regarding health issues

healthgate.com
HealthGate: gateway to health information

hospice-cares.com
Additional information for hospice care with links to other hospice sites and related care

hypnosis.com
Online reference source, up-to-date information on the study of hypnosis

infoventures.com/cancer
CancerWeb: a monthly publication of the latest information appearing in recent medical journals on cancer-related research

interact.withus.com/interact/mbc
Internet Male Breast Cancer Group

jcrt.harvard.edu/hcog.htm
Harvard Collaborative Oncology Group: mutual assistance among institutions affiliated with Harvard Medical School

kidscope.org
KidsCope: helps families and kids better understand cancer

lbbc.org
Living Beyond Breast Cancer: focuses on issues faced after completing primary treatment for breast cancer

lymphnet.org
National Lymphedema Network: gives education and guidance to lymphedema patients and healthcare providers

med.stanford.edu/bca
Breast Cancer Action: grassroots group of ordinary people educating themselves on breast cancer

medsch.wisc.edu/bca
Breast Cancer Answers: gives accurate and up-to-date information on breast cancer research and treatments

napbc.org:80
National Action Plan on Breast Cancer: promotes communication, cooperation, and collaboration of all engaged in the fight against breast cancer

natlbcc.org
National Breast Cancer Coalition: a network of activists whose goal is to eradicate breast cancer through action and advocacy

ncbi.nlm.nih.gov/pubmed
National Library of Medicine: medically related databases

noah.cuny.edu/cancer/breastcancer.html
New York Online Access to Health

nysernet.org/bcic
Breast Cancer Information Clearinghouse

trfn.clpgh.org/bcis
Breast Cancer Information Service

tricaresw.af.mil/breastcd
Interactive Site on Breast Cancer Awareness—"Breast Health—Your Decision"

wcn.org
Women's Cancer Network

webmed.org
Provides online medical and healthcare information

wehealnewyork.org/healthinfo/breastcancer/bctoc.html
Continuum Health Partners Cancer Services

women.com
A potpourri of women's issues and topics, including health

www2.ari.net:80/icare
International Cancer Alliance: nonprofit organization providing cancer information

Index

361

P

pain medications, taking during recovery, 96

palpable lumps, 6

parents, telling diagnosis to, 21

partial mastectomy, 76-77

participating in advocacy, 317-318

partner/husband
  ending relationship with, 235-236
  helping to cope, 233-234
  sexual intimacy, 234-235
  telling diagnosis to, 17-19

pathologists, 9

pathology reports, 97, 101
  interpreting
    hormone receptor test, 103-104
    invasive cancer, 103
    negative lymph nodes, 102
    negative margins, 102
    positive lymph nodes, 102
    positive margins, 102
  process, 84

PCBs (polychlorinated biphenyls), 185

pelvic exams, importance of, 169

Pension and Welfare Benefits Administration Web site, 353

people as support tools, 224-227

personal history (risk factor), 181-184

personal risk factors, determining, 181

personal strength, importance of, 217-218

personality of doctors/ surgeons, 42-43

phantom feelings, 98

phases of grief
  Phase 1 (denial/shock/ isolation), 304
  Phase 2 (anger), 305
  Phase 3 (bargaining), 305
  Phase 4 (depression), 306
  Phase 5 (acceptance), 306

physical exams, importance of, 169

physical life changes, 269
  buying a wig, 270-271
  exercise, 273
  hair care, 271
  nutrition, 269-270
  skin tone, 272

physical therapy, 172

plastic surgeons, 40, 243-245

platelets, 121

pneumonia shots, 173

political campaigns, raising research funds, 322

polychlorinated biphenyls (PCBs), 185

population group (risk factor), 181

portacaths (ports), 107, 116
  advantages, 107-108
  disadvantages, 108
  implanting, 107

positive lymph nodes, 29-30, 84, 102

positive margins, 53, 84, 102

post-surgery instructions/ precautions
  lumpectomies, 82-83
  lymph node removal, 100-101

post-surgical bras, 260-261, 284-285

post-surgical clothing (manufacturers/ distributors), 343-349

prayer, 216-217

pre-cancerous conditions. *See also* cancer
  ductal carcinoma in situ, 28-29
  intraductal carcinoma, 29
  lobular cancer in situ, 28-29
  noninvasive carcinoma, 28-29

preexisting conditions, 236

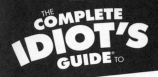